AF342127

Clinical Syndromes in
VETERINARY NEUROLOGY

Clinical Syndromes in
VETERINARY NEUROLOGY

Kyle G. Braund

DVM, MS, PhD, FRCVS
Dip. ACVIM-SPECIALTY NEUROLOGY

Professor, Scott-Ritchey Research Program
and Department of Small Animal Surgery & Medicine
College of Veterinary Medicine
Auburn University
Auburn, Alabama

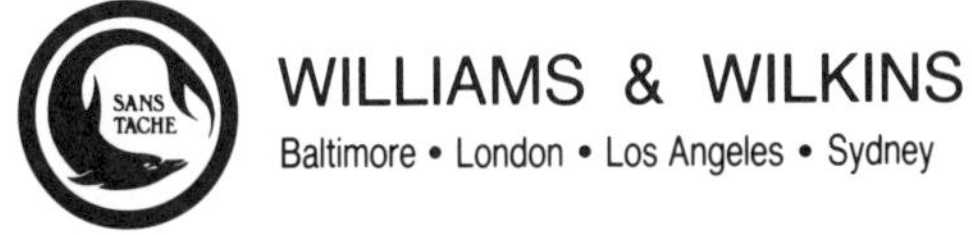

WILLIAMS & WILKINS
Baltimore • London • Los Angeles • Sydney

Editor: Jonathan W. Pine, Jr.
Associate Editor: Carol Eckhart
Copy Editor: Deborah K. Tourtlotte
Design: Bob Och
Illustration Planning: Lorraine Wrzosek
Production: Anne G. Seitz

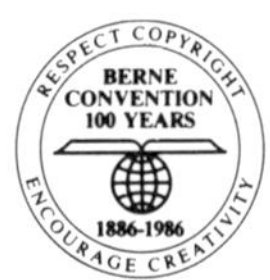

Accurate indications, adverse reactions, and dosage schedules for drugs are provided in this book, but it is possible that they may change. The reader is urged to review the package information data of the manufacturers of the medications mentioned.

Printed in the United States of America

Library of Congress Cataloging-in-Publication Data

Braund, Kyle G.
    Clinical syndromes in veterinary neurology.

    Includes index.
    1. Dogs—Diseases. 2. Cats—Diseases. 3. Veterinary neurology. 4. Syndromes in animals. I. Title. SF992.N3B73 1986   636.7′08968   85-26591
ISBN 0-683-01015-8

Composed and printed at the
Waverly Press, Inc.

86 87 88 89 90
10 9 8 7 6 5 4 3 2 1

For Kathryn, Mandy, Stuart,
Knobby, and Darwin

Foreword

Modern radiographic imaging techniques and electrodiagnostic methods are changing the scope of neurological diagnosis, but the fundamental wisdom of Gowers' words is not diminished. The signs of disease remain the most meaningful evidence of lesions of the nervous system. As the neurologists of Gowers' era established, thorough clinical examination provides the basis for anatomical diagnosis, while historic data provide the clues to the nature of the disease process.

In this new textbook, Dr. Braund relies heavily on the significance of signs. He has illustrated the technique of the neurological examination (the orderly collection of the signs of disease) and grouped the signs into syndromes that call attention to anatomical divisions of the nervous system. For each syndrome, he has provided a list of diseases tabulated according to both pathological process and clinical course. Each listed disease is described; a complete bibliography is provided for those who seek the original reports. Finally, there is a discussion of diagnostic methods that can be used to arrive at a specific diagnosis (or to limit the differential diagnoses).

The design of this book will provide a practical solution to most of the diagnostic challenges that clinicians face. It will be especially well suited to those whose background in neuroanatomy and neurophysiology is limited. The diagnosis of neurological disease is often a source of frustration and is approached with reluctance. By simplifying the approach to neurodiagnosis, Dr. Braund's book facilitates diagnostic success. Buoyed by this success, students and clinicians may well be inspired to explore in greater depth the mechanisms and disorders of the nervous system.

Sheldon A. Steinberg, V.M.D

Preface

The purpose of this book is to provide a simplified and logical approach to neurological diseases of dogs and cats based on a concept of readily identifiable neurological syndromes.

Clinical neurology continues to be taught in most veterinary teaching institutions using a global approach, usually with accent on disease etiology and pathology. Indeed, clinical signs are often treated as a perfunctory component of the disorder, and there is often no orderly, sequential framework established for disease diagnosis. For example, by discussing all of the infectious diseases or developmental disorders of the central nervous system, it is incorrectly assumed that the student knows how to localize the lesion.

It is evident that a new approach is needed in order to overcome the data "overkill" acquired by students, interns, residents, and practitioners following their travels through neuroanatomy, neurophysiology, and clinical neurology. Since it is now established that specific lesions within the CNS, peripheral nervous system (PNS), and skeletal muscle result in predictable, specific, clinical signs, it naturally follows that through the recognition of certain key clinical signs, a lesion can be localized within any of these areas. This concept of neurological syndromes provides the basis for lesion localization, without which differential diagnosis of disease cannot be logically pursued.

Once a lesion has been localized, it is a simple chore to categorize various disorders that have a known predilection for a given area or region of the CNS, PNS, or muscle, and that produce a recognizable clinical syndrome. In order to facilitate a differential diagnosis, the various diseases can be tabulated according to rapidity of onset and to their progressive or nonprogressive course. These diseases also can be categorized according to the nature of the disease process, e.g., degenerative, neoplastic, traumatic, etc. From this clinical "data base," the diagnosis can be logically attained using a combination of signalment (age, breed, sex) and historical information, and such appropriate ancillary procedures as radiography, cerebrospinal fluid analysis, and electrodiagnostic tests.

It is hoped that this sequential method removes the stigma of complexity and, sometimes, irrationality from clinical neurology. Experience has shown that students, interns, residents, and practitioners can use this easily recognizable syndrome approach immediately without the need for detailed knowledge of neuroanatomy, neurophysiology, or neuropathology. This syndrome approach is designed to be a practical guide to help the practitioner with the immediate case in hand rather than to be a substitute for these areas of discipline. I believe that the syndrome approach to localization will prove to be an invaluable aid for the practitioner in his or her quest to provide the best care possible for the patient.

Chapter 1 covers the neurological examination. Chapter 2 is concerned with the neurological syndromes and localization. In Chapter 3, specific neurological diseases are discussed alphabetically. Diagnostic techniques are contained in Chapter 4.

K.G.B.

Acknowledgment

I thank Mrs. Karen Amling for her tireless efforts in helping with all stages of preparation of this book.

Contents

1
Neurological Examination

Introduction

The neurological examination is the basic and most important tool of clinical neurology. It is through the neurological examination that abnormal clinical signs are noted. These abnormal signs will form the building blocks of the neurological syndromes discussed in Chapter 2. Within the 10- to 15-minute period that it takes to conduct a detailed neurological examination, the clinician will be able to determine the presence or absence of nervous system disorders, support or confirm the information collected from the history, locate the site(s) of involvement and thereby determine if the disease is focal or multifocal, determine the severity of the dysfunction, arrive at a tentative differential diagnosis and treatment, and, finally, provide a short- and long-term prognosis. The neurological examination thus forms an integral part of the overall diagnostic process and provides a foundation for further ancillary investigations (1–6). Not only is it of value in understanding the nature of the disease process, but it also provides information concerning the state of the disease (progressive or static) and the efficacy of subsequent medical or surgical management. An outline summary of the complete neurological examination is shown in Table 1.1.

Diagnostic Equipment

A minimum of special equipment is required for the clinical examination. Basic needs are: (*a*) reflex hammer; (*b*) 18-gauge hypodermic needle; (*c*) penlight or other source of focal beam of light; (*d*) nonirritating volatile oil or food; (*e*) blindfold; and (*f*) hemostatic forceps. At the conclusion of the examination, it may be apparent that specialized tests are required to substantiate a clinical diagnosis—e.g., electroencephalography (EEG), electromyography (EMG), nerve conduction velocity studies (NCV), spinal fluid analysis, radiography, myelography, etc.

Historical Information

An important adjunct to the neurological examination is a complete and chronological history taking, which in itself may suggest a tentative diagnosis. One should not, however, ignore other possible causes of the signs described by the owner or observed by the clinician. Certain disorders are often related to (*a*) breed—e.g., intervertebral disk disease in the dachshund, epilepsy in the poodle, hydrocephalus in the Chihuahua, and spinal dysraphism in the Weimaraner (Table 1.2); (*b*) age—e.g., hereditary and inflammatory disease in young animals and certain degenerative and neoplastic disorders in older animals; (*c*) functional use of the animal—e.g., hypoglycemia-related central nervous system (CNS) disturbances in pointers.

Table 1.1. Summary of Neurological Examination

A. **History:**	Differential diagnosis:
	(Degenerative) (anomalous) (autoimmune)
B. **Mental status:**	(Metabolic) (neoplastic) (nutritional)
	(Idiopathic) (inflammatory) (traumatic)
C. **Locomotion:**	(Toxic)

D. **Postural reactions:**	(9. Glossopharyngeal)
1. Wheelbarrowing: L R	(10. Vagus)
2. Hemistanding: L R	(12. Hypoglossal)
3. Hemiwalking: L R	
4. Hopping: LF RF LH RH	F. **Muscle tone:** LF RF LH RH
5. Proprioception: LF RF LH RH	Atrophy:
6. Extensor postural thrust:	
LF RF LH RH	G. **Spinal reflexes:**
7. Righting: L R	Bicipital: L R
8. Placing: Tactile:	Tricipital: L R
LF RF LH RH	Extensor carpi radialis: L R
Visual:	Patellar: L R
LF RF LH RH	Cranial tibial: L R
9. Tonic neck:	Gastrocnemius: L R
	Flexor: LF RF LH RH
E. **Cranial nerves:**	Anal:
(1. Olfactory)	Panniculus:
(2. Optic)	
Menace: L R	H. **Pain perception:**
Following:	Head/face:
Obstacle:	Thoracic limb: L R
(3. Oculomotor) L R	Pelvic limb: L R
Direct:	Trunk:
Consensual:	Perineal:
Strabismus:	Tail:
(5. Trigeminal)	
Palpebral: L R	
Corneal: L R	
Masticatory atrophy: L R	
(6. Abducens)	
Strabismus: L R	
(7. Facial)	
(8. Cochlear)	
(Vestibular)	**Grading scale:**
Nystagmus—	0 = absent
Physiologic:	1 = decreased
Spontaneous:	2 = normal
Positional:	3 = exaggerated

The rapidity of onset of an abnormality may be important in the differential diagnosis. For example, acute onset may suggest (*a*) toxicosis, (*b*) trauma, (*c*) vascular accident, or (*d*) a fulminating inflammatory etiology. On the other hand, a more chronic course will suggest a degenerative, neoplastic, or low grade inflammatory process. It is important to ascertain whether the condition has progressed, as in German shepherd myelopathy; remained static, as in a post-traumatic condition; or demonstrated periodic relapses, as in intervertebral disk disease.

Information related to the first abnormal signs and any subsequent signs noted in a patient may differentiate between a focal and a multifocal disease process. In an animal in which the first signs are pelvic limb paresis or paralysis with subsequent thoracic limb involvement, a multifocal progressive process is suggested—e.g., ascending viral myelitis.

Table 1.2. Breed- and Species-Related Neurological Disorders

Breed	Age	Disorder
Akita	Birth	Deafness
Afghan	3–13 mo	Hereditary myelopathy
Australian heeler	Birth	Deafness
Australian shepherd	Birth	Deafness
Australian silky terrier	<1 yr	Glucocerebrosidosis
Bassett hound	Adult	Disk disease
	Adult	Globoid leukodystrophy
Beagle	<6 mo	Globoid leukodystrophy
	<1 yr	Narcolepsy
	Adult	Seizures
	Adult	Hound ataxia
	Adult	Disk disease
Border collie	<3 mo	Cerebellar degeneration
	Birth	Deafness
Boston terrier	Birth	Hydrocephalus
	Birth	Deafness
	Any age	Hemivertebra
	Adult	Brain tumors
Bouvier des Flandres	<1 yr	Laryngeal paralysis
Boxer	<6 mo	Boxer neuropathy
	Adult	Brain tumors
Brittany spaniel	<>1 yr	Hereditary spinal muscular atrophy
Bulldog	<1 yr	Spina bifida
	<1 yr	Hemivertebra
Bull mastiff	<3 mo	Cerebellar degeneration
Bull terrier	Birth	Deafness
Burmese cat	<3 mo	Deafness/vestibular disease
Cairn terrier	<6 mo	Globoid leukodystrophy
Chihuahua	Birth	Hydrocephalus
	Adult	Ceroid lipofuscinosis
Chow Chow	Birth	Hypomyelinogenesis
	Birth	Myotonic myopathy
Cocker spaniel	Birth	Deafness
	Adult	Idiopathic facial paralysis
	Adult	Disk disease
	Adult	Ceroid lipofuscinosis
Collie	Birth	Deafness
	<6 mo	Dermatomyositis
Collie sheepdog	Adult	Neuroaxonal dystrophy
Dalmation	Birth	Deafness
	<6 mo	Dalmation leukodystrophy
	<1 yr	Narcolepsy
	<1 yr	Cramping
Dachshund	Birth	Sensory neuropathy
	<1 yr	Narcolepsy
	Adult	Disk disease
	Adult	Ceroid lipofuscinosis
Doberman pinscher	<3 mo	Deafness/vestibular disease
	<1 yr	Narcolepsy
	Any age	Cervical malformation/malarticulation
	Adult	Dancing Doberman disease
	Adult	Masticatory myositis/atrophic myopathy
	Adult	Sensory neuronopathy
English pointer	<1 yr	Mutilating neuropathy
English setter	Adult	Ceroid lipofuscinosis
	Birth	Deafness
Eygptian Mau cat	Birth	Spongiform degeneration
Fox hound	Adult	Hound ataxia

Table 1.2.—*Continued*

Breed	Age	Disorder
Fox terrier (smooth)	<3 mo	Deafness/vestibular disease
	<6 mo	Hereditary ataxia
	<6 mo	Myasthenia gravis
Fox terrier (wirehaired)	<6 mo	Esophageal hypomotility
	<1 yr	Lissencephaly
German shepherd	<3 mo	Deafness/vestibular disease
	<6 mo	Esophageal hypomotility
	<1 yr	Glycogenosis
	Adult	Seizures
	Adult	Masticatory myositis/atrophic myopathy
	Adult	Infarction
	Adult	Degenerative myelopathy
	Adult	Fibrotic myopathy
	Adult	Giant axonal neuropathy
	Adult	Myasthenia gravis
German shorthaired pointer	Adult	Gangliosidosis
Golden retriever	<6 mo	Myotonic myopathy
	Adult	Sensory neuronopathy
Gordon setter	<>1 yr	Cerebellar degeneration
Great Dane	Any age	Cervical malformation/malarticulation
	<6 mo	Esophageal hypomotility
	Adult	Infarction
Harrier hound	Adult	Hound ataxia
Hound	Adult	Coonhound paralysis
	<1 yr	Globoid leukodystrophy
	Adult	Hypoglycemia
Irish setter	Birth	Hereditary quadriplegia and amblyopia
	<6 mo	Esophageal hypomotility
	<1 yr	Lissencephaly
	Adult	Seizures
Irish terrier	<6 mo	Myotonic myopathy
Jack Russell terrier	<1 yr	Myasthenia gravis
	<6 mo	Hereditary ataxia
Japanese spaniel	Adult	Gangliosidosis
Kerry blue terrier	<6 mo	Cerebellar degeneration
Korat cat	<6 mo	Gangliosidosis
Labrador retriever	Birth	Familial reflex myoclonus
	<6 mo	Hereditary myopathy
	<6 mo	Spongiform degeneration
	<1 yr	Fibrinoid leukodystrophy
	<1 yr	Narcolepsy
Lhasa apso	Birth	Hydrocephalus
	<1 yr	Lissencephaly
Maltese terrier	Birth	Hydrocephalus
Manx cat	Birth	Sacrococcygeal dysgenesis
Old English sheepdog	Birth	Deafness
Pekingese	Adult	Disk disease
Persian cat	<1 yr	Mannosidosis
Pointer	<1 yr	Spinal muscular atrophy
	Adult	Pyogranulomatous meningoencephalomyelitis
Pomeranian	Birth	Hydrocephalus
	<>1 yr	Globoid leukodystrophy
Poodle	Birth	Hydrocephalus
	<6 mo	Sphingomyelinosis
	<1 yr	Hypoglycemia
	<1 yr	Atlantoaxial luxation
	<1 yr	Narcolepsy
	<1 yr	Demyelinating myelopathy
	<1 yr	Globoid leukodystrophy

Table 1.2.—*Continued*

Breed	Age	Disorder
	Adult	Seizures
	Adult	Disk disease
Pug	Adult	Encephalitis
Rhodesian Ridgeback	Any age	Dermoid sinus
Rottweiler	Adult	Leukoencephalomyelopathy
	Adult	Neuroaxonal dystrophy
Rough-coated collie	<3 mo	Cerebellar degeneration
Saint Bernard	<1 yr	Narcolepsy
	Adult	Seizures
	Adult	Infarction
Saluki	Adult	Ceroid lipofuscinosis
Samoyed	Birth	Spongiform degeneration
Schnauzer	<6 mo	Esophageal hypomotility
	Adult	Seizures
	Adult	Infarction
Scottish terrier	Any age	Scotty cramp
	Adult	Sensory neuronopathy
Sheltie	<6 mo	Dermatomyositis
Shih Tzu	Adult	Disk disease
Shropshire terrier	Birth	Deafness
Siamese cat	<6 mo	Gangliosidosis
	<6 mo	Deafness/vestibular disease
	<6 mo	Esophageal hypomotility
	<6 mo	Sphingomyelinosis
	<1 yr	Mucopolysaccharidosis
	<1 yr	Ceroid lipofuscinosis
Siberian husky	<1 yr	Laryngeal paralysis
	Adult	Degenerative myelopathy
	Adult	Sensory neuronopathy
Silky terrier	Birth	Spongiform degeneration
Springer spaniel	Birth	Hypomyelinogenesis
	<6 mo	Myasthenia gravis
	Adult	Fucosidosis
Staffordshire terrier	<6 mo	Myotonic myopathy
Swedish Lapland	<3 mo	Spinal muscular atrophy
	<1 yr	Glycogenosis
Tibetan mastiff	<6 mo	Hypertrophic neuropathy
Walker American foxhound	Birth	Deafness
Weimaraner	<6 mo	Spinal dysplasia
Welsh corgi	Adult	Disk disease
West Highland white terrier	<1 yr	Globoid leukodystrophy
Whippet	Adult	Sensory neuronopathy
Yorkshire terrier	Birth	Hydrocephalus

Some diseases, such as idiopathic epilepsy in poodles and German shepherds, have a familial relationship. Accordingly, detailed information about the pedigree may establish a basis for a suspected hereditary disorder.

Behavioral and personality changes or abnormalities should be ascertained when taking the history as an aid in differential diagnosis; for instance, sudden onset periods of fear or aggression may suggest a psychomotor-like epilepsy or a space-occupying mass of the forebrain.

Method of Examination

The examination should be undertaken in a systematic manner. A routine should be established and adhered to so that no part of the examination is omitted. One method is to evaluate the nervous system from the higher to the lower centers of integration.

The examination should include assessment of (*a*) mental status, (*b*) gait, (*c*) postural reactions, (*d*) craniospinal reflexes, and (*f*) muscle tonus (Tables 1.1, 1.3, 1.4). The order of the examination may depend upon the clinical condition and the cooperative attitude of the patient. Tests which may cause undue excitation (such as response to painful stimuli, e.g., withdrawal reflex) should not be performed on anxious patients early in the examination.

Mental Status (Level of Consciousness)

The level of consciousness is influenced by the functional relationship between the active brainstem and the higher cortical centers. Normal mental status is present in animals which are bright and alert and react to visual, auditory, and tactile stimuli. Abnormal or altered mental status is usually indicative of a lesion in the cerebral cortex, hypothalamus, or midbrain and may be characterized by hysteria, depression, confusion, delirium, or coma. The mental status in individual cases will depend upon the duration and severity of the disease, and may be altered by previous medical treatment. Mental status is sometimes altered by a lower brainstem lesion.

Locomotion

In dogs and cats, body movements are initiated by the cerebral cortex and midbrain. The cerebellum coordinates these movements and the vestibular system maintains body posture when the movements are being performed. The spinal cord acts as a conduit for motor messages (from brain to peripheral nerve and muscle) and for sensory messages (from skin, muscle, and joints to the brain) for further coordination of body movements. It is obvious that many areas of the nervous system are functioning simultaneously during locomotion and that it requires additional testing in order to localize a lesion.

The owner or an assistant should induce the animal to walk, run, and if possible, ascend and descend steps. In addition, the animal can be led or directed toward objects it must avoid by visual means. This portion of the examination allows the clinician to evaluate the function of four systems: (*a*) visual, (*b*) motor, (*c*) vestibular, and (*d*) cerebellar.

Signs of dysfunction can include the following:

1. Bumping into objects or reluctance to ambulate suggests a disease of the visual system.

2. Paresis or paralysis of one or more limbs suggests motor dysfunction due to brainstem, spinal cord, or peripheral nerve disease.

3. Loss of balance, circling, and/or falling to one side suggests a disease of the vestibular system.

4. Head bobbing, hypermetria, hypometria, or lack of coordination indicates disease of the cerebellum or its pathways.

These observations serve to focus attention on the specific systems that must be evaluated carefully as the examination is continued.

Postural Reactions

Postural reactions, such as wheelbarrowing, hemistanding, hemiwalking, hopping, righting, and placing, assess reflex pathways (including touch-pressure, stretch receptors in joints, muscles, and tendons) as well as ascending and

Table 1.3. Cranial Nerve Dysfunction

Nerve	Clinical Signs	Clinical Tests	Normal Response	Abnormal Response
1. Olfactory	Hyposmia or anosmia	Smell of food or nonirritating, volatile substance	Interest in food; Sniff, recoil, or nose lick with volatile substance	No reaction
2. Optic	Visual impairment and hesitancy in moving	1. Obstacle test 2. Visual placing reaction 3. Menace reaction 4. Following movement test	1. Avoidance of obstacle 2. Visual placing of limbs 3. Eye blink 4. Eyes follow objects	1. Bumping objects 2–4. No reaction
	Dilated pupil (mydriasis)	Point source of light in each eye	Direct and consensual pupillary light reflexes	On affected side, direct and consensual reflexes are absent; but they are present on unaffected side
3. Oculomotor	Ventrolateral strabismus Paralysis of upper eyelid (ptosis) Mydriasis	1. Ocular movements in horizontal and vertical planes 2. Point source of light in each eye	1. Normal and ocular excursion 2. Direct and consensual pupillary light reflexes	1. Impaired movements of affected eye 2. On affected side, direct pupillary reflex absent, consensual reflex present; on normal side, direct pupillary reflex present, consensual reflex absent
	Sympathetic control of pupillary function	Constricted pupil (miosis) Enophthalmos Prolapse of third eyelid Ptosis of upper lid		
4. Trochlear	Usually not noted			

Nerve	Clinical Signs	Clinical Tests	Normal Response	Abnormal Response
5. Trigeminal (motor and sensory)	Atrophy of masticatory muscles Inability to close mouth	1. Jaw tone 2. Palpate/observe masticatory muscles 3. Palpebral reflex 4. Corneal reflex 5. Probe nasal mucosa 6. Touch face	1. Resistance to opening jaws 2. Normal muscle contour and resilience 3. Eyeblink 4. Eyeblink/globe retraction 5. Recoil 6. No reaction	1. Lack of resistance 2. Atrophy, hypotonia 3–5. No reaction 6. Intense discomfort
6. Abducens	Medial strabismus	Ocular movements in horizontal plane	Normal ocular excursion	Impaired lateral movement of affected eye
7. Facial	Asymmetry of facial expression Inability to close eyelids Lip commissure paralysis Ear paralysis	1. Palpebral reflex 2. Corneal reflex 3. Menace reaction 4. Tickle ear	1–3. Eyeblink 4. Ear flick	1–4. No reaction
8. Vestibulocochlear				
Vestibular	Nystagmus Head tilt Circling Falling/rolling	1. Ocular movements in horizontal/vertical planes 2. Caloric/rotatory test 3. Righting reactions	1–2. Normal physiological hystagmus 3. Normal righting	1–3. No reaction Ventrolateral strabismus on dorsal extension of head
Cochlear	Deafness	1. Handclap	2. Startle reaction, blink, ear contraction	No reaction
9. Glossopharyngeal	Dysphagia	Gag reflex	Swallowing response	No reaction
10. Vagus	Dysphagia Abnormal vocalizing Inspiratory dyspnea Megaesophagus	1. Gag reflex 2. Laryngeal reflex 3. Oculocardiac reflex	1. Swallow 2. Cough 3. Bradycardia	1–3. No reaction
11. Spinal accessory	Usually not noted			
12. Hypoglossal	Deviation of tongue	1. Tongue stretch 2. Rub nose	1. Retraction 2. Lick response	1–2. No reaction

Table 1.4. Spinal Cord Reflexes

Reflex	Peripheral Nerve	Spinal Cord Origin
Thoracic limb		
1. Flexor	Axillary	C7-C8
	Musculocutaneous	C6-C8
	Median and ulnar	C8-T2
2. Bicipital	Musculocutaneous	C6-C8
3. Tricipital	Radial	C7-T2
4. Extensor carpi radialis	Radial	C7-T2
Pelvic limb		
1. Flexor	Sciatic	L6-S1
2. Patellar	Femoral	L4-L6
3. Cranial tibial	Common peroneal	L6-L7
4. Gastrocnemius	Tibial	L7-S1
Other spinal cord reflexes		
1. Anal (perineal)	Pudendal	S1-S3
2. Panniculus	Spinal nerves (sensory)	C8-T1
	Thoracodorsal nerve (motor)	
3. Defecation	Pelvic	S1-S3
4. Micturition	Pelvic	S1-S3

descending fiber tracts in the spinal cord and brain. The main value of postural reaction testing is to detect subtle asymmetrical deficiencies that may go unnoticed in the gross examination of locomotion. Animals with cerebral and/or midbrain lesions may have a normal gait; however, careful postural reaction testing will often reveal deficits. Postural reaction deficits will be noted on the side opposite (contralateral) the cerebral or midbrain lesion. Lesions in the pons and medulla usually produce gait and postural reaction deficits in limbs on the same side (ipsilateral) as the lesion.

The most reliable postural reactions are hopping, wheelbarrowing, proprioception, and extensor postural thrust. Placing reactions and hemiwalking (especially in cats) tend to produce variable results.

Wheelbarrowing

Normal walking reactions may be tested by supporting the patient under the abdomen so that the pelvic limbs do not touch the ground and forcing the patient to walk using the thoracic limbs (Fig. 1.1). Normal animals will walk with a symmetrical, alternate, thoracic limb movement with the head extended in a normal position. Patients with lesions of the peripheral nerves, cervical spinal cord, brainstem, or higher centers may show asymmetrical movements, stumbling, or knuckling. More severe lesions involving the cervical spinal cord produce a tendency to carry the head flexed with the nose close to and occasionally touching the ground for support. This test is useful in differentiating disease of the brachial plexus and cervical spinal cord from those associated with the thoracolumbar cord. In the latter, the wheelbarrowing reaction should be symmetrical and normal. If deficits in wheelbarrowing are mild, extension of the head may exaggerate the problem.

Hemistanding and Hemiwalking

Hemistanding and hemiwalking reactions test the patient's ability to stand or walk with the pelvic and thoracic limbs on one side only. These can be evaluated

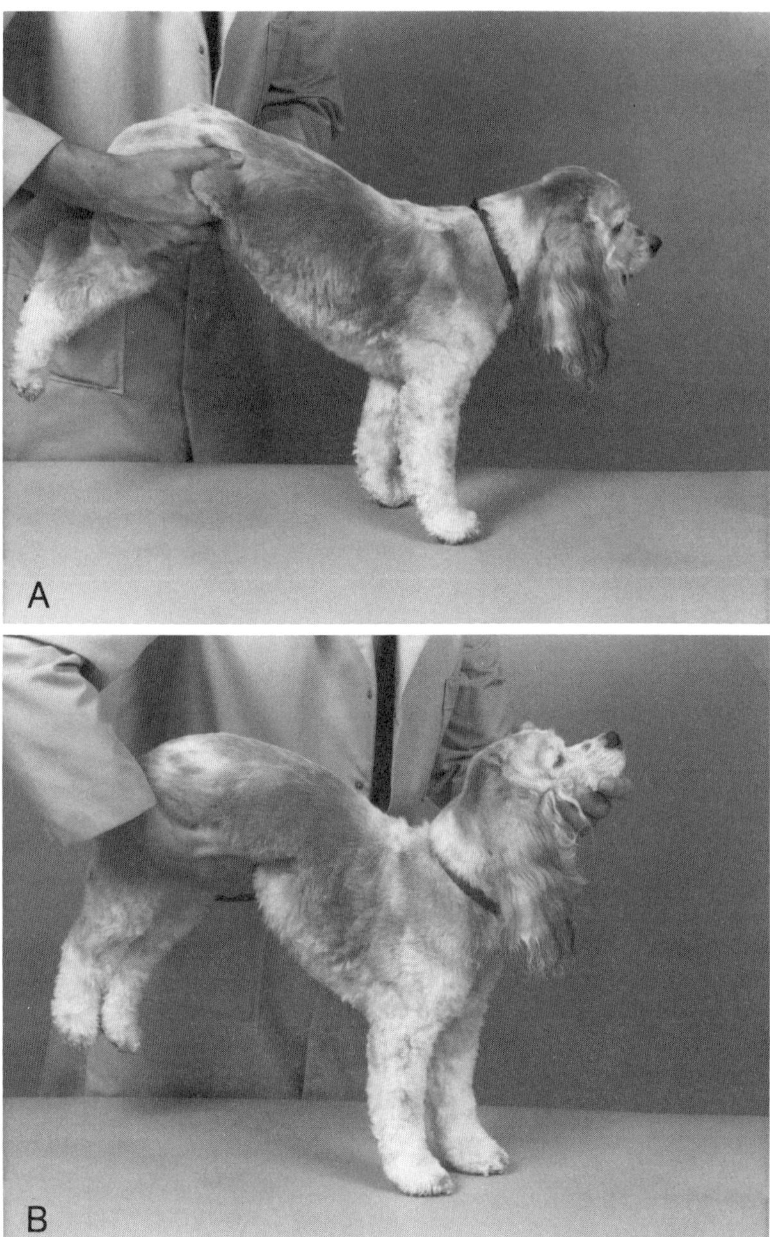

Figure 1.1. Wheelbarrowing postural reactions. (*A*) Normal posture. (*B*) With extended neck.

by holding the pelvic and thoracic limbs of the same side off the ground and forcing the patient to move either forward or sideways (Fig. 1.2). This particular test determines the functional integrity of the motor cortex and the spinal cord. The animal's normal response is to postion the limbs vertical to the axial plane of the body and to move them in a symmetrical fashion when forced to move. A patient with a unilateral lesion in the cerebrum may have a normal gait when all four limbs are used but during hemiwalking will frequently show a contralateral deficit—e.g., scuffing of the limb, knuckling, or a delayed limb positioning reaction. With severe cervical and thoracic cord lesions, the limbs on the same (ipsilateral) side may be unable to support the animal when it is in a hemistanding position. An exaggerated or hypermetric response may be observed in animals with disorders of the cerebellum.

Hopping Reactions

These reactions depend upon a great number of CNS structures and are some of the most complex of the reactions tested. They involve the cerebrum, cerebellum, brainstem, spinal cord, and touch-pressure/pressure-stretch receptors in the joints, muscles, and tendons.

These reactions are tested by holding the animal in a horizontal position. Three of the limbs should be elevated so that they do not touch the examination table or floor, and the animal is supporting its weight on one limb. Move the animal forward and to each side (Fig. 1.3). The animal should hop on the supporting leg in the direction of the displacement, keeping the foot directly under its body to support its weight. This reaction should be attempted on each of the four limbs. A variety of abnormal responses similar to those in the hemiwalking test may be observed.

Proprioception

Proprioceptive positioning tests evaluate the sensory system that determines the patient's ability to recognize the position of the limb when it has been flexed or extended, and the motor response that returns the limb to a normal position. The animal's paw is placed in a flexed position so that the dorsal surface is on the floor, and the response is observed (Fig. 1.4). A normal animal should return the paw to its usual position so that it will support itself against gravity. The reaction time is considered normal when the response occurs within 1 to 3 seconds. Patients with peripheral nerve pathology or unilateral lesions of the spinal cord or higher ascending and descending pathways may fail to show the proprioceptive positioning reaction.

Extensor Postural Thrust Reaction

This reaction involves touch, pressure, and stretch receptors. The cerebrum, vestibulocerebellar system, and spinal cord must be intact for this reaction to occur. The animal is held by the axillae and lowered until its hind limbs touch the floor or a solid supporting surface (Fig. 1.5). The limbs should stiffen in extension and support weight. Animals often take one or two steps backward after the pelvic limbs touch the floor. If the lesion is in the spinal cord but is incomplete and unilateral, only one limb will react. If the lesion is complete, there will be no extension on either side. If there is a cerebral lesion, the contralateral side may be abnormal; if the dog has a vestibulocerebellar lesion, the ipsilateral side may be abnormal. This reaction is assessed in the thoracic limbs by supporting the dog by the pelvis.

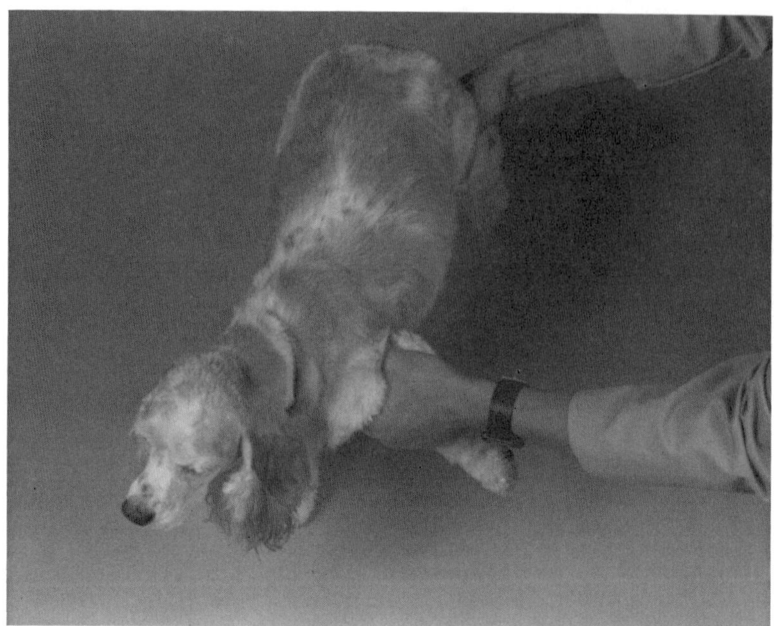

Figure 1.2. Hemistanding/hemiwalking postural reactions.

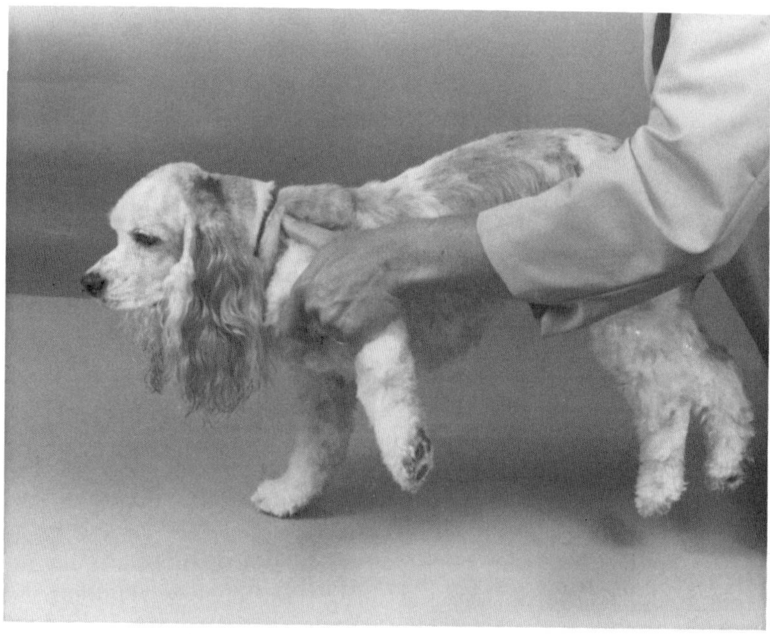

Figure 1.3. Hopping postural reactions.

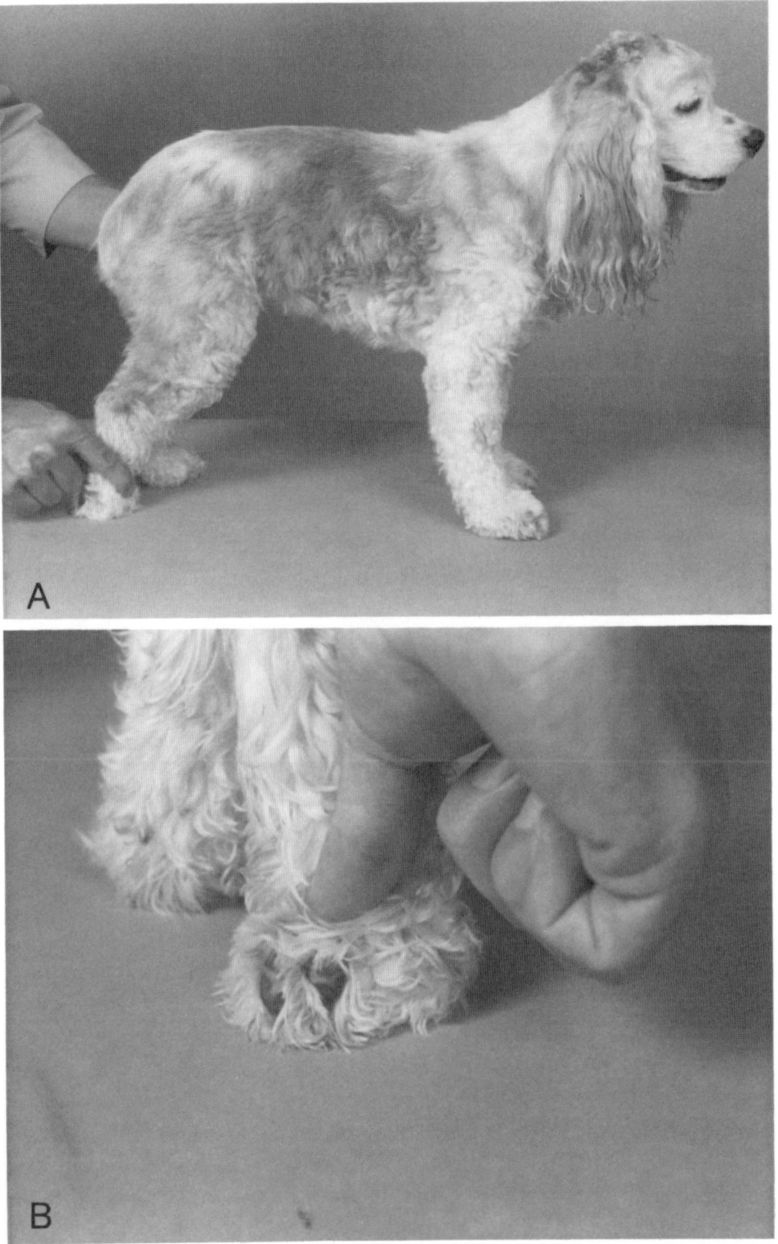

Figure 1.4. (*A* and *B*) Dorsal knuckling of paw for testing proprioception.

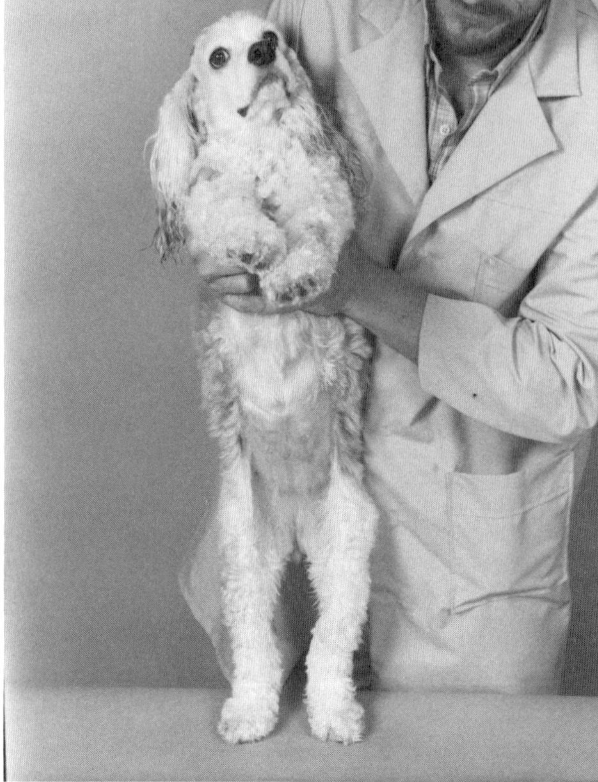

Figure 1.5. Extensor postural thrust.

Righting Reactions

The ability of an animal to maintain its normal position in relation to gravity and during motion involves three physiological mechanisms: the visual system, the vestibular system, and the contact-pressure proprioceptive system. When evaluating righting reactions, it is necessary to eliminate one or two of the three remaining systems.

Test.

1. The animal is suspended by the pelvis and the position of the head is observed. The head should assume a position in space at approximately a 45° angle to the horizontal and in a line with its body, not rotating to one side or the other, and the limbs should be held in an extended position (Fig. 1.6). To test vestibular function alone, the animal should be blindfolded.

2. The animal is placed in a lateral recumbent position on each side, and the animal's ability to right itself is noted. The contact-pressure receptors on the side of the body will be stimulated, and the animal should right itself normally by extension and flexion of uppermost and lowermost limbs, respectively. If unilateral vestibular pathology is present, this righting reaction will be abnormal on the ipsilateral side.

Placing Reactions

Placing reactions involve both tactile and visual pathways. In the former, the reactions are initiated by touch and pressure stimulation, and with the latter the initiating stimulus originates in the visual centers.

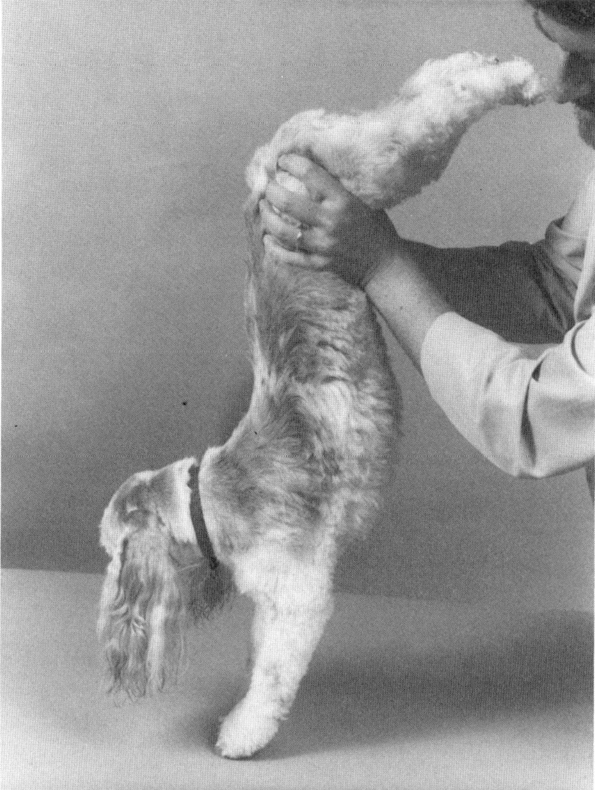

Figure 1.6. Righting reaction.

Tactile Placing Reactions (Animal Blindfolded). The blindfolded animal is grasped under the thorax and held in a horizontal position in the air with the thoracic limbs hanging. It is then moved toward the edge of a solid object, such as a table edge, in order to initiate contact with the dorsal surface of the distal extremities of the thoracic limbs. The slightest contact should result in accurate and immediate placing of the paws in a supporting position on the table surface (Fig. 1.7). The thoracic limb response is tested in both limbs at the same time and then in each limb separately. The pelvic limb responses are tested in a similar manner. These reactions, especially in the pelvic limbs, may be difficult to elicit upon repeated testing.

Visual Placing Reaction. The animal is supported in the same way as for the tactile placing reaction test (Fig. 1.7). As the table is approached the animal's normal response is to place both paws on the surface. Each limb should be tested individually.

Tonic Neck Reactions

The dog is placed in a standing position and the head is raised. The normal dog will extend the thoracic limbs and partially flex the pelvic limbs. When the head is flexed downward, semiflexion of the thoracic limbs and extension of the pelvic limbs are normal responses. When the head is rotated to the right and to the left, limb extension on the side to which the head is rotated is a normal response. These complex responses are a result of the coordination of the vestibular centers with neck muscle and joint receptors.

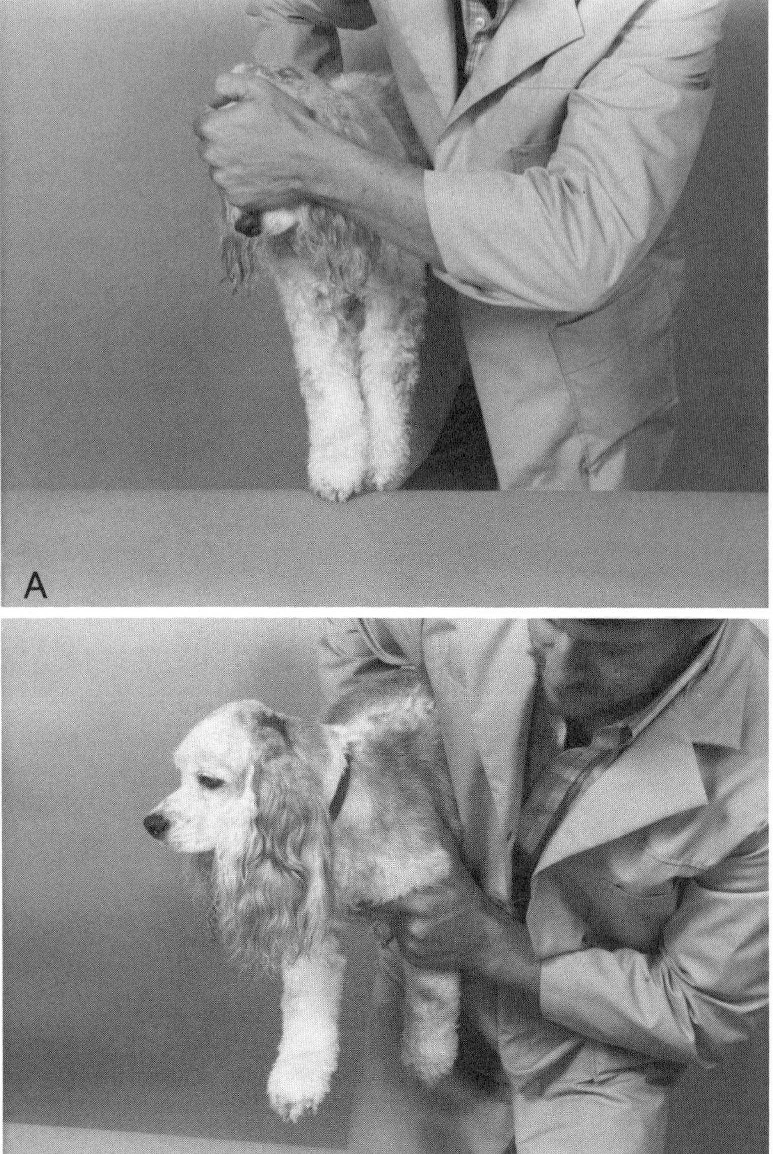

Figure 1.7. Placing reactions. (*A*) Tactile. (*B*) Visual.

Cerebral lesions may cause contralateral abnormalities, and vestibular lesions may cause ipsilateral abnormalities. A patient with cervical spinal cord and/or brainstem disease may fail to extend the thoracic limbs, and these joints may passively flex so that the weight is borne on the dorsal surface of the paw.

The occurrence of two or more postural reaction deficits in any limb(s) is indicative of a significant deficit. Postural reaction deficits provide regional rather than specific lesion localization. For example, deficits in limbs on the same side suggest an ipsilateral cervical cord or brainstem lesion or a contralateral cerebral lesion. In another animal, if postural reactions are abnormal in pelvic limbs but normal in thoracic limbs, the lesion is located somewhere behind the T2 spinal cord level.

Thus, postural reactions provide a guide for more definitive neurological localization using cranial and spinal nerve examinations.

Examination of the Cranial Nerves

The cranial nerves, which are conventionally numbered 1 through 12, comprise (*a*) those that are attached to the brainstem, (*b*) the olfactory nerve (cranial nerve 1) fibers which enter the olfactory bulb of the hemispheres, and (*c*) the spinal accessory nerve (Cr. n. 11), which is attached to the cervical spinal cord but enters the skull and re-emerges from it (Table 1.3). The optic nerve (Cr. n. 2) is not a true peripheral nerve developmentally, structurally, or in its pathological manifestations. Cranial nerves may be motor or sensory or may contain fibers for both functions. Parasympathetic fibers are carried in oculomotor (Cr. n. 3), facial (Cr. n. 7), glossopharyngeal (Cr. n. 9), and vagus (Cr. n. 10) nerves. The cranial nerves should be examined in sequence from 1 to 12 so that none are omitted.

Olfactory Nerve (Cr. n. 1)

A nonirritating volatile substance may be used to test the functional integrity of the olfactory system. Most animals will recoil and lick their noses after sniffing the substance when it is placed near the external nares. However, some animals will not respond sufficiently for diagnostic purposes. The ability of a hungry animal to detect the smell of food is frequently a more reliable reaction of olfactory acuity. Disorders of the sense of smell (hyposmia-anosmia) are relatively rare in the dog but do occur. They may be caused by conditions that affect the primary olfactory receptors in the nasal mucosa, such as severe bacterial infections. Occasionally, the virus of distemper may destroy these cells. The neurons of the olfactory bulb and tract may also be affected; however, this is relatively rare. Lesions of the uncus, a part of the olfactory system, may cause hallucinations of smell, and the owner may report that the animal continually appears to be smelling something that is not present.

Optic Nerve (Cr. n. 2) and Associated Pathways

For normal sight the retina, optic nerves, optic tracts, lateral geniculate bodies, optic radiations, and occipital lobes must all be functional. Determination of the visual acuity of an animal is sometimes difficult because of tactile or auditory sense compensation. The fundus should be examined by either direct or indirect ophthalmoscopy. In addition, the following tests may be used to evaluate the visual pathways.

Menace Reaction. A threatening gesture toward the eye will result in a blink response of the eye and some head recoil (Fig. 1.8). The eyes should be tested individually. The menace reaction is mediated by the optic and facial nerves. This test can be conducted using a sheet of transparent material between the examiner and the animal to prevent air currents and the possible induction of another blink reflex mediated by the trigeminal and facial nerves. Demented animals, young animals less than 3 months of age, and animals with severe cerebellar disease may not show a menace response but can see.

Following Movements. The following movement test evaluates the integrity of the visual centers. (*a*) Move the hand in front of the animal and note

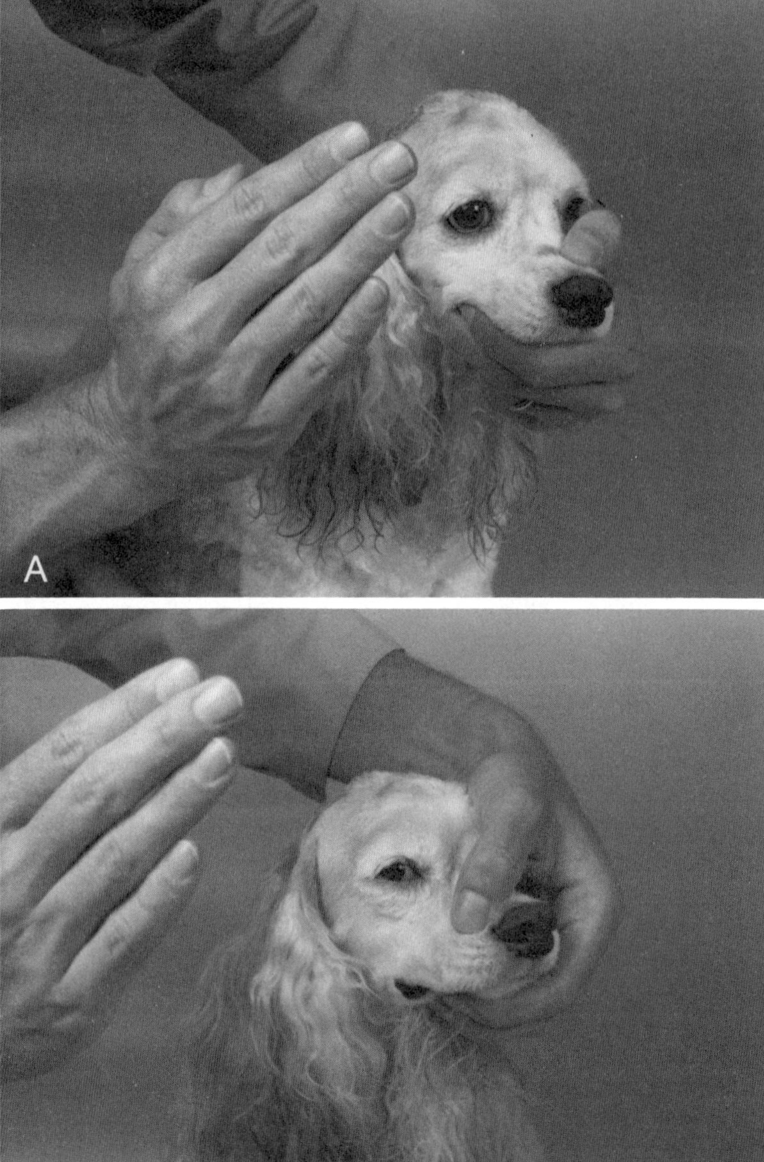

Figure 1.8. Menace reaction. (*A*) Threatening gesture. (*B*) Blink response.

whether its eyes follow the hand. (*b*) Cotton balls may be tossed toward or in front of the animal's face. The normal animal will follow the trajectory of the cotton ball once it has entered its visual field (Fig. 1.9).

Obstacle Test. Lead the animal through an obstacle course in both bright and reduced light conditions.

Visual Placing Reactions. See the earlier discussion of placing reactions.

Pupillary Light Reflex. Evaluation of the pupillary light reflex tests the function of optic and oculomotor nerves. As a strong light is directed into one eye (Fig. 1.10), the pupil of that eye should constrict (direct pupillary reflex), as

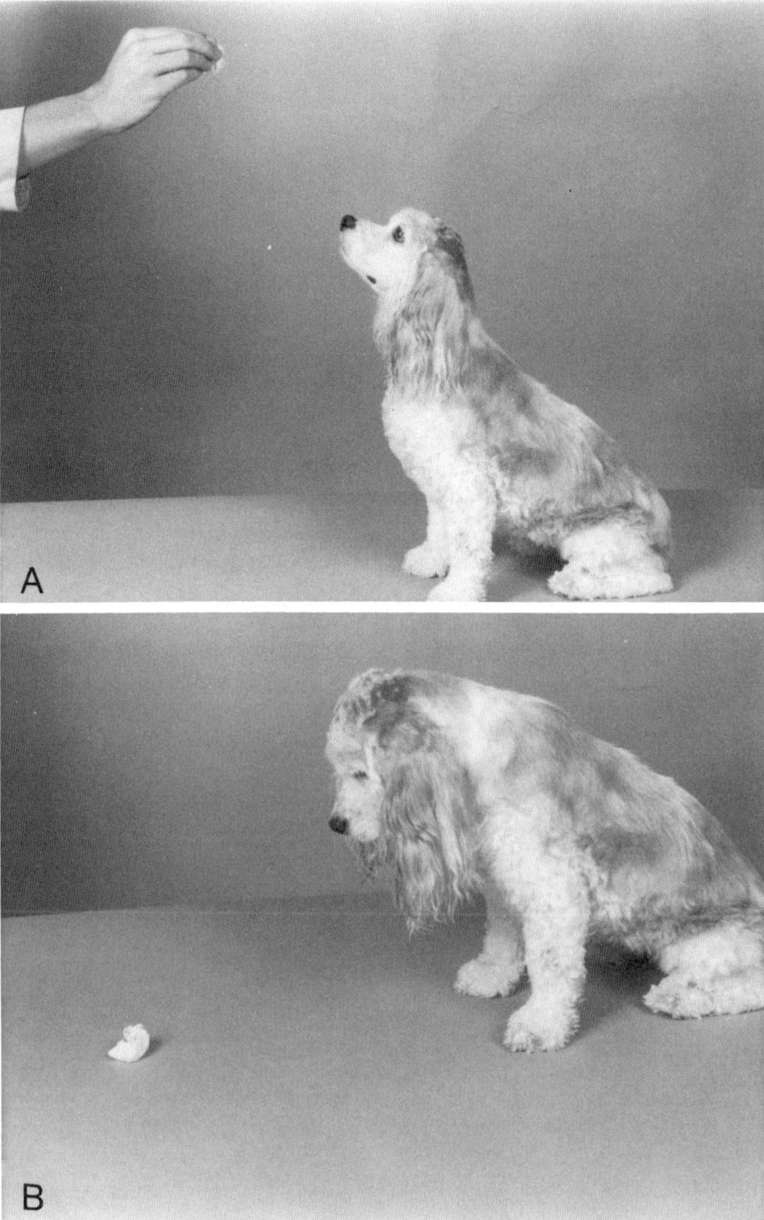

Figure 1.9. (*A* and *B*) Visual following movements.

well as that of the opposite pupil (indirect or consensual response) (see "Oculo-motor Nerve," below).

Clinical Signs of Optic Nerve Dysfunction. These signs include (*a*) visual impairment and (*b*) mydriasis, in which the iris is dilated and unresponsive to stimulation by bright light and there is no consensual response in the normal eye. However, light detected at the opposite eye will result in pupillary constriction of the affected eye as a result of the consensual response.

It is also possible to have visual impairment with normal pupillary light reflexes (7). This would indicate a lesion in the central visual pathways (lacteral geniculate

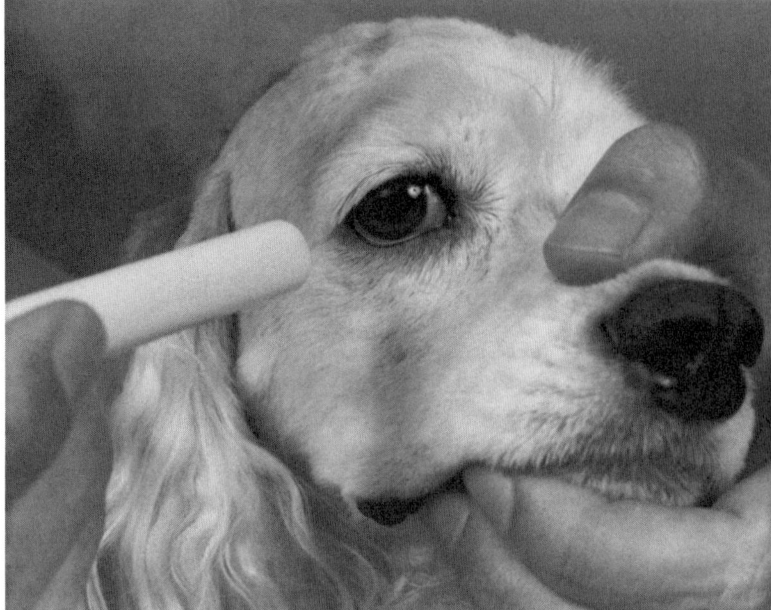

Figure 1.10. Pupillary light reflex.

body, optic radiation, or visual cortex). Since most of the fibers cross in the optic chiasm, the lesion would be contralateral to the eye with the menace deficit.

Oculomotor Nerve (Cr. n. 3)

The motor portion of the oculomotor nerve innervates all of the extrinsic ocular muscles except for the lateral rectus, retractor bulbi, and dorsal oblique. In addition, this nerve has a parasympathetic component which is concerned with pupillary-motor control and accommodation.

Motor Function. Motor function can be tested by slowly rotating the head in both horizontal and vertical planes and observing ocular movement. By moving the patient's head side to side and up and down, symmetrical eyeball movements and brief normal horizontal and vertical nystagmus should occur with the fast phase in the direction of movement. These normal ocular movements that result from movement of the head are referred to as the oculocephalic reflex. They are dependent upon normal head-eye coordination which is controlled by the nerves that supply the eyeballs (oculomotor, trochlear, and abducens) and the vestibular system.

Abnormalities of Motor Function of the Oculomotor Nerve. These may include (*a*) ventrolateral strabismus, (*b*) reduced or absent adduction of the eye in the horizontal plane and reduced ocular movement of the eye, and (*c*) paralysis of the upper eyelid of the affected side (ptosis), resulting in a narrowed palpebral fissure.

Pupillary Light Reflexes. The parasympathetic fibers in the oculomotor nerve respond to the amount of light received by the retinas of each eyeball. Activity of these fibers is decreased in diminished light and the pupils dilate. In bright light, these fibers are activated and pupillary constriction (miosis) occurs.

Pupil size also can be influenced by the sympathetic nervous system. Factors that stimulate this system include excitement, fear, or anger. Normally, pupillary size is modulated by parasympathetic and sympathetic systems. The pupillary light reflexes depend upon the functional integrity of the oculomotor nerve and the optic nerve together with the midbrain and sympathetic pathways. Inequality in resting pupil diameter is called anisocoria.

Test. When light is focused on the retina using a brillant point-surface of light, the normal iris constricts, causing the pupil to become smaller (direct pupillary reflex). When the light is withdrawn, the iris relaxes and the pupil becomes larger. Because of the neuronal cross-connections in the optic chiasm and midbrain, the opposite pupil should also respond to the light in a similar manner, even though the light is directed into only one eye. This response is called the consensual or indirect pupillary reflex.

Abnormalities of Parasympathetic Function of the Oculomotor Nerve. (*a*) There is an unresponsive, dilated pupil in the eye tested but a normal consensual response in the contralateral eye. Stimulation of the contralateral eye will result in a normal direct response but an absent consensual response in the affected eye. (*b*) Transient unilateral or bilateral miosis possibly due to midbrain compression may be seen early in the acute phase of cranial trauma. Later, as midbrain compression progresses, the pupils may become dilated and unresponsive to direct light stimulation. In such cases the consensual response will be absent bilaterally.

The sympathetic pathways begin in the hypothalamus and pass through the brainstem and cervical cord to synapse with cell bodies located in the intermediolateral gray matter of the spinal cord in T1 and T2 segments. Fibers from these neurons travel via the vagosympathetic trunk to the cranial cervical ganglia where synapse occurs. Postganglionic fibers continue through the middle ear eventually to innervate the dilator pupillae muscle and the smooth muscle of the lids and periorbita.

Lesions at any level of the sympathetic pathways (but especially at T1-T2 cord segments and in the middle ear) may produce a group of signs known as Horner's syndrome.

Abnormalities of Sympathetic Control. These abnormalities include (*a*) pupillary miosis; (*b*) ptosis (the result of loss of tone in the smooth muscle of the eyelids); the ptosis noted in sympathetic dysfunction is the least reliable of the signs and is less than that which occurs with oculomotor nerve dysfunction; (*c*) enophthalmos (the result of loss of tone in the periorbital smooth muscle); (*d*) prolapse of the third eyelid (the result of loss of innervation of its smooth muscle and of retraction of the globe caused by denervation of the periorbital smooth muscle).

Trochlear Nerve (Cr. n. 4)

Disorders of this nerve or of its central nuclei rarely produce clinical signs in animals. There may be a slight dorsomedial rotation of the affected eye due to paresis or paralysis of the dorsal oblique muscle.

Trigeminal Nerve (Cr. n. 5)

The trigeminal nerve is both motor and sensory. The motor portion innervates the muscles of mastication (temporalis, masseter, medial and lateral pterygoid muscles, and anterior portion of the digastric muscle). The sensory portion supplies the face, eyelids, pinnae, cornea, oral cavity structures, and mucosa of the nasal septum inside the nares.

Sensory Tests. (*a*) Corneal reflex: stimulation of the cornea with a moistened cotton swab will induce an ipsilateral blink reflex. The eyeball may also retract into the orbit, indicating a functional abducent nerve. (*b*) Palpebral reflex: stimulation of the margins of the palpebral fissure will also produce an ipsilateral blink response (Fig. 1.11).

Both reflex tests are mediated via the trigeminal nerve (sensory) and the facial nerve (motor). The ability of the animal to perceive pain sensation is tested by blunt, gentle probing of the nasal mucosa (Fig. 1.12). The normal response is abrupt withdrawal of the head from the stimulus. The menace reaction (via cranial nerves 2 and 7) may be elicited if these tests are performed too aggressively.

Sensory Abnormalities. These include (*a*) absence of the previously mentioned reflexes, (*b*) reduced (hypesthesia) or absent (anesthesia) sensation of the affected side, and (*c*) hyperesthesia (a trigeminal neuralgia-like syndrome) with intense discomfort induced by mild sensory stimulation.

Motor Tests. Open and close the dog's mouth and note the resistance. Normal trigeminal nerve motor control will be evident by resistance to opening the mouth.

Motor Abnormalities. Abnormalities may manifest as (*a*) an inability to close the jaw, as seen in the early phase of bilateral trigeminal motor paralysis, e.g., rabies, or idiopathic trigeminal neuritis; unilateral trigeminal lesions do not appear to interfere with normal jaw function; or (*b*) unilateral or bilateral atrophy of masticatory muscles.

Abducens Nerve (Cr. n. 6)

The abducens nerve is the remaining cranial nerve associated with extrinsic ocular muscle innervation. This nerve supplies the lateral rectus muscle and the retractor bulbi muscle.

Abnormalities. These include (*a*) medial strabismus of the affected side, (*b*) impaired abduction of the globe of the affected side when the head is rotated, and (*c*) impaired retraction of the eyeball when the cornea is lightly touched.

Facial Nerve (Cr. n. 7)

This nerve supplies motor innervation to the muscles of facial expression and the posterior portion of the digastric muscle. It also supplies the anterior two-thirds of the tongue for taste sensation and all major exocrine glands of the head (lacrimation, salivation) except the parotid and zygomatic salivary glands.

Tests. (*a*) The menace response (via cranial nerves 2 and 7) and (*b*) corneal and palpebral reflexes (via cranial nerves 5 and 7) are used to test the facial nerve.

Abnormalities. Facial nerve abnormalities may be (*a*) an inability to close the eye, (*b*) paresis or paralysis of the lip commissure of the affected side, (*c*) impaired ear movement on the affected side, and (*d*) widening of the palpebral fissure (due to lack of tone in the orbicularis oculi muscle) on the affected side.

Clinical signs will depend upon the level of the lesion. If the lesion is external to the stylomastoid foramen, the above signs will be seen; however, if it is more centrally located (at or before the level of the geniculate ganglion in the genu of the facial canal), these signs together with reduced or absent lacrimation will lead to dryness of the eye with potential keratitis sicca of the cornea. Schirmer's tear test can be used to determine if the parasympathetic fibers supplying the lacrimal gland are functional. Also, there may be no immediate response to the

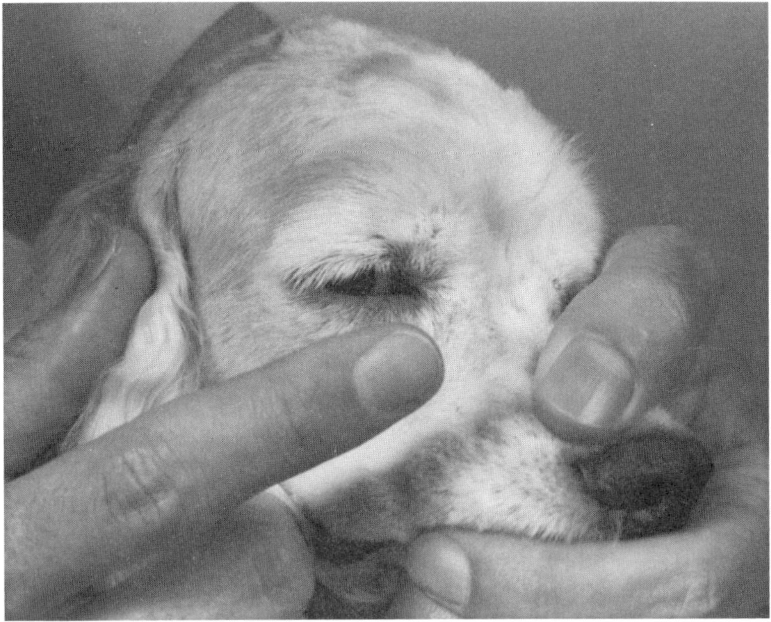

Figure 1.11. Blink response associated with the palpebral reflex.

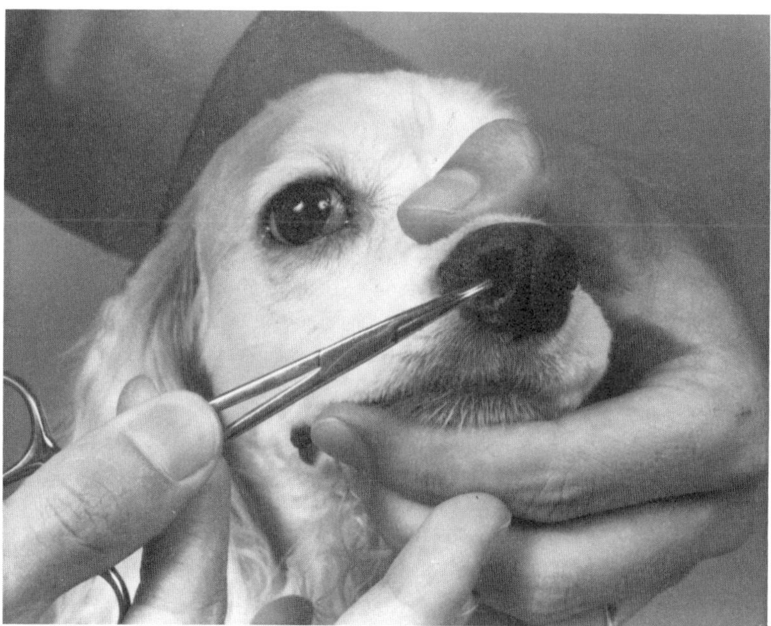

Figure 1.12. Sensory examination of the nasal mucosa.

bitter taste of atropine solution applied to the tongue with a cotton-tipped applicator.

Trauma to the facial nerve where it curves around the mandible is the most common cause of facial paralysis. Extension of inflammatory conditions from the external to the middle ear may also involve the facial nerve. Occasionally, space-occupying lesions (tumors) in the pons may be responsible for facial paralysis. When this occurs, however, usually some other cranial nerve abnormality will also be observed.

Brainstem lesions and/or irritations of facial nerves are believed occasionally to induce hemifacial spasms or hypertonicity of facial muscles. The eyelid margins, ears, and lip commissures may be pulled caudally. Spasms may be intermittent (8, 9).

Vestibulocochlear Nerve (Cr. n. 8)

This nerve has two subdivisions and serves two functions. The cochlear nerve serves in a sensory capacity for hearing, and the vestibular nerve is proprioceptive for equilibrium and posture control.

COCHLEAR NERVE

Tests. The cochlear nerve may be tested by (*a*) clapping the hands behind the head of the animal. Normally, the animal responds by turning the head toward the source of the sound, blinking the eyes, and moving the ears. (*b*) Electroencephalographic audiometry, a test used in veterinary teaching institutions, is more definitive for a partial auditory impairment.

Abnormalities. If the cochlear nerve is impaired, the animal may show lack of startle response or turning toward the source of the sound.

VESTIBULAR NERVE

The vestibular system of each side consists of the end organs (utricle, saccule, and three semicircular canals), the vestibular nerve, and four brainstem nuclei, all of which regulate normal posture of the eyes, head/neck, trunk, and limbs.

Tests. (*a*) Rapid movement of the head in horizontal and vertical planes normally produces a physiological nystagmus in each plane. (*b*) The caloric test—the installation of cold or warm water into the ear canal for 3 to 5 minutes—will produce physiological nystagmus. (*c*) The postrotatory nystagmus test is conducted by spinning the animal on a rotatable object, such as a swivel chair, for 30 to 60 seconds and then stopping suddenly. Upon cessation of rotation a nystagmus will appear with the fast component toward the direction opposite that of body rotation. (*d*) To perform the vestibular righting test the animal is supported by the pelvis and held suspended for a period of 20 to 30 seconds. The normal response noted is thoracic limb extension, and the head is held at approximately a 45° angle with the nose directed vertically (Fig. 1.6). The caloric and postrotatory tests can be cumbersome and are rarely performed.

Abnormalities. Vestibular nerve abnormalities may cause the following reactions: (*a*) lack of induction of physiological nystagmus when the animal's head is moved toward the side of the vestibular lesion. (*b*) Spontaneous nystagmus—vertical, horizontal, or oscillating. In the dog the most common type is horizontal. It may have an equal rate of ocular movement in each direction (pendular nystagmus), or it may be unequal with fast-slow components (jerking nystagmus). In jerking nystagmus the direction of the quick phase is by convention the direction of the nystagmus. In vestibular disorders the direction of the quick phase is opposite the side of involvement. In these disorders the slow component is abnormal, and the fast phase is compensatory. The nystagmus may be present at rest, or it may be induced by manipulation of the head (positional nystagmus). (*c*) Head tilt toward the side of the vestibular disease (ipsilateral). (*d*) Falling or rolling or both (ipsilateral). (*e*) Tight circling toward the side of the lesion. (*f*) Vestibular strabismus on the same side as the abnormality. This is a ventrolateral strabismus which may be apparent when the head is dorsally extended.

Central (brainstem) and peripheral (receptors in inner ear and vestibular nerve) vestibular disease have similar clinical signs. Cranial nerve abnormalities, other than those of the facial nerve or Horner's syndrome, such as trigeminal nerve dysfunction, usually indicate a central vestibular disorder. The presence of vertical nystagmus or a change in direction of nystagmus with varying head positions also indicates a central brainstem lesion.

Glossopharyngeal Nerve (Cr. n. 9)

The glossopharyngeal nerve innervates the musculature of the pharyngeal and palatine structures; and the zygomatic and parotid salivary glands, and provides sensory innervation to the posterior third of the tongue (taste).

Test. Gag reflex: When pressure is applied externally to the pharyngeal area, swallowing is the normal response (Fig. 1.13). This reflex can also be initiated

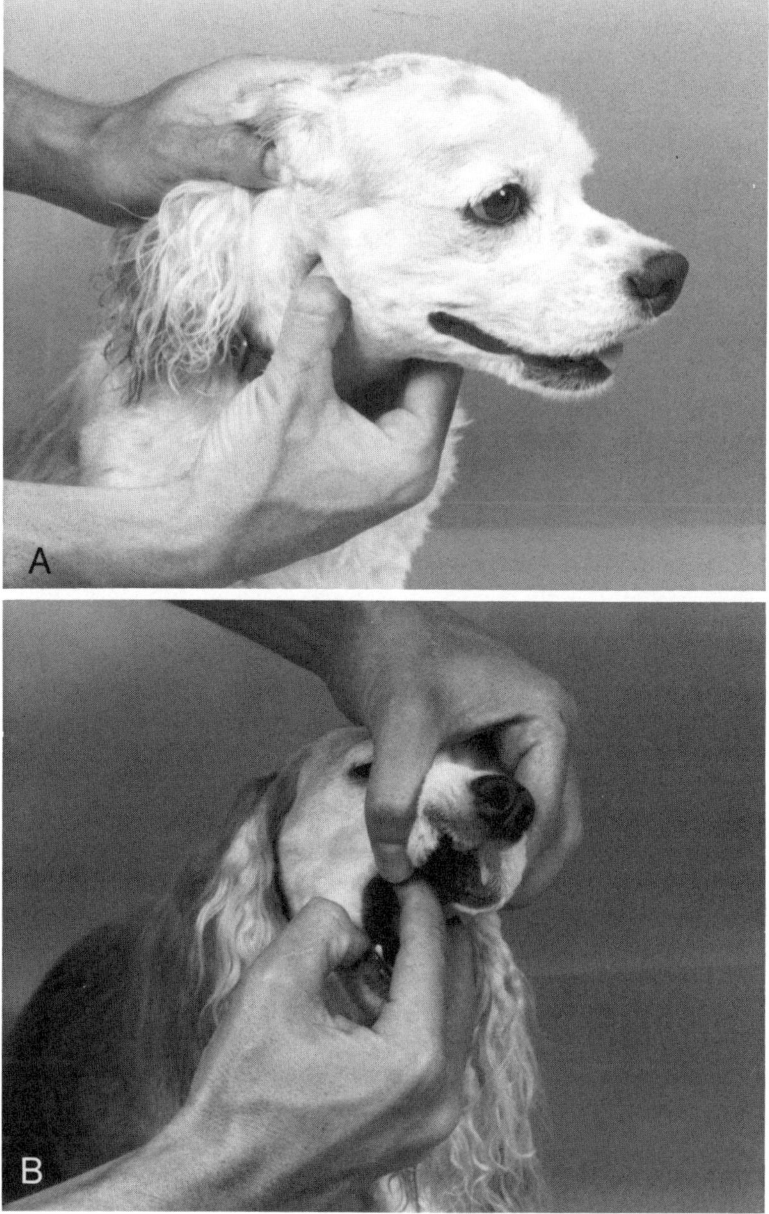

Figure 1.13. Gag reflex. (*A*) External stimulation. (*B*) Direct digital stimulation.

by direct digital pharyngeal stimulation (Fig. 1.13). The reflex is mediated by glossopharyngeal and vagus nerves.

Abnormalities. These include (*a*) absence of the gag reflex, (*b*) reduced pharyngeal tone, and (*c*) dysphagia.

Vagus Nerve (Cr. n. 10)

The sensory and motor functions of the vagus nerve are similar to those of the glossopharyngeal nerve with regard to swallowing and the gag reflex. In addition, vocalization is controlled by the vagus nerve. The autonomic function of the vagus is cardioregulation and innervation of the thoracic and abdominal viscera.

Tests. The vagus nerve is tested by the (*a*) gag reflex, (*b*) laryngeal reflex—moderate external pressure over the laryngeal area normally results in a slight coughing response, and (*c*) oculocardiac reflex—direct pressure applied to both eyeballs simultaneously results in reflex bradycardia (this reflex is mediated by cranial nerves 5 and 10).

Abnormalities. Vagus nerve abnormalities are indicated by (*a*) absence of the above reflexes, (*b*) dysphagia, and (*c*) altered vocalization. (*d*) In bilateral vagal disorders in dogs and cats, inspiratory dyspnea due to laryngeal paralysis and megaesophagus due to esophageal paralysis may also be noted.

Spinal Accessory Nerve (Cr. n. 11)

This nerve supplies innervation to certain muscles of the neck (trapezius and parts of the sternocephalicus and brachiocephalicus muscles). Paralysis of these muscles is rarely a clinical problem.

Hypoglossal Nerve (Cr. n. 12)

The hypoglossal nerve is the motor nerve to the musculature of the tongue.

Test. Rubbing or moistening the nose will induce the animal to lick, which allows examination of the tongue. Manual stretching of the tongue induces a voluntary retraction.

Abnormalities. These include (*a*) lack of retraction in response to stretch (*b*) lateral deviation of the tongue. In the early stage of unilateral hypoglossal paralysis, the deviation is on the side opposite the lesion (flaccid paralysis of the muscles of the diseased side enables the contralateral muscles to act unopposed). In chronic paralysis, atrophy and fibrotic contraction result in a corrugated appearance of the tongue, and the deviation occurs on the affected side.

Spinal Cord Reflexes

Spinal reflexes form the basic unit of CNS investigation and function. In most cases reflex testing does not test any other portion of the CNS except those cord segments in which the reflexes are involved (Table 1.4). It should be realized that all reflexes are influenced by higher centers of control.

Spinal reflexes may be elicited when the animal is either in a lateral recumbent position or supported upright by an assistant. When the animal is supported, it may become excited, and this will interfere with the reactions. The animal must be relaxed if the reflexes are to be elicited in their normal form. It is best to start with the reflexes least likely to disturb the animal and then proceed to those initiated by pain. Spinal reflexes are more easily elicited in the larger breeds.

Tendon Reflexes (Myotatic)

Tendon reflexes are initiated by stimulation of muscle spindle activity through muscle stretch.

Patellar Reflex. The patellar reflex is the most reliable tendon reflex in the dog and is mediated via the cord segments L4 to L6. With the hind limb in a relaxed, semiflexed position, the straight patellar ligament is lightly tapped with a percussion hammer (Fig. 1.14). The normal response is a quick extension of the stifle joint.

Abnormalities. These include (*a*) absence of response (areflexia), (*b*) depressed response (hyporeflexia), (*c*) increased response (hyperreflexia), and (*d*) repetitive response (clonus). The first two abnormal reflexes are indicative of peripheral nerve disorders and/or of the spinal cord segments in which the reflexes are involved, while increased reflexes are usually seen with lesions of the brainstem or of the spinal cord rostral to the level of the limbs being tested.

Gastrocnemius Reflex. This reflex is mediated via tibial branches of the sciatic nerve and cord segments L7 and S1. Using the reflex hammer, a sharp tap is applied to the examiner's forefinger, which is placed over the gastrocnemius tendon (Fig. 1.15). The normal response is a reflex extension of the hock.

Abnormalities. These are the same as those for the patellar reflex.

Cranial Tibial Reflex. This reflex is mediated by the peroneal nerve and cord segments L6-L7 and is elicited by tapping the belly of the muscle (Fig. 1.16). The normal response is a slight flexion of the hock.

Bicipital, Tricipital, and Extensor Carpi Radialis Reflexes. In the thoracic limb these reflexes can be elicited in dogs that are lying relaxed in a lateral recumbent position.

The bicipital reflex is mediated by the musculocutaneous nerve and cord segments C6 to C8. It is elicited by placing the forefinger on the biceps tendon on the anterior-medial aspect of the elbow and tapping the finger with a percussion hammer (Fig. 1.17). A slight flexion of the elbow will occur in a normal animal.

The tricipital reflex is mediated by the radial nerve and cord segments C7-C8 and T1-T2. It is tested by tapping the tendon of insertion of the triceps proximal

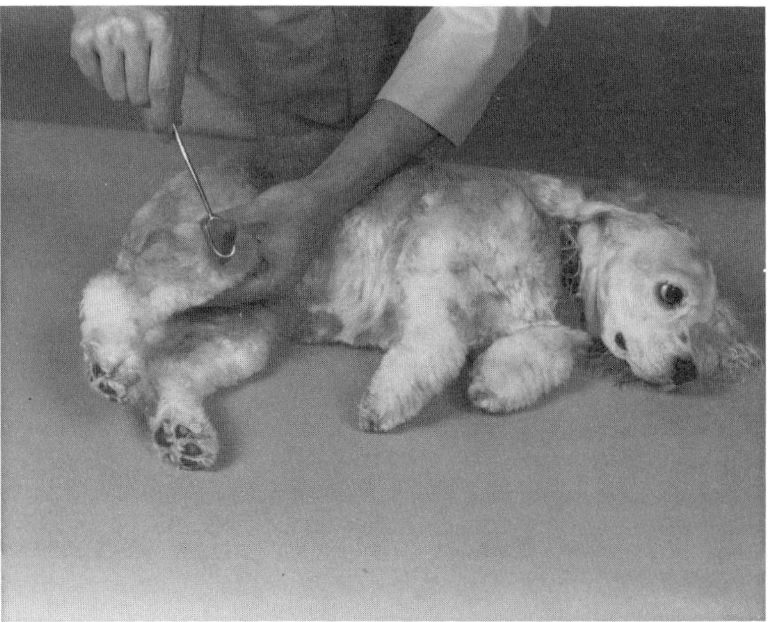

Figure 1.14. Patellar reflex.

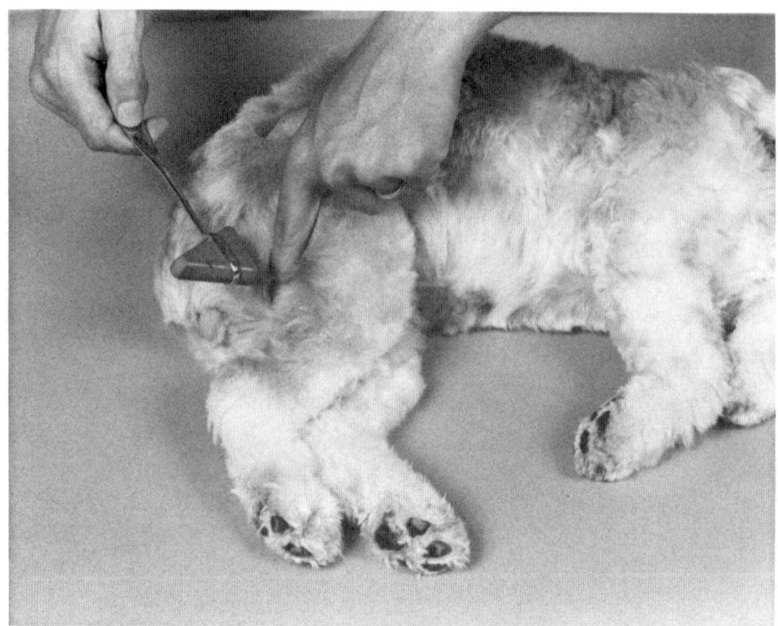

Figure 1.15. Gastrocnemius reflex.

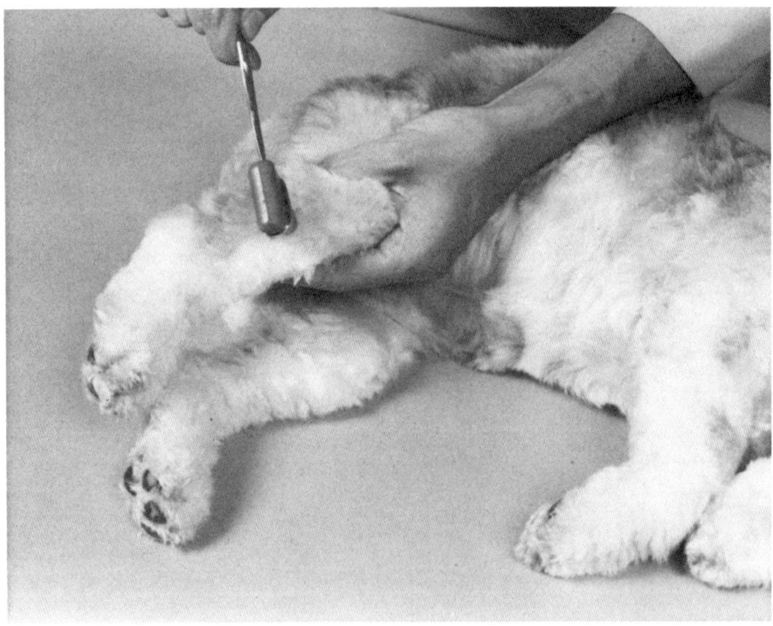

Figure 1.16. Cranial tibial reflex.

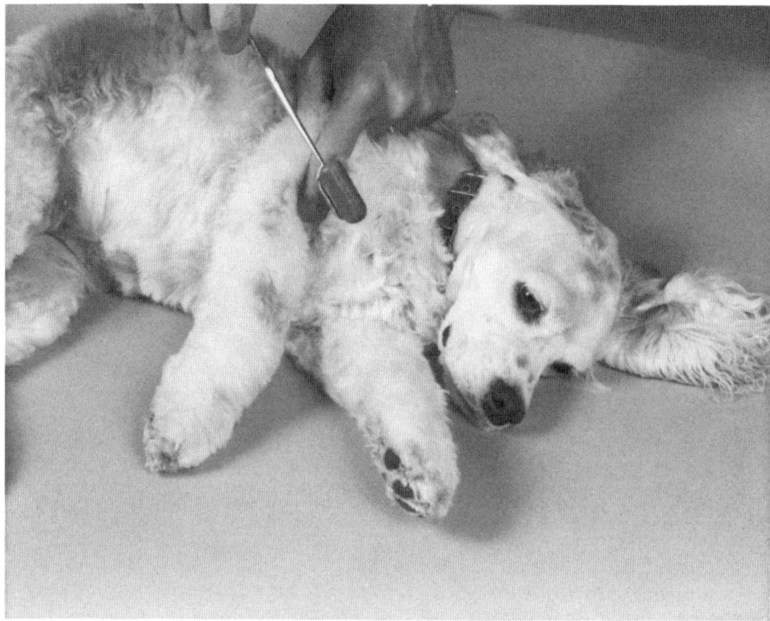

Figure 1.17. Bicipital reflex.

to the olecranon or by placing the forefinger or thumb on the tendon and tapping the finger or thumb with the hammer (Fig. 1.18). The normal response is a slight extension of the elbow.

The extensor carpi radialis reflex is mediated by the radial nerve. It is elicited by tapping the belly of the muscle just distal to the elbow (Fig. 1.19). The response is an extension of the carpus.

At times it is difficult to see these thoracic limb reactions; however, if the respective muscles are palpated during the test, the contraction may be felt.

Abnormalities. These are the same as those for the pelvic limb tendon reflexes.

Flexor Reflexes

The flexor reflexes are initiated by painful stimuli and determine the integrity of the reflex arc and the spinal cord centers, as well as the pathways in the CNS that are concerned with the patient's response to a painful stimulus.

The pelvic limb flexor reflex is mediated by the sciatic nerve and its branches and by cord segments L6-L7 and S1.

The thoracic limb flexor reflex is mediated by the axillary, musculocutaneous, and medial/ulnar nerves and by cord segments C6-C8 and T1-T2.

Stimulation of pain receptors by compression of foot pads (Fig. 1.20), interdigital tissue, or the nail-skin junction results in reflex flexion of the appropriate limb. Intense stimulation will result in vocalization and turning of the head toward the stimulus (see "Sensory Evaluation," below).

Abnormalities. (*a*) Areflexia, (*b*) hyporeflexia, (*c*) hyperreflexia, (*d*) clonus, and (*e*) crossed extensor reflex may be noted.

Crossed Extensor Reflex

When a painful stimulus is applied to one limb, the opposite (contralateral) limb will extend. The crossed extensor reflex is not seen in a normal animal. Its presence is indicative of spinal cord pathology above the spinal cord segments controlling the reflex.

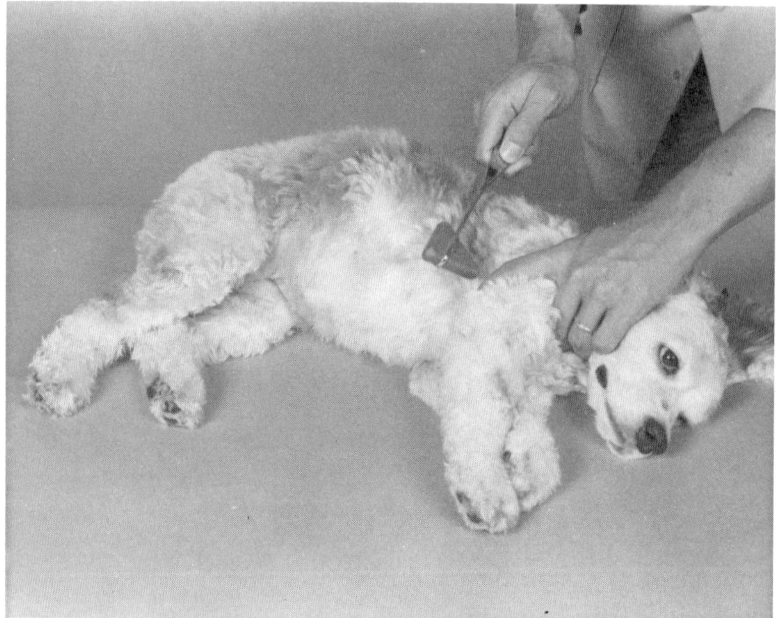

Figure 1.18.   Tricipital reflex.

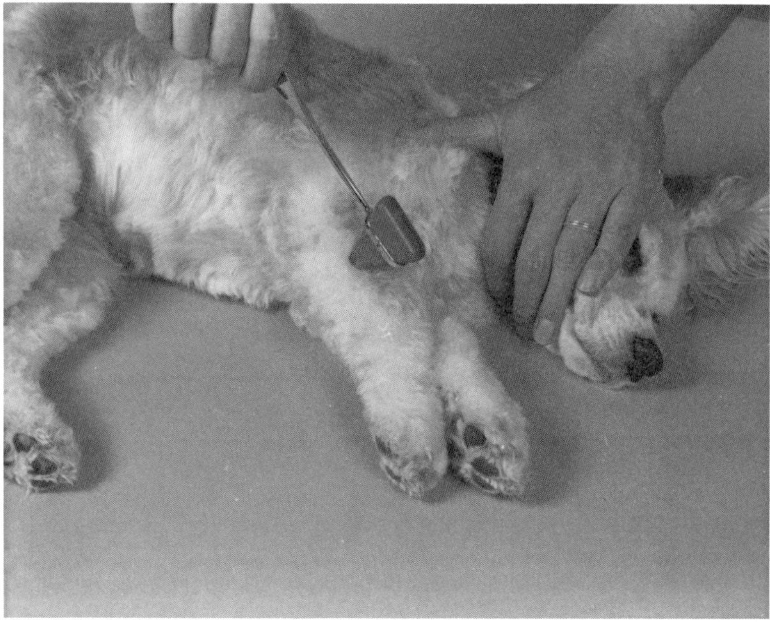

Figure 1.19.   Extensor carpi radialis reflex.

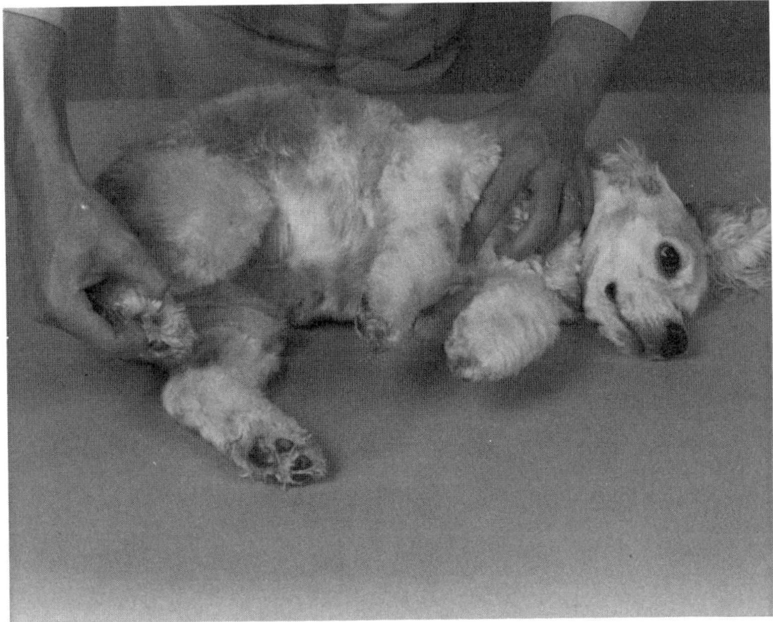

Figure 1.20. Flexor reflex.

Anal (Perineal) Reflex

The anal or perineal reflex is mediated via the pudendal nerve and cord segments S1-S3. It can be elicited by (*a*) tactile stimulation of the perianal region (Fig. 1.21) or (*b*) compression of the glans of the penis in males. The normal response is a contraction of the external anal sphincter.

Abnormalities. Abnormal responses include (*a*) areflexia and (*b*) hyporeflexia.

Panniculus Reflex

The panniculus reflex tests the integrity of the innervation of the musculature of the subcutaneous trunk. The afferent limb of this reflex is mediated via the segmental sensory nerves, and the efferent component is mediated via C8 and T1 motor nerves.

To elicit the panniculus reflex, a tactile stimulus is applied to the dorsal midline of the thoracolumbar region with a blunt, pointed instrument or by pinching the skin with hemostats (Fig. 1.22). The test is usually started over the lumbosacral region and continues rostrally to the cervicothoracic area. The normal response is a reflex contraction of the subcutaneous musculature at the point of stimulation.

Abnormalities. One may note (*a*) an absent/depressed reflex caudal to the level of a thoracolumbar spinal lesion or (*b*) exaggerated muscle contraction and increased pain sensation (hyperesthesia) at the level of, or immediately above, the area of cord involvement. The panniculus reflex can be a valuable test for localizing a focal lesion in the thoracolumbar cord region.

Visceral Reflexes

Two important reflex functions that are mediated by sacral nerves are defecation and micturition.

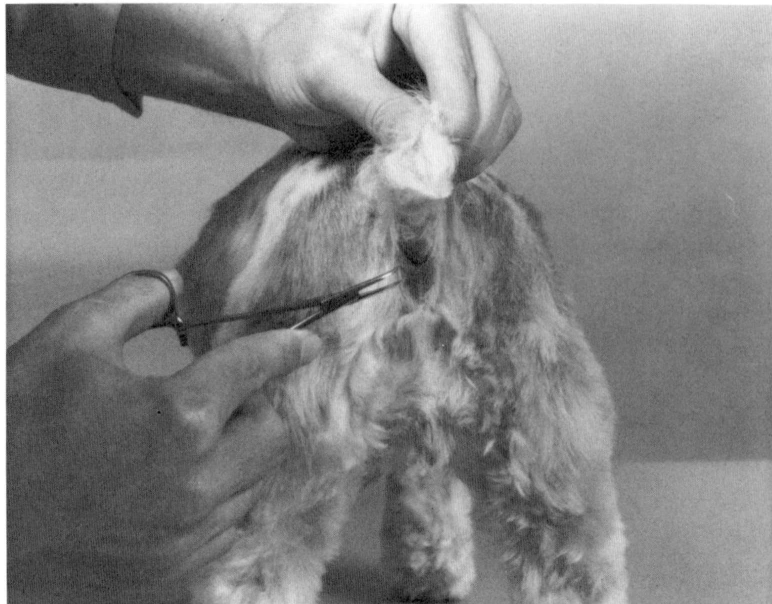

Figure 1.21. Anal (perineal) reflex.

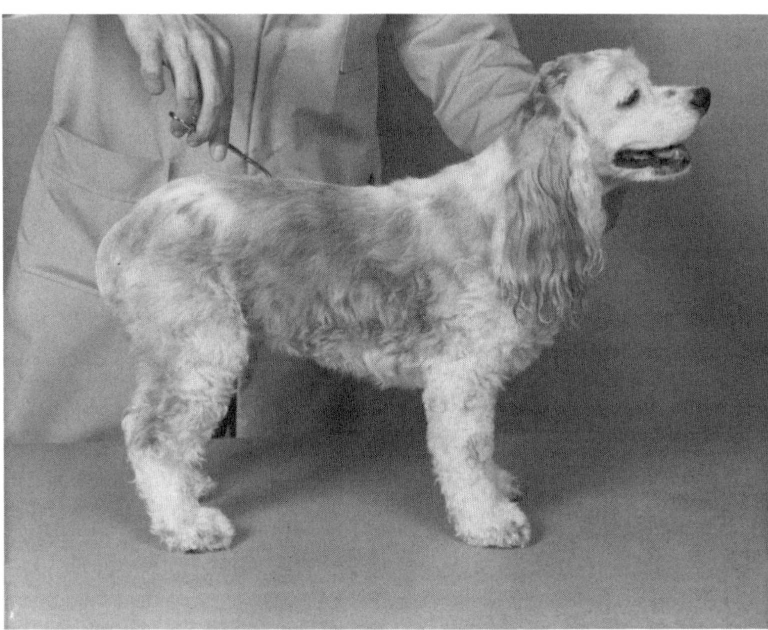

Figure 1.22. Panniculus reflex.

Defecation. Voluntary control of defecation is mediated by pathways from the brain to the sacral cord segments. Although the rectum is innervated by the pelvic (parasympathetic) nerves, which originate in the sacral segments, emptying of the rectum can occur even with disruption of sacral innervation due to intrinsic innervation within the bowel wall. Since the external anal sphincter is innervated by the pudendal nerve, which also originates in the sacral segments, the perineal (anal) reflex provides a good assessment of sacral spinal cord function.

Micturition. Unlike the bowel, the bladder is dependent on its extrinsic (outside) innervation for function. When the bladder is distended, sensory impulses from the bladder pass to the brainstem. Motor fibers then pass back to the sacral cord segments with activation of the pelvic (parasympathetic) nerves which cause the bladder to contract. Normal micturition also requires synchronized contraction of the urethral smooth muscle, which is supplied by pelvic and hypogastric (sympathetic) nerves, and relaxation of the urethral skeletal muscle, which is innervated by the pudendal nerve. The micturition reflex will be abolished by lesions of the pelvic nerves, sacral cord segments, or pathways to and from the brainstem. Consequently, the bladder will distend with urine and eventually overflow. Lesions of the sacral segments will also result in loss of innervation to the skeletal muscle of the urethra. This renders the bladder easy to express manually with little urethral resistance. Thus, animals with sacral cord lesions may suffer from continual overflow incontinence. In contrast, spinal cord lesions cranial to the sacral segments can result in increased tone in the urethral skeletal muscle, making the bladder very difficult to express manually; catheterization is usually required. The incontinence is often characterized by sporadic spurting of urine.

In animals with spinal cord lesions above the sacral segments, the micturition reflex tends to be lost about the same time that voluntary motor function is lost. With recovery, both functions generally return together.

Muscle Tone

Muscle tone is maintained by the muscle spindles and their spinal cord connections and modulated largely by brainstem nuclei. Muscle tone is usually examined when spinal cord reflexes are evaluated with the animal lying in lateral recumbency.

Muscle tone can be easily tested by (*a*) passive manipulation of limbs (flexion and extension) and/or (*b*) individual muscle palpation (paraspinal, appendicular, etc). Normal response to manipulation is an increase in resistance. Normal muscles exhibit a degree of resilience and tension when palpated (normotonia).

Abnormalities. (*a*) Absence of tone (atonia), (*b*) reduced tone (hypotonia), (*c*) increased tone (hypertonia), (*d*) exaggerated tone (spasticity/clasp-knife effect), or (*e*) the Schiff-Sherrington phenomenon may be noted. The first two abnormalities are often observed in animals with disease of the peripheral nerve(s) and/or associated spinal cord segments. Neurogenic segmental muscular atrophy may be associated with these signs. Hypertonia and spasticity may be present with lesions of the brainstem or of the spinal cord rostral to the level of the limbs being tested. The Schiff-Sherrington phenomenon is characterized by extensor hypotonus of the thoracic limbs. It is usually observed in animals with severe spinal cord injury from T2 to L4, and it is due to interruption of pathways running between the lumbar spinal cord and thoracic limb cord segments. Thoracic limb postural reactions remain intact. Muscle tone may be reduced in pelvic limbs, but reflexes are present. The presence of the Schiff-Sherrington phenomenon often bespeaks a guarded prognosis.

Sensory Evaluation

Apart from conscious proprioception (the tests for which have already been discussed under "Postural Reactions"), evaluation of the sensory system in animals is largely dependent upon tests for pain perception. Other sensory

Table 1.5. Dermatomal Evaluation

Dermatomal Area	Sensory Nerve	Nerve Origin
Head		
Face, nasal cavity, oral cavity	Sensory trigeminal	Brainstem and upper cervical cord
Thoracic limb		
Lateral surface of brachium	Axillary	C7-C8
Medial surface of forearm	Musculocutaneous	C6-C8
Dorsal surface of paw, craniolateral surface of forearm	Radial	C7-T2
Palmer surface of paw	Median and ulnar	C8-T2
Caudal surface of forearm	Ulnar	C8-T2
Pelvic limb		
Caudolateral surface of hock, stifle, and thigh	Sciatic	L6-S1
Medial surface of paw, hock, stifle, and thigh	Saphenous	L4-L6
Craniodorsal surface of paw, hock, and stifle	Common peroneal	L6-L7
Plantar surface of paw	Tibial	L7-S1
Trunk, perineum, and tail		
Paraspinal surface of trunk	Spinal	C1-S1
Perineum	Pudendal	S1-S3
Tail	Coccygeal	Cy1...(n)

modalities, such as heat, cold, and touch-pressure, are extremely difficult to assess objectively and quantitatively. Assessment of pain sensation is important for the localization of a spinal cord lesion and for the prognosis.

Deep and superficial pain sensations are easily tested. Superficial pain sensation is elicited by pinching or pricking the skin and subcutaneous tissues using a blunt needle or forceps. Deep pain sensation is tested by pinching the digits with the fingers or forceps.

Normal Response. Retraction of the limb, head recoil, vocalization, and turning of the head toward the site of stimulus comprise the animal's normal response to pain.

Abnormalities. Included are (*a*) absence of pain (anesthesia)—this usually carries a poor prognosis, (*b*) reduced pain sensation—this usually carries a guarded prognosis, (*c*) increased pain sensation (hyperesthesia), and (*d*) muscle spasms (e.g., paraspinal).

Testing for pain perception over recognized dermatomal areas also will provide useful information about the integrity of the sensory nerves and associated spinal cord segments (Table 1.5) (10–14).

References

1. Redding RW, Braund KG: Neurologic examination. In Hoerlein BF (ed): *Canine Neurology—Diagnosis and Treatment*, ed 3. Philadelphia, WB Saunders, 1978, p 53.
2. de Lahunta A: *Veterinary Neuroanatomy and Clinical Neurology*, ed 2. Philadelphia, WB Saunders, 1983.
3. Shell L: Cranial nerve disorders in dogs and cats. *Comp Cont Ed* 4:458–466, 1982.
4. Greene CE, Oliver JE: Neurologic examination. In Ettinger SJ (ed): *Textbook of Veterinary Internal Medicine*, ed 2. Philadelphia, WB Saunders, 1983, p 419.
5. McGrath JT: *Neurologic Examination of the Dog*, ed 2. Philadelphia, Lea and Febiger, 1960.

6. Palmer AC: *Introduction to Animal Neurology*, ed 2. London, Blackwell Scientific Publications, 1976.
7. Braund KG, Vandevelde M, Albert RA, Higgins RJ: Central (post-retinal) visual impairment in the dog—a clinical-pathological study. J Small Anim Pract 18:395–405, 1977.
8. Roberts SR, Vainisi SJ: Hemifacial spasms in dogs. *J Am Vet Med Assoc* 150:381–385, 1967.
9. Parker AJ, Cusick PK, Park RD, Small E: Hemifacial spasms in a dog. *Vet Rec* 93:514–516, 1973.
10. Fletcher TF, Kitchell RL: The lumbar, sacral and coccygeal tactile dermatomes of the dog. *J Comp Neurol* 128:171–180, 1966.
11. Bailey CS: Patterns of cutaneous anesthesia associated with brachial plexus avulsion in the dog. *J Am Vet Med Assoc* 185:889–899, 1984.
12. Bailey CS, Kitchell RL: Clinical evaluation of the cutaneous innervation of the canine thoracic limb. *J Am Anim Hosp Assoc* 20:939–950, 1984.
13. Bailey CS, Kitchell RL, Johnson RD: Spinal nerve root origins of the cutaneous nerves arising from the canine brachial plexus. *Am J Vet Res* 43:820–825, 1982.
14. Bailey CS, Kitchell RL, Haghighi SS, Johnson RD: Cutaneous innervation of the thorax and abdomen of the dog. *Am J Vet Res* 45:1689–1698, 1984.

2
Localization Using Neurological Syndromes

Introduction

The neurological examination is a tool used for compiling a list of clinical neurological abnormalities. A complete neurological and clinical examination should be performed on each animal to avoid missing important clinical signs. In some instances, however, the clinical status of the animal may dictate the extent of the examination. For example, pelvic limb postural reaction testing could be wisely omitted in an animal presenting with acute spinal cord trauma so as to avoid excessive spinal manipulation and possible aggravation of the injury. Since it is now established that specific lesions within the CNS, peripheral nervous system (PNS), and skeletal muscle result in predictable, specific, clinical signs, it naturally follows that through the recognition of certain key clinical signs, a lesion can be localized within any of these areas. This concept of neurological syndromes provides the basis for lesion localization, without which differential diagnosis of disease cannot be logically pursued (1–4). Each neurological syndrome has an associated table that includes a comprehensive list of diseases known to produce that given syndrome. Each disease is categorized according to the nature of the disease process (e.g., degenerative, neoplastic, traumatic, etc), the rapidity of onset of clinical signs, and its progresive or nonprogressive course. Specific diseases are alphabetically arranged in Chapter 3. Since many neurological diseases are breed- and/or species-related, the tables include such information, whenever applicable. From this clinical "data base," the diagnosis can be logically attained using a combination of key diagnostic aids, including signalment data (age, breed, sex), historical information, and such appropriate ancillary procedures as radiography, cerebral spinal fluid analysis, electrodiagnostics, etc.

This sequential method may help to remove much of the stigma of complexity and, sometimes, irrationality from clinical neurology. Experience has shown that students, interns, residents, and practitioners can use this easily recognizable syndrome approach immediately, without the need for detailed knowledge of neuroanatomy, neurophysiology, or neuropathology.

When reading through a given syndrome it is important to understand that it is not necessary for all of the clinical signs listed to be observed. A sufficient number of key clinical signs will still be present to permit the clinician to define that syndrome accurately. The concept of neurological syndromes is based on the truism: **"We remember 20% of what we hear but 80% of what we see."**

Myopathic Syndrome

In general, myopathic disorders are uncommon and are reported more often in dogs than in cats. Myopathies tend to have a bilaterally symmetrical distribution. Reflexes are usually preserved, and sensory perception of pain is not impaired.

The myopathic syndrome is characterized by generalized weakness, exercise intolerance, and stiff, stilted gait. While gait disturbance is worsened by exercise in the majority of myopathies, in certain myotonic disorders, such as those reported in Chows and Staffordshire terriers, stiffness becomes less apparent with exercise. Also, in these breeds, muscle mass is increased (hypertrophy), whereas in many other myopathies, muscle wasting (atrophy) tends to be a feature. A temporary dimple contracture in the muscle (e.g., limb muscle or tongue) can be induced in certain myotonic myopatheis, such as myotonia congenita, following a sudden tap with the hand or percussion hammer. Muscle pain, induced by palpation, is often present in animals with polymyositis. Limited joint movement resulting from contracture is the hallmark of certain myopathies, e.g., pelvic limb hyperextension in puppies with toxoplasmosis.

The principal clinical signs of the myopathic syndrome are listed in Figure 2.1, and the diseases known to produce this syndrome are outlined in Table 2.1.

Common causes of the myopathic syndrome seen in practice: Polymyositis; masticatory myositis; atrophic myopathy; steroid myopathy; toxoplasmosis.

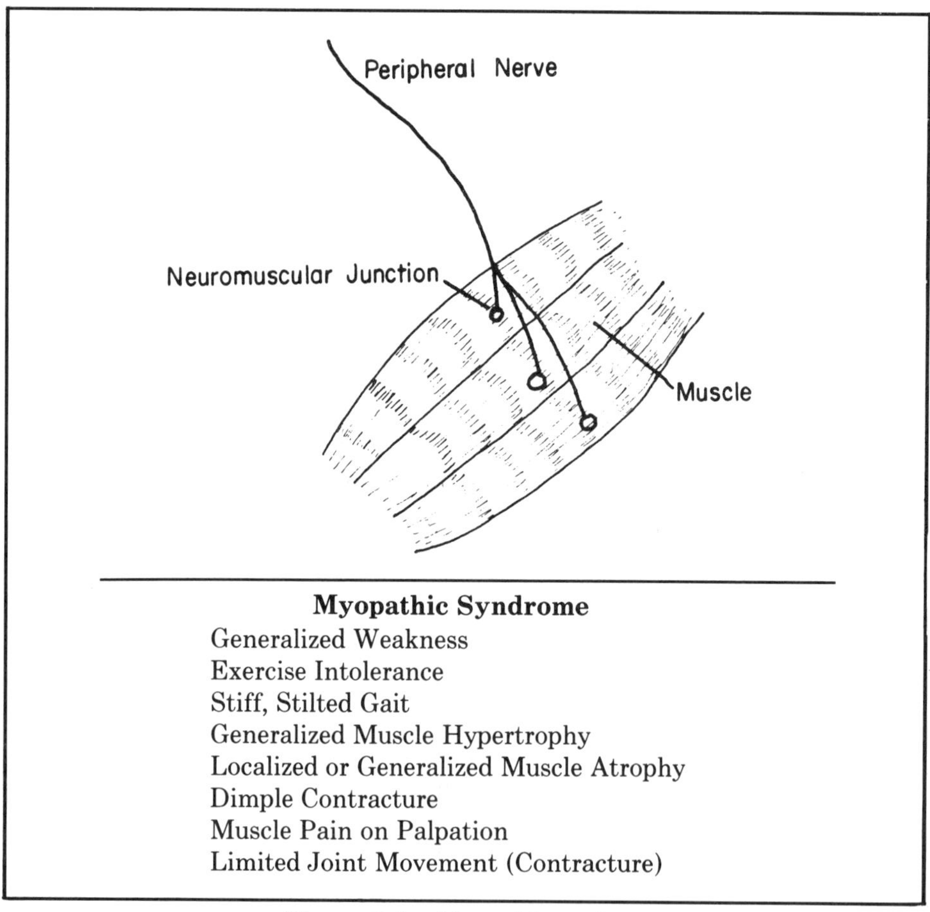

Myopathic Syndrome

Generalized Weakness
Exercise Intolerance
Stiff, Stilted Gait
Generalized Muscle Hypertrophy
Localized or Generalized Muscle Atrophy
Dimple Contracture
Muscle Pain on Palpation
Limited Joint Movement (Contracture)

Figure 2.1. Myopathic syndrome.

Table 2.1. Myopathies in Dogs and Cats

Category of Disease	Acute Onset		Chronic Onset
	Progressive	Nonprogressive	
Degenerative	None	Ischemic neuromyopathy—cat	1. Myotonic myopathy—Chow; Staffordshire terrier; Irish terrier; golden retriever 2. Hereditary myopathy of Labrador retrievers 3. Congenital myasthenia gravis*—smooth fox terrier; Jack Russell terrier; springer spaniel 4. Paraneoplastic neuromyopathy 5. Glycogenosis—Swedish Lapland; German shepherd 6. Atrophic myopathy 7. Immobilization myopathy 8. Ossifying myopathy 9. Fibrotic myopathy—German shepherd
Autoimmune/immune-mediated	1. Polymyositis 2. Masticatory myositis	None	1. Polymyositis 2. Masticatory myositis 3. Acquired myasthenia gravis* 4. Dermatomyositis—collie; sheltie
Metabolic	1. Malignant hyperthermia 2. Hyperkalemia 3. Hypokalemia	1. Exertional myopathy	1. Hyperadrenocortical myopathy 2. Steroid myopathy 3. Hypothyroid myopathy
Nutritional	None	None	1. Vitamin E/selenium-responsive myopathy
Inflammatory/infectious	1. Toxoplasmosis	None	1. Toxoplasmosis 2. Idiopathic feline polymyopathy
Toxic	1. None	None	1. Drug toxicities*

* Refers to disorders of the neuromuscular junction ("junctionopathies").

Neuropathic Syndrome

The neuropathic syndrome is one of the most commonly observed syndromes in clinical practice. It is frequently associated with trauma of peripheral and, sometimes, cranial nerves. The hallmarks of this syndrome are reduced or absent reflexes (hyporeflexia, areflexia), flaccid weakness (paresis), reduced muscle tone (hypotonia), paralysis of appendicular or head muscles, and after 1 to 2 weeks, neurogenic muscle atrophy. A variable degree of loss of sensation may be detected upon cutaneous (dermatomal) testing, since most nerves contain motor and sensory components. In animals with primary sensory neuropathies (e.g., mutilating neuropathy and sensory neuronopathy), the syndrome may include loss of pain sensation and/or proprioception, abnormal sensitivity about the face or trunk (paresthesia), and hyporeflexia without muscle atrophy.

Peripheral neuropathies most commonly involve a single nerve (mononeuropathy), such as common peroneal, radial, or facial nerves. Polyneuropathies involve several nerves, are usually bilaterally symmetrical, and are best exemplified by coonhound paralysis. Other less common degenerative polyneuropathies may have a proximal limb muscle distribution, e.g., hereditary spinal muscular atrophy in Brittany spaniels, or a distal limb muscle distribution, e.g., giant axonal neuropathy in German shepherds. The majority of neuropathies are insidious in onset and have a chronic course. Signs of autonomic nerve dysfunction are rarely observed in animals with polyneuropathies. Similarly, cranial nerve dysfunction is uncommon, with the exception of the facial nerve (Cr. n. 7) in coonhound paralysis and occasionally in hypothyroid neuropathy, and the vagus nerve (Cr. n. 10) resulting in dysphagia and megaesophagus in giant axonal neuropathy.

Certain disorders of the neuromuscular junction, namely botulism and tick paralysis, produce signs that mimic those observed in a diffuse polyneuropathy.

The principal clinical signs of the neuropathic syndrome are listed in Figure 2.2, and the diseases known to produce this syndrome are outlined in Table 2.2.

Common causes of the neuropathic syndrome seen in practice: **Traumatic neuropathies; coonhound paralysis; tick paralysis; ischemic neuromyopathy; idiopathic facial paralysis.**

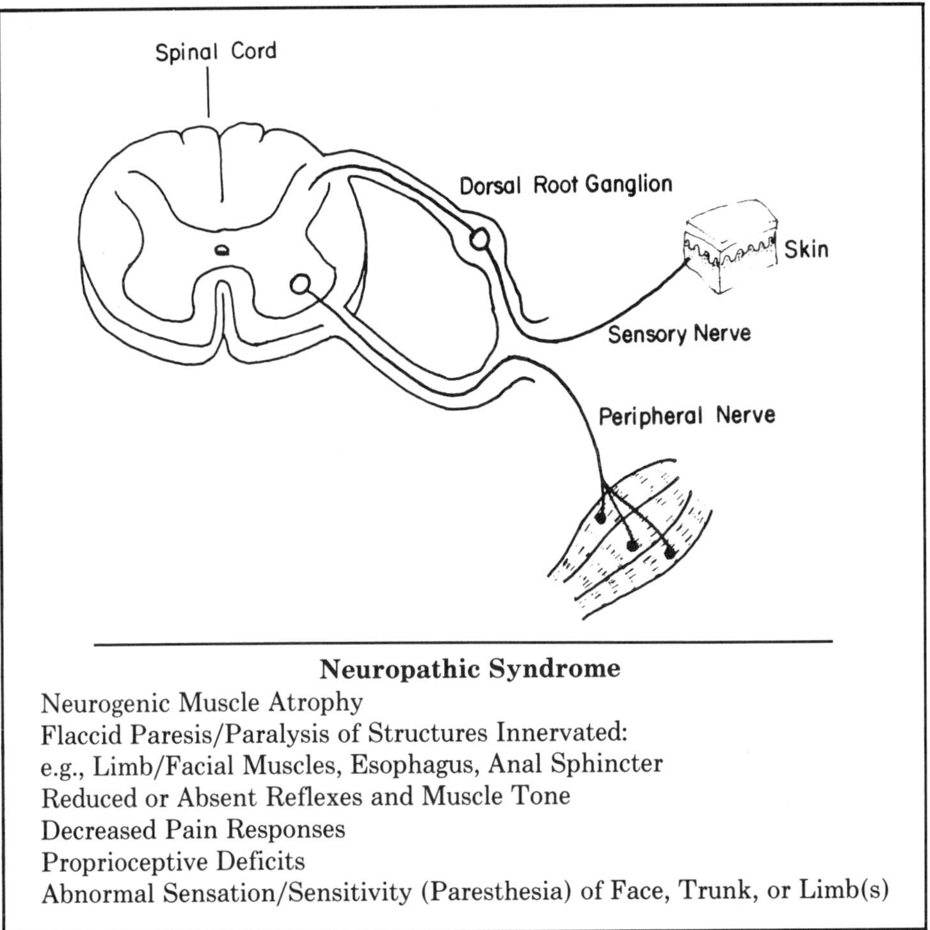

Neuropathic Syndrome
Neurogenic Muscle Atrophy
Flaccid Paresis/Paralysis of Structures Innervated:
e.g., Limb/Facial Muscles, Esophagus, Anal Sphincter
Reduced or Absent Reflexes and Muscle Tone
Decreased Pain Responses
Proprioceptive Deficits
Abnormal Sensation/Sensitivity (Paresthesia) of Face, Trunk, or Limb(s)

Figure 2.2.   Neuropathic syndrome.

Table 2.2.   Neuropathies in Dogs and Cats

Category of Disease	Acute Onset		Chronic Onset
	Progressive	Nonprogressive	
Degenerative	1. Progressive diffuse myelomalacia*—dog	1. Infarction* 2. Ischemic neuromyopathy—cat	1. Distal symmetrical polyneuropathy 2. Distal denervating disease 3. Spinal muscular atrophy*—Brittany spaniel; pointer; Swedish Lapland; giant-breed crosses 4. Deafness 5. Giant axonal neuropathy—German shepherd 6. Boxer neuropathy 7. Hypertrophic neuropathy—Tibetan mastiff 8. Dachshund sensory neuropathy 9. Mutilating neuropathy—English pointer 10. Laryngeal paralysis—Siberian huskie; Bouvier des Flanders 11. Esophageal hypomotility 12. Globoid leukodystrophy 13. Sensory neuronopathy 14. Dancing Doberman disease 15. Feline dysautonomia 16. Idiopathic facial paralysis 17. Paraneoplastic neuromyopathy 18. Sensory trigeminal neuropathy
Anomalous	None	1. Optic nerve (Cr. n. 2)	1. Deafness
Autoimmune/immune-mediated	1. Coonhound paralysis 2. Brachial plexus neuropathy	None	1. Coonhound paralysis 2. Chronic relapsing polyradiculoneuritis
Metabolic	1. Diabetic neuropathy 2. Hypocalcemia	1. Hypocalcemia	1. Diabetic neuropathy

Table 2.2—*Continued*

Category of Disease	Acute Onset		Chronic Onset
	Progressive	Nonprogressive	
Neoplastic	None	None	1. Nerve sheath tumors (see Chapter 3, "Neoplasia")
Inflammatory/infectious	1. Optic neuritis 2. Labyrinthitis 3. Idiopathic feline polyneuritis	1. Trigeminal neuritis	1. Labyrinthitis
Traumatic	1. Spinal trauma* 2. Brachial plexus avulsion	1. Traumatic neuropathy	None
Toxic	1. Botulism† 2. Tick paralysis†	None	1. Drug toxicities†

* Indicates involvement of ventral horn cells within the spinal cord.
† Refers to disorders of neuromuscular junction ("junctionopathies").

Lumbosacral Syndrome

This syndrome represents the first of four spinal cord syndromes. The lumbosacral syndrome reflects various degrees of involvement of the pelvic limbs, bladder, anal sphincter, and tail. Clinical signs will range from flaccid weakness to paralysis of pelvic limbs and tail. Patellar and withdrawal reflexes (as well as gastrocnemius and cranial tibial reflexes) may be depressed (hyporeflexia) or absent (areflexia) in pelvic limbs, as may perineal (anal) and bulbocavernosus (in male dogs) reflexes. Tone in pelvic limb muscles may be reduced (hypotonia) or absent (atonia or flaccid). After 1 to 2 weeks, muscle atrophy will be observed. Pelvic limb postural reactions, such as hopping and placing, may be depressed. Thoracic limb function is normal. Pain perception in pelvic limbs, tail, and perineum may be reduced (hypalgesia) or absent (analgesia). Pelvic limb lameness and pain on manipulation may be observed in animals with lumbosacral disk extrusion that compresses and entraps nerve roots. The anal sphincter may be flaccid and dilated, resulting in fecal incontinence. The bladder is frequently paralyzed, resulting in urine retention and passive overflow incontinence. With this syndrome, the flaccid bladder is easily evacuated manually.

It is important to note that some animals with the lumbosacral syndrome will be paretic or paralyzed in the pelvic limbs, with reduced reflexes and muscle tone, but have normal anal sphincter function. In other animals, anal sphincter and bladder dysfunction may be the principal clinical signs, with only mild pelvic limb weakness. Both groups of animals have the lumbosacral syndrome, but the lesion occurs at slightly different levels of the lumbosacral spinal cord.

The principal clinical signs of the lumbosacral syndrome are listed in Figure 2.3, and the diseases known to produce this syndrome are outlined in Table 2.3.

***Common causes of the lumbosacral syndrome seen in practice:* Pelvic fractures and luxations; fibrocartilaginous emboli; lumbosacral stenosis; disk disease; sacrococcygeal dysgenesis.**

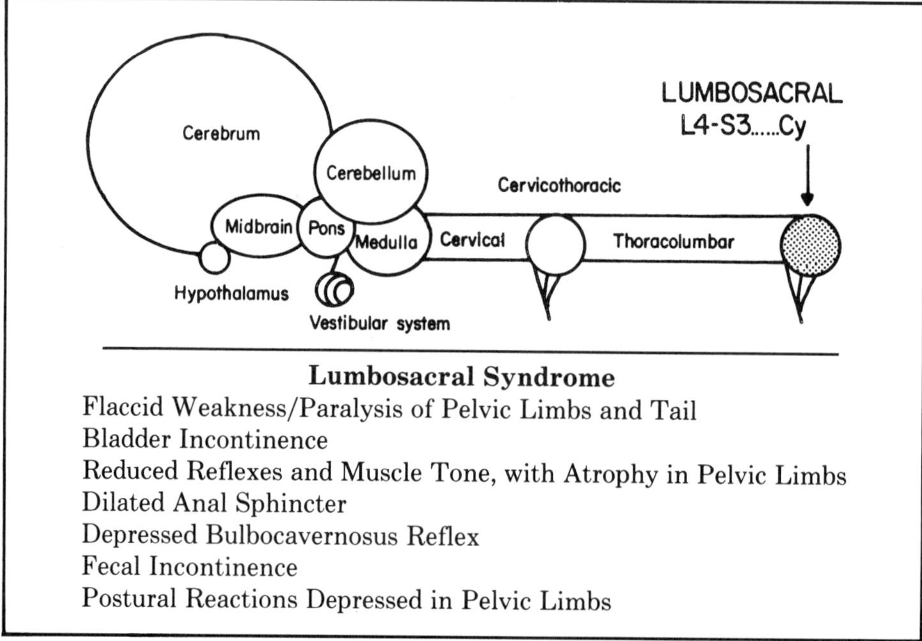

Lumbosacral Syndrome
Flaccid Weakness/Paralysis of Pelvic Limbs and Tail
Bladder Incontinence
Reduced Reflexes and Muscle Tone, with Atrophy in Pelvic Limbs
Dilated Anal Sphincter
Depressed Bulbocavernosus Reflex
Fecal Incontinence
Postural Reactions Depressed in Pelvic Limbs

Figure 2.3. Lumbosacral syndrome.

Table 2.3. Lumbosacral Syndrome (L4-S3 + Coccygeal)

Category of Disease	Acute Onset		Chronic Onset
	Progressive	Nonprogressive	
Degenerative	1. Disk disease 2. Progressive diffuse myelomalacia	1. Infarction	1. Disk disease 2. Spondylosis deformans 3. Dural ossification 4. Degenerative myelopathy
Anomalous	None	None	1. Spinal dysplasia—weimaraner 2. Spina bifida—brachycephalic breeds; Manx cat 3. Sacrococcygeal dysgenesis—Manx cat 4. Lumbosacral stenosis 5. Hemivertebra—brachycephalic breeds 6. Dermoid sinus—Rhodesian ridgeback
Neoplastic	Metastatic (see Chapter 3, "Neoplasia")	None	1. Primary; secondary tumors (see Chapter 3, "Neoplasia")
Infectious	1. Distemper 2. Rabies 3. Meningitis 4. Diskospondylitis 5. Toxoplasmosis 6. Parasitic migration 7. Mycotic diseases	None	1. Refer to Acute Onset Progressive 2. Abscessation 3. Feline infectious peritonitis 4. Granulomatous meningoencephalomyelitis 5. Postvaccinal rabies
Traumatic	Progressive, diffuse myelomalacia (ascending/descending)	1. Spinal trauma	None

Thoracolumbar Syndrome

A spinal cord lesion between cervical and lumbar enlargements (intumescences), i.e., between T3 and L3 cord segments, will produce a thoracolumbar syndrome. This is the most commonly encountered spinal cord syndrome in dogs and cats. The thoracolumbar syndrome is characterized by spastic (increased muscle tone, especially extensor muscles) weakness or paralysis of pelvic limbs. Pelvic limb reflexes are intact (normal or increased); however, postural reactions, such as hopping and placing, are depressed in pelvic limbs. Thoracic limb function is normal. Animals with thoracolumbar disk disease may keep their backs slightly arched ("kyphosis"). Often, there is reduced cutaneous sensation along the dorsal spine behind the lesion site, but sensation is increased at, or immediately above, the level of the lesion. Animals are usually incontinent, with a characteristic inadequate spurting urination of brief duration ("spastic bladder"). It is difficult (and may be dangerous) to express the bladder manually.

An acute, compressive lesion of the thoracolumbar spinal cord occasionally may be accompanied by a Schiff-Sherrington posture, which is observed as rigid extension of the thoracic limbs with the animal in lateral recumbency. Voluntary movement (with support) and postural reactions, such as wheelbarrowing and hopping, however, are normal in thoracic limbs. The wheelbarrow reaction especially is a useful test of thoracic limb function. It is usually depressed in animals with cervicothoracic or cervical syndromes.

The principal clinical signs of the thoracolumbar syndrome are listed in Figure 2.4, and the diseases known to produce this syndrome are outlined in Table 2.4.

***Common causes of the thoracolumbar syndrome seen in practice:* Disk disease; spinal fractures; degenerative myelopathy; distemper myelitis; diskospondylitis; metastatic lymphosarcomas in cats; progressive, diffuse myelomalacia; hemivertebra.**

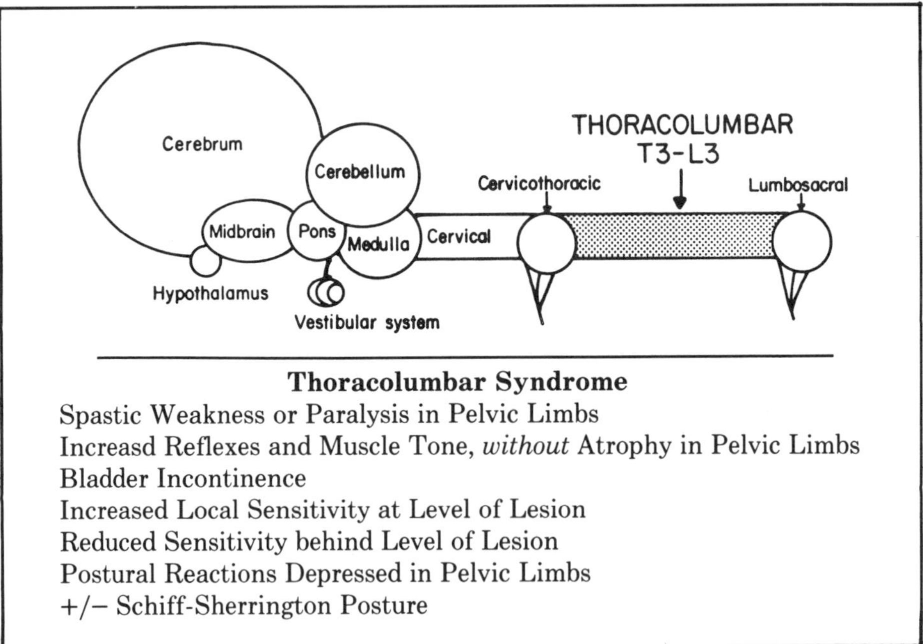

Thoracolumbar Syndrome
Spastic Weakness or Paralysis in Pelvic Limbs
Increasd Reflexes and Muscle Tone, *without* Atrophy in Pelvic Limbs
Bladder Incontinence
Increased Local Sensitivity at Level of Lesion
Reduced Sensitivity behind Level of Lesion
Postural Reactions Depressed in Pelvic Limbs
+/− Schiff-Sherrington Posture

Figure 2.4. Thoracolumbar syndrome.

Table 2.4. Thoracolumbar Syndrome (T3-L3)

Category of Disease	Acute Onset		Chronic Onset
	Progressive	Nonprogressive	
Degenerative	1. Disk disease 2. Progressive, diffuse myelomalacia	None	1. Degenerative myelopathy—German shepherd 2. Disk disease 3. Spondylosis deformans 4. Dural ossification 5. Hereditary myelopathy of Afghan hounds 6. Multiple cartilaginous exostotis 7. Hereditary ataxia—smooth fox terrier; Jack Russell terrier 8. Demyelinating myelopathy—miniature poodle
Anomalous	None	None	1. Spinal dysplasia—weimaraner 2. Hemivertebra—brachycephalic breeds 3. Arachnoid cyst 4. Dermoid sinus
Neoplastic	Metastic (see Chapter 3, "Neoplasia")	None	1. Primary and secondary tumors (see Chapter 3, "Neoplasia")
Nutritional	None	None	1. Hound ataxia—foxhound; beagle; harrier hound
Inflammatory/infectious	1. Distemper 2. Rabies 3. Meningitis 4. Diskospondylitis 5. Toxoplasmosis 6. Mycotic diseases 7. Parasitic migration	None	1. Refer to Acute Onset, Progressive 2. Abscessation 3. Feline infectious peritonitis 4. Granulomatous meningoencephalomyelitis 5. Postvaccinal rabies 6. Feline polioencephalomyelitis
Traumatic	Progressive, diffuse myelomalacia	1. Spinal trauma	None

Cervicothoracic Syndrome

The hallmarks of the cervicothoracic syndrome are depressed or absent reflexes (tricipital, bicipital, withdrawal) and tone in thoracic limb(s). Muscle atrophy becomes apparent after 1 to 2 weeks. In pelvic limbs, reflexes are intact and may be increased (brisk), and there is no atrophy. Animals may be weak in all limbs (tetraparesis), weak or paralyzed only in thoracic and pelvic limbs on the same side (hemiparesis to hemiplegia), or paralyzed in all limbs (tetraplegia). Postural reactions, such as hopping and placing, may be depressed in all limbs, especially in the thoracic. In some instances, animals will clumsily propel themselves on their chins, using their pelvic limbs, with thoracic limbs drawn to their flanks. The panniculus reflex may be depressed unilaterally or bilaterally, depending on the extent and location of the lesion. Bladder incontinence is usually observed. Many animals will have signs of a Horner's syndrome, namely, miosis (small pupil), ptosis (upper lid droop), enophthalmos (sunken globe), and prolapse of the third eyelid.

A common cause of the cervicothoracic syndrome is traumatic avulsion of the brachial plexus. Animals with this disorder may show evidence of areflexia, muscle atrophy, and weakness/paralysis (monoparesis/monoplegia) of one thoracic limb together with signs of a partial Horner's syndrome, in which only miosis is observed. The miosis will be ipsilateral, i.e., on the same side as the paralyzed thoracic limb.

The principal clinical signs of the cervicothoracic syndrome are listed in Figure 2.5, and the diseases known to produce this syndrome are outlined in Table 2.5.

Common causes of the cervicothoracic syndrome seen in practice: **Brachial plexus avulsion; neurofibromas; fibrocartilaginous emboli; cervical malformation-malarticulation; disk disease.**

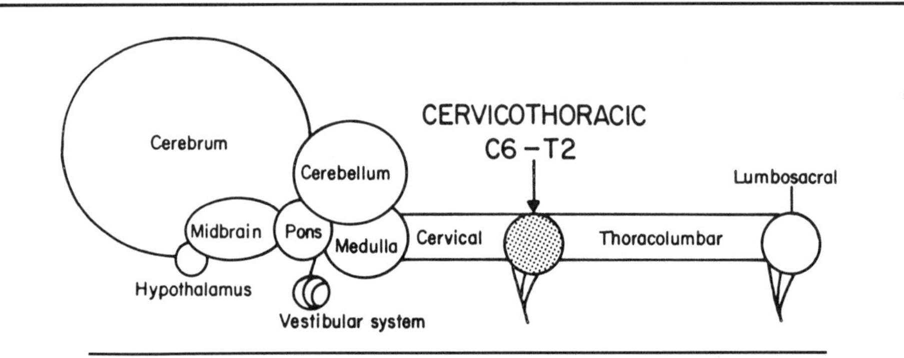

Cervicothoracic Syndrome

Monoparesis(-plegia), Hemiparesis(-plegia), or Tetraparesis(-plegia)
Depressed Reflexes and Muscle Tone, *with* Atrophy in Thoracic Limbs
Increased Reflexes and Muscle Tone, *without* Atrophy in Pelvic Limbs
Postural Reactions Depressed in All Limbs
Bladder Incontinence
Increased Local Sensitivity at Level of Lesion
Reduced Sensitivity behind Level of Lesion
Horner's Syndrome:
    Miosis
    Enophthalmos
    Ptosis
    Protrusion of Third Eyelid
Depressed Panniculus Reflex (Unilateral or Bilateral)

Figure 2.5. Cervicothoracic syndrome.

Table 2.5. Cervicothoracic Syndrome (C6-T2)

Category of Disease	Acute Onset		Chronic Onset
	Progressive	Nonprogressive	
Degenerative	1. Disk disease 2. Progressive, diffuse myelomalacia	1. Infarction	1. Cervical malformation/malarticulation—Great Dane; Doberman 2. Disk disease 3. Hereditary myelopathy of Afghan hounds 4. Spondylosis deformans 5. Dural ossification 6. Demyelinating myelopathy—miniature poodle
Anomalous	None	None	1. Spinal dysplasia—weimaraner 2. Hemivertebra—brachycephalic breeds 3. Arachnoid cyst 4. Dermoid sinus—Rhodesian ridgeback
Neoplastic	Metastatic (see Chapter 3, "Neoplasia")	None	1. Primary and secondary tumors (see Chapter 3, "Neoplasia")
Nutritional	None	None	Hypervitaminosis A—cats
Inflamamtory/infectious	1. Distemper 2. Rabies 3. Meningitis 4. Diskospondylitis 5. Parasitic migration 6. Toxoplasmosis 7. Mycotic diseases	None	1. Refer to Acute Onset, Progressive 2. Abscessation 3. Feline infectious peritonitis 4. Granulomatous meningoencephalomyelitis
Traumatic	Progressive, diffuse myelomalacia	1. Spinal trauma 2. Brachial plexus avulsion	None

Cervical Syndrome

With a cervical syndrome, clinical signs may range from spastic (rigid) hemiparesis, to tetraparesis, to tetraplegia. Reflexes and muscle tone are intact in all limbs, and there is no evidence of atrophy. Cervical spasms, pain on palpation, and cervical rigidity will be present in some animals, e.g., dogs with cervical disk disease. Such animals also may assume an abnormal posture with the nose held close to the ground and the back arched. In some dogs with cervical disk disease, one thoracic limb may be held in partial flexion, or a repetitive "stamping" motion may be observed. These animals frequently show considerable pain on manipulation of the limb and neck. This combination of signs is termed "root signature" and is believed to be associated with nerve root entrapment by a fragment of extruded disk material.

The wheelbarrow reaction is usually depressed, and hopping and placing reactions may be deficient in thoracic and pelvic limbs. Bladder incontinence is often present. Occasionally, an animal may manifest a variable degree of respiratory difficulty. Rarely, in an animal with a severe, destructive lesion in the cervical cord, e.g., infarction secondary to fibrocartilaginous embolization, Horner's syndrome may be present.

The principal clinical signs of the cervical syndrome are listed in Figure 2.6, and the diseases known to produce this syndrome are outlined in Table 2.6.

***Common causes of the cervical syndrome seen in practice:* Disk disease; cervical malformation-malarticulation; meningitis; atlantoaxial subluxation; diskospondylitis.**

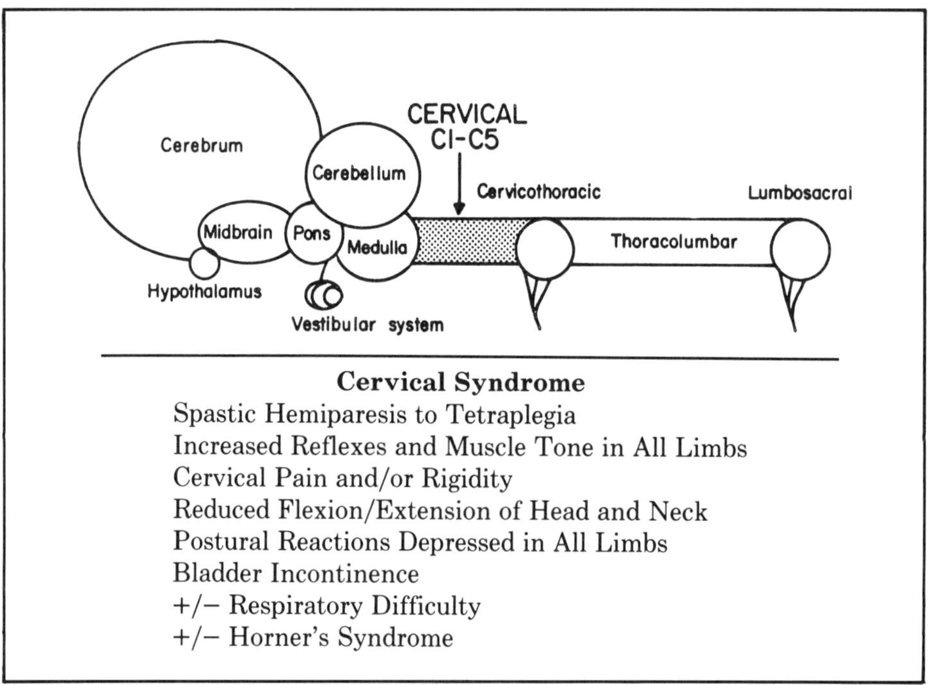

Cervical Syndrome
Spastic Hemiparesis to Tetraplegia
Increased Reflexes and Muscle Tone in All Limbs
Cervical Pain and/or Rigidity
Reduced Flexion/Extension of Head and Neck
Postural Reactions Depressed in All Limbs
Bladder Incontinence
+/− Respiratory Difficulty
+/− Horner's Syndrome

Figure 2.6. Cervical syndrome.

Table 2.6. Cervical Syndrome (C1-C5)

Category of Disease	Acute Onset		Chronic Onset
	Progressive	Nonprogressive	
Degenerative	1. Disk disease 2. Progressive, diffuse myelomalacia	1. Infarction	1. Disk disease 2. Hereditary ataxia—smooth fox terrier; Jack Russell terrier 3. Cervical malformation/malarticulation—Great Dane; Doberman; bassett hound
Anomalous	None	None	1. Atlantoaxial luxation—miniature and toy breeds 2. Spinal dysplasia 3. Demyelinating myelopathy—miniature poodle 4. Arachnoid cyst 5. Dermoid sinus—Rhodesian ridgeback
Neoplastic	Metastatic (see Chapter 3, "Neoplasia")	None	1. Primary and secondary tumors (see Chapter 3, "Neoplasia")
Nutritional	None	None	Hypervitaminosis A—cats
Inflammatory/ infectious	1. Distemper 2. Rabies 3. Meningitis 4. Diskospondylitis 5. Toxoplasmosis 6. Parasitic migration 7. Mycotic diseases 8. Pyogranulomatous meningoencephalomyelitis—pointers	None	1. Refer to Acute Onset, Progressive 2. Abscessation 3. Feline infectious peritonitis 4. Granulomatous meningoencephalomyelitis
Traumatic	Progressive, diffuse myelomalacia	1. Spinal trauma	None

Pontomedullary Syndrome

This syndrome is characterized by the presence of multiple cranial nerve deficits in an animal showing signs of hemiparesis, tetraparesis, or tetraplegia. Postural reactions can be depressed in all limbs or in limbs on one side only. Reflexes are intact in all limbs. Cranial nerve deficits may include jaw paralysis, decreased facial sensation, and depressed palpebral reflex (cranial nerve 5; trigeminal); medial strabismus (cranial nerve 6; abducens); inability to close eyelid(s), lip paralysis, ear droop, facial spasms (cranial nerve 7; facial); head tilt, rolling, nystagmus (cranial nerve 8, vestibular); pharyngeal, laryngeal, and esophageal paralysis resulting in dysphonia, dysphagia, megaesophagus, and depressed gag reflex (cranial nerves 9 and 10; glossopharyngeal and vagus); and tongue paralysis (cranial nerve 12; hypoglossal). Respiration is often irregular and apneic, or rapid and shallow. Mental depression may be observed.

The principal clinical signs of the pontomedullary syndrome are listed in Figure 2.7, and the diseases known to produce this syndrome are outlined in Table 2.7.

***Common causes of the pontomedullary syndrome seen in practice:* Cranial trauma; distemper encephalitis; granulomatous meningoencephalitis (reticulosis); rabies, pseudorabies; feline infectious peritonitis; choroid plexus papilloma.**

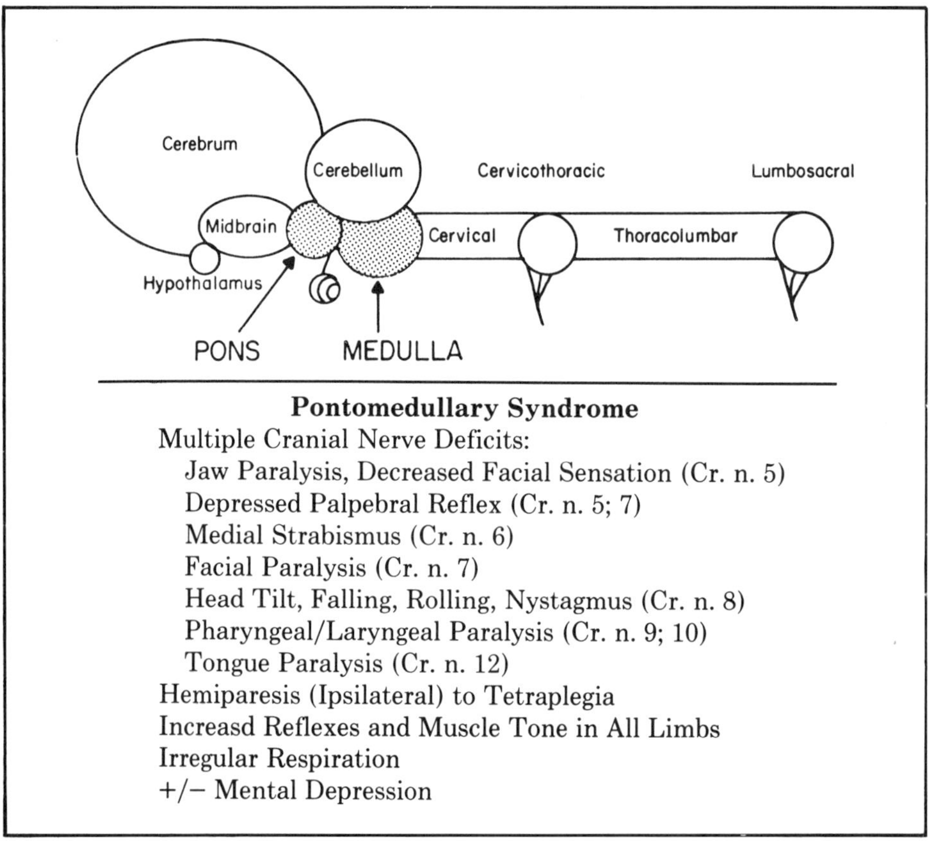

Pontomedullary Syndrome
Multiple Cranial Nerve Deficits:
    Jaw Paralysis, Decreased Facial Sensation (Cr. n. 5)
    Depressed Palpebral Reflex (Cr. n. 5; 7)
    Medial Strabismus (Cr. n. 6)
    Facial Paralysis (Cr. n. 7)
    Head Tilt, Falling, Rolling, Nystagmus (Cr. n. 8)
    Pharyngeal/Laryngeal Paralysis (Cr. n. 9; 10)
    Tongue Paralysis (Cr. n. 12)
Hemiparesis (Ipsilateral) to Tetraplegia
Increasd Reflexes and Muscle Tone in All Limbs
Irregular Respiration
+/− Mental Depression

Figure 2.7. Pontomedullary syndrome.

Table 2.7. Pontomedullary Syndrome

Category of Disease	Acute Onset		Chronic Onset
	Progressive	Nonprogressive	
Degenerative	None	1. Infarction 2. Hemorrhage	1. Globoid leukodystrophy—West Highland white terrier; cairn terrier 2. Demyelinating diseases—miniature poodle
Anomalous	None	None	1. Occipital dysplasia—miniature and toy breeds 2. Hydrocephalus—miniature and toy breeds
Neoplastic	Metastatic (see Chapter 3, "Neoplasia")	None	1. Primary and secondary tumors (see Chapter 3, "Neoplasia")
Inflammatory/ infectious	1. Distemper 2. Rabies 3. Meningitis 4. Diskospondylitis 5. Toxoplasmosis 6. Parasitic migration 7. Mycotic diseases 8. Pyogranulomatous meningoencephalomyelitis—mature pointers 9. Pseudorabies	None	1. Refer to Acute Onset, Progressive 2. Abscessation 3. Feline infectious peritonitis 4. Granulomatous meningoencephalomyelitis 5. Protothecosis
Traumatic	None	1. Cranial trauma	None

Cerebellar Syndrome

This is one of the most readily recognizable syndromes in veterinary practice. Clinical signs include exaggerated limb responses (hypermetria) when a movement is initiated, such as "goose-stepping" when walking or during postural reaction testing, such as hopping and placing, and overshooting a food bowl when attempting to eat. All limb movements are spastic (rigid), clumsy, faltering, and jerky. The animal assumes a broad-based stance at rest, and swaying of the trunk (truncal ataxia) may be observed when the animal is walking. Initiation of movement is delayed and is often accompanied by tremors (intention tremors). Tremors are especially noticeable in the head. Fine, pendular, or oscillatory eye movements also may be present. Menace response (a threatening gesture toward the animal's head that results in an eye blink) may be absent. If the lesion involves only one side of the cerebellum, the menace deficit will be ipsilateral (i.e., on the same side as the lesion). Vision is not affected.

The principal clinical signs of the cerebellar syndrome are listed in Figure 2.8, and the diseases known to produce this syndrome are outlined in Table 2.8.

***Common causes of the cerebellar syndrome seen in practice:* Cerebellar malformation (hypoplasia) in cats; canine distemper encephalitis; hypomyelinogenesis; feline infectious peritonitis; cerebellar degeneration; choroid plexus papilloma; hexachlorophene toxicity.**

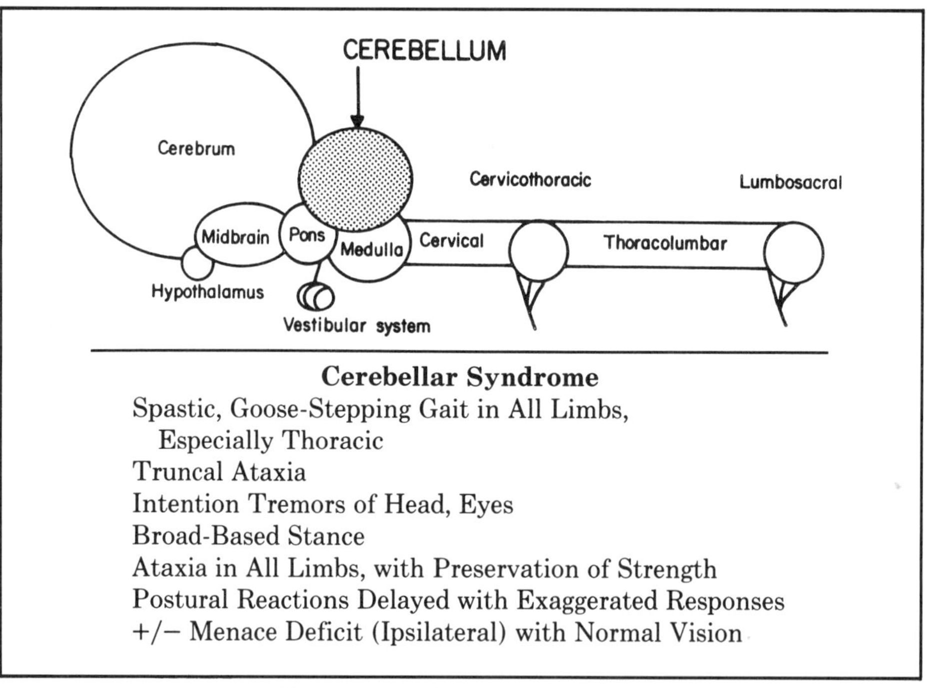

Cerebellar Syndrome
Spastic, Goose-Stepping Gait in All Limbs,
   Especially Thoracic
Truncal Ataxia
Intention Tremors of Head, Eyes
Broad-Based Stance
Ataxia in All Limbs, with Preservation of Strength
Postural Reactions Delayed with Exaggerated Responses
+/− Menace Deficit (Ipsilateral) with Normal Vision

Figure 2.8. Cerebellar syndrome.

Table 2.8. Cerebellar Syndrome

Category of Disease	Acute Onset		Chronic Onset
	Progressive	Nonprogressive	
Degenerative	None	1. Infarction 2. Hemorrhage	1. Cerebellar degeneration—Kerry blue terrier; Gordon setter; rough-coated collie; border collie; bull mastiff 2. Leukoencephalomyelopathy—rottweiler 3. Neuroaxonal dystrophy—rottweiler; collie sheepdog 4. Gangliosidosis—Siamese, Korat, domestic cats; German short-haired pointer 5. Sphingomyelinosis—Siamese cat 6. Glucocerebrosidosis—Australian silky terrier 7. Globoid leukodystrophy—West Highland white terrier; cairn terrier 8. Mannosidosis—Persian cat 9. Spongiform degeneration—Egyptian Mau cat; silky terrier; samoyed; Labrador retriever
Anomalous	None	None	1. Cerebellar hypoplasia (see Chapter 3, "Cerebellar Malformation") 2. Hypomyelinogenesis—chow chow; springer spaniel
Neoplastic	1. Metastatic (see Chapter 3, "Neoplasia")	None	1. Primary and secondary tumors (see Chapter 3, "Neoplasia")
Inflammatory/ infectious	1. Distemper 2. Rabies 3. Meningitis 4. Toxoplasmosis 5. Parasitic migration 6. Mycotic diseases 7. Pyogranulomatous meningoencephalo-myelitis—pointer	None	1. Refer to Acute Onset, Progressive 2. Abscessation 3. Feline infectious peritonitis 4. Granulomatous meningoencephalomyelitis 5. Herpes virus encephalitis 6. Feline Parvovirus (see Chapter 3, "Cerebellar Malformation")
Traumatic	None	1. Cranial trauma	None
Toxic	1. Hexachlorophene	None	None

Vestibular Syndrome

The vestibular syndrome is another commonly recognized syndrome in clinical practice. Clinical signs may include head tilt, falling, rolling, or walking in tight circles, and nystagmus. Nystagmus is present in the acute stages of most vestibular diseases and is usually jerking or rotational in nature with fast and slow components. The quick phase of horizontal or rotational nystagmus is in a direction away from the side of the lesion. Sometimes in animals with vestibular disease, nystagmus can be initiated by moving and holding the head in a different position (positional nystagmus). Normal, physiological nystagmus can be induced by rapid head movements in vertical or horizontal planes. The fast phase of the nystagmus is in the direction of the head movement. This response may be depressed or absent in animals with vestibular disease when the head is moved toward the side of the lesion. A ventrolateral strabismus (abnormal position of the eyeball) may be elicited in affected animals by elevating the head. The strabismus is ipsilateral.

The above signs may occur with central (brainstem) and peripheral (middle or inner ear) vestibular disease. Central vestibular disease is suggested by the presence of vertical and positional nystagmus, altered mental status, and evidence of other cranial nerve dysfunction,e.g., trigeminal nerve (jaw weakness, decreased facial sensation, depressed palpebral reflex) and/or abducent nerve (medial strabismus). Horner's syndrome and facial paralysis are frequently observed with

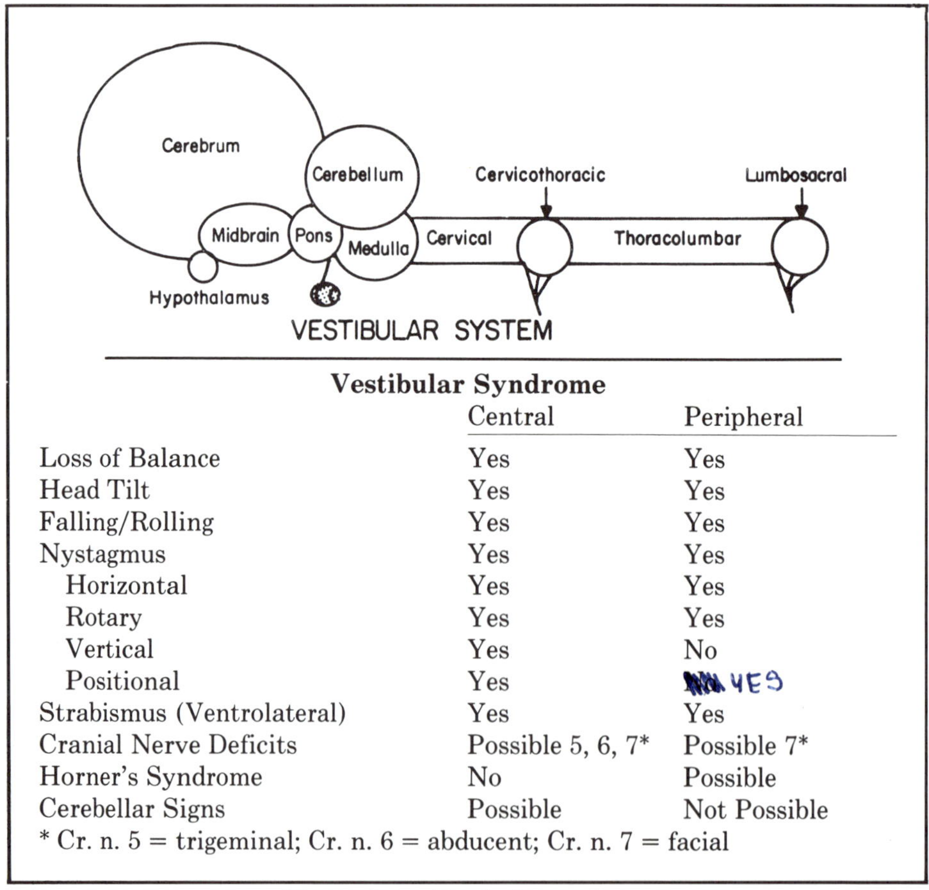

Vestibular Syndrome

	Central	Peripheral
Loss of Balance	Yes	Yes
Head Tilt	Yes	Yes
Falling/Rolling	Yes	Yes
Nystagmus	Yes	Yes
Horizontal	Yes	Yes
Rotary	Yes	Yes
Vertical	Yes	No
Positional	Yes	No
Strabismus (Ventrolateral)	Yes	Yes
Cranial Nerve Deficits	Possible 5, 6, 7*	Possible 7*
Horner's Syndrome	No	Possible
Cerebellar Signs	Possible	Not Possible

* Cr. n. 5 = trigeminal; Cr. n. 6 = abducent; Cr. n. 7 = facial

Figure 2.9. Vestibular syndrome.

peripheral vestibular diseases that are associated with otitis media since both facial and sympathetic nerves pass through the middle ear. Hemifacial spasms may rarely occur in dogs in association with brainstem scarring or facial nerve irritation. Eyelid margins, ears, and lip commissures on one side of the face are spasmodically pulled caudally. A Horner's syndrome and vestibular signs may accompany the spasms. Peripheral vestibular diseases are more common than central disorders.

The principal clinical signs of the vestibular syndrome are listed in Figure 2.9, and the diseases known to produce this syndrome are outlined in Table 2.9.

Common causes of the vestibular syndrome seen in practice: Peripheral: Otitis media/otitis interna; feline and canine idiopathic vestibular disease; aminoglycoside toxicity. Central: Granulomatous meningoencephalitis; choroid plexus papilloma; distemper encephalitis; toxoplasmosis; cryptococcosis.

Table 2.9. Vestibular Syndrome

Category of Disease	Acute Onset		Chronic Onset
	Progressive	Nonprogressive	
Degenerative	None	1. Infarction 2. Hemorrhage	None
Neoplastic	1. Metastatic (see Chapter 3, "Neoplasia")	None	1. Primary and Secondary tumors (see Chapter 3, "Neoplasia")
Nutritional	None	None	1. Thiamine deficiency—cat
Idiopathic	None	1. Idiopathic vestibular disease	None
Inflammatory/ infectious	1. Distemper 2. Labyrinthitis 3. Toxoplasmosis 4. Granulomatous meningoencephalomyelitis 5. Pyogranulomatous meningoencephalomyelitis 6. Abscessation 7. Parasitic migration 8. Feline infectious peritonitis 9. Mycotic diseases	None	1. Refer to Acute Onset, Progressive
Traumatic	None	1. Cranial trauma	None
Toxic	None	None	1. Aminoglycosides (see Chapter 3, "Drug Toxicities")

Midbrain Syndrome

This is a relatively uncommon syndrome. Animals may be depressed or comatose, and there may be rigid extension of all limbs (opisthotonus). If the lesion is located on one side of the midbrain, limbs on the contralateral (opposite) side will show signs of spastic weakness (hemiparesis). Most animals will have a ventrolateral strabismus, mydriatic (widely dilated) pupils that are unresponsive to light stimulation, and ptosis (drooping) of the upper eyelids. These signs will be ipsilateral or bilateral, depending on the location and extent of the lesion. Vision is normal. Animals may hyperventilate.

The principal clinical signs of the midbrain syndrome are listed in Figure 2.10, and the diseases known to produce this syndrome are outlined in Table 2.10.

***Common causes of the midbrain syndrome seen in practice:* Thiamine deficiency in cats; cranial trauma with midbrain hemorrhage; distemper encephalitis; granulomatous meningoencephalomyelitis.**

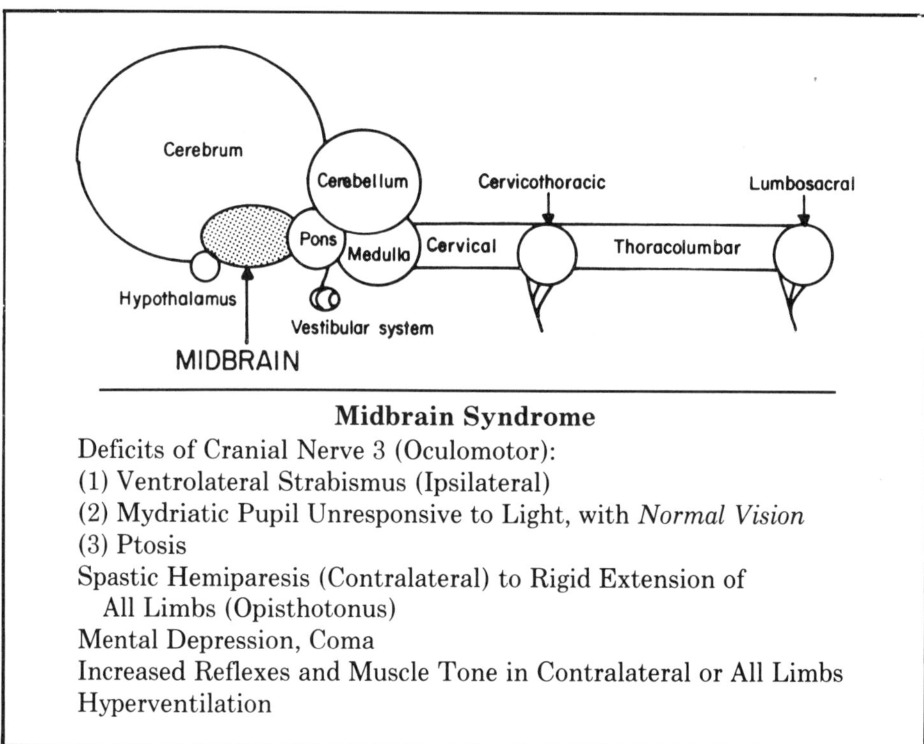

Midbrain Syndrome

Deficits of Cranial Nerve 3 (Oculomotor):
(1) Ventrolateral Strabismus (Ipsilateral)
(2) Mydriatic Pupil Unresponsive to Light, with *Normal Vision*
(3) Ptosis
Spastic Hemiparesis (Contralateral) to Rigid Extension of
    All Limbs (Opisthotonus)
Mental Depression, Coma
Increased Reflexes and Muscle Tone in Contralateral or All Limbs
Hyperventilation

Figure 2.10. Midbrain syndrome.

Table 2.10. Midbrain Syndrome

Category of Disease	Acute Onset		Chronic Onset
	Progressive	Nonprogressive	
Degenerative	None	1. Infarction 2. Hemorrhage	None
Anomalous	None	None	1. Hydrocephalus—miniature and toy breeds
Metabolic	Hepatic encephalopathy	None	1. Hepatic encephalopathy
Neoplastic	1. Metastatic (see Chapter 3, "Neoplasia")	None	1. Primary and secondary tumors (see Chapter 3, "Neoplasia")
Nutritional	None	None	1. Thiamine deficiency
Inflammatory/Infectious	1. Distemper 2. Rabies 3. Meningitis 4. Infectious canine hepatitis 5. Toxoplasmosis 6. Meningitis 7. Mycotic diseases 8. Granulomatous meningoencephalomyelitis	None	1. Refer to Acute Onset, Progressive 2. Feline infectious peritonitis 3. Abscessation 4. Idiopathic feline polioencephalomyelitis 5. Pyogranulomatous meningoencephalomyelitis—pointers 6. Protothecosis
Traumatic	None	1. Cranial trauma	None

Hypothalamic Syndrome

This, also, is a relatively uncommon syndrome. Animals may manifest altered behavior or mental status, such as aggression, disorientation, hyperexcitability, or coma. Vision is frequently impaired if the lesion extends to involve the optic chiasm and/or optic tracts, in which case pupils may be dilated and weakly responsive or nonresponsive to light stimulation. Endocrine disturbances may include diabetes insipidus or hyperadrenocorticism. Abnormal temperature regulation may be manifested as hyperthermia, hypothermia, or poikilothermia. Abnormalities in appetitie are seen as hyperphagia and obesity or as anorexia and cachexia. Gait is usually normal.

The principal clinical signs of the hypothalamic syndrome are listed in Figure 2.11, and the diseases known to produce this syndrome are outlined in Table 2.11.

Common causes of the hypothalamic syndrome seen in practice: **Pituitary adenomas; extension of nasal adenocarcinomas; granulomatous masses, e.g., toxoplasmosis, mycoses (cryptococcosis, blastomycosis).**

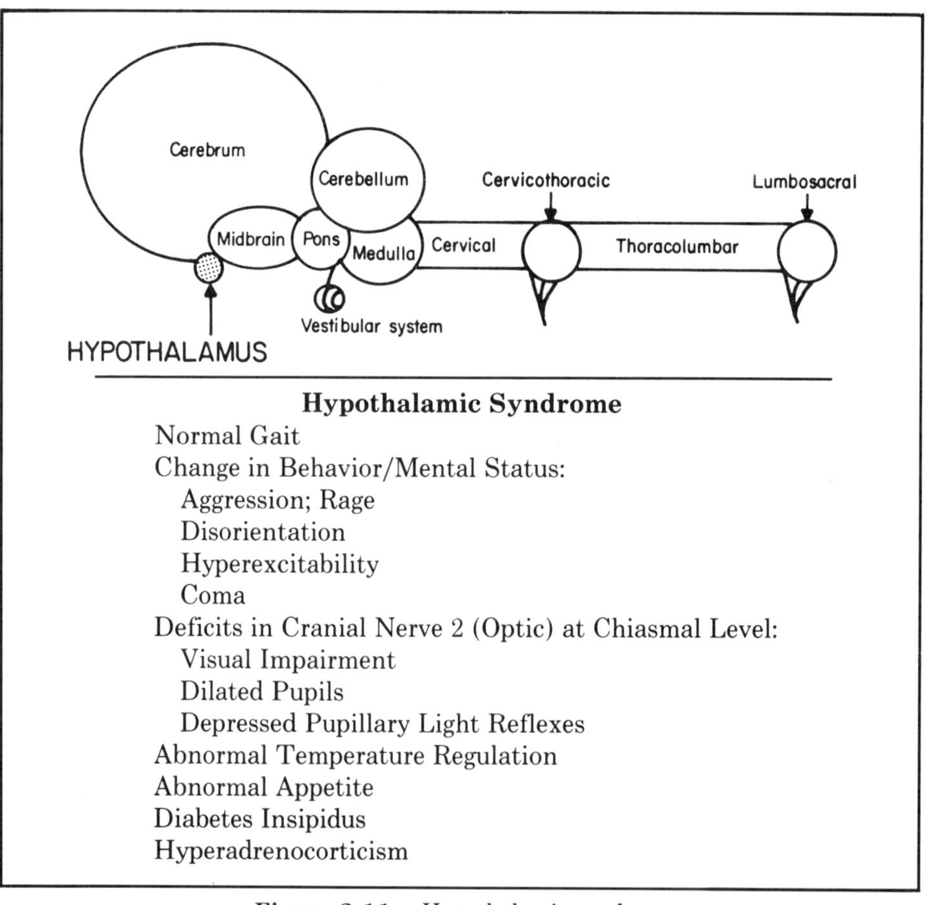

Hypothalamic Syndrome

Normal Gait
Change in Behavior/Mental Status:
    Aggression; Rage
    Disorientation
    Hyperexcitability
    Coma
Deficits in Cranial Nerve 2 (Optic) at Chiasmal Level:
    Visual Impairment
    Dilated Pupils
    Depressed Pupillary Light Reflexes
Abnormal Temperature Regulation
Abnormal Appetite
Diabetes Insipidus
Hyperadrenocorticism

Figure 2.11. Hypothalamic syndrome.

Table 2.11. Hypothalamic Syndrome

Category of Disease	Acute Onset		Chronic Onset
	Progressive	Nonprogressive	
Neoplastic	1. Metastatic (see Chapter 3, "Neoplasia")	None	1. Primary tumors—pituitary adenoma; craniopharyngioma; gliomas (see Chapter 3, "Neoplasia") 2. Extension tumors—nasal adenocarcinoma (see Chapter 3, "Neoplasia")
Inflammatory/infectious	None	None	*Granulomatous Masses* (see individual diseases) 1. Mycotic diseases—cryptococcosis; blastomycosis 2. Toxoplasmosis 3. Granulomatous meningoencephalomyelitis 4. Feline infectious peritonitis 5. Abscessation 6. Parasitic migration

Cerebral Syndrome

This commonly occurring syndrome is characterized by abnormal movement and/or abnormal postures, such as circling (usually to the same side as the lesion), continual pacing, head pressing into a wall or cage, and, sometimes, with the body bent to one side (pleurothotonus). Altered behavior and mental status are frequently observed: apathy or depression, disorientation, sometimes aggression, or hyperexcitability. Vision may be impaired (bumping into objects, depressed menace reflex) on the side opposite the lesion; however, pupillary light reflexes are normal. Seizures and papilledema may be observed. While animals may have a normal gait, postural reactions, such as hopping, placing, and hemiwalking, are usually depressed in contralateral limbs (opposite the side of the lesion). In comatose animals, breathing may be characterized by waxing and waning of the depth of respiration, with regularly recurring periods of apnea (Cheyne-Stokes respiration).

The principal clinical signs of the cerebral syndrome are listed in Figure 2.12, and the diseases known to produce this syndrome are outlined in Table 2.12.

Common causes of the cerebral syndrome seen in practice: **Cranial trauma; hydrocephalus; distemper encephalitis; rabies; meningitis; meningiomas in cats; gliomas (astrocytomas, oligodendrogliomas) in brachycephalic dogs; hepatic encephalopathy; feline ischemic encephalopathy.**

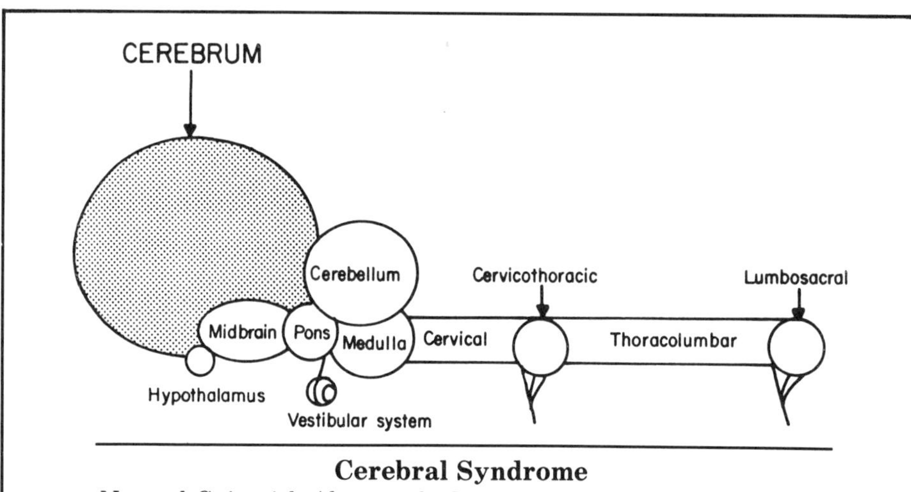

Cerebral Syndrome

Normal Gait with Abnormal Movement/Postures:
    Circling (Frequently to Side of Lesion)
    Pacing
    Head Pressing
    Pleurothotonus (Body Bent to One Side)
Change in Behavior/Mental Status:
    Apathy/Depression
    Disorientation
    Aggression
    Hyperexcitability
Visual Impairment (Contralateral)–Pupillary Reflexes *Normal*
Seizures
Papilledema
Postural Reactions Depressed in Contralateral Limbs

Figure 2.12. Cerebral syndrome.

Table 2.12. Cerebral Syndrome

Category of Disease	Acute Onset		Chronic Onset
	Progressive	Nonprogressive	
Degenerative	None	1. Infarction 2. Hemorrhage	1. Dalmation leukodystrophy 2. Fucosidosis—springer spaniel 3. Gangliosidosis—German shorthaired pointer; Siamese, Korat, domestic cats 4. Ceroid lipofuscinosis—English setter; dachshund; saluki; cocker spaniel; Siamese cat
Anomalous	None	1. Lissencephaly 2. Porencephaly 3. Hydranencephaly	1. Hydrocephalus—miniature and toy breeds
Metabolic	1. Hepatic encephalopathy 2. Hypoglycemia	None	1. Hepatic encephalopathy
Neoplastic	1. Metastatic (see Chapter 3, "Neoplasia")	None	1. Primary and secondary tumors (see Chapter 3, "Neoplasia")
Inflammatory/ infectious	1. Distemper 2. Granulomatous meningoencephalomyelitis 3. Rabies 4. Postvaccinal distemper 5. Babesiosis 6. Pseudorabies 5. Meningitis 7. Encephalitozoonosis 8. Parasitic migration 9. Toxoplasmosis 10. Mycotic diseases 11. Parvovirus encephalitis	None	1. Refer to Acute Onset, Progressive 2. Old dog encephalitis (see Chapter 3, "Distemper") 3. Feline infectious peritonitis 4. Abscessation 5. Protothecosis 6. Pug encephalitis
Traumatic	None	1. Cranial trauma	None

Multifocal Syndromes

In all of the preceding syndromes, a single lesion is presumed to account for the clinical signs. However, a situation may arise in which an animal has signs that reflect two or more different syndromes, e.g., cerebral and lumbosacral syndromes. This indicates that more than one lesion site is present, and this is termed a "multifocal syndrome."

Multifocal syndromes are usually seen in animals with infectious diseases of the nervous system. Multifocal syndromes also tend to be the hallmark of the rare, degenerative storage diseases (e.g., gangliosidosis, globoid cell leukodystrophy, etc), which, in the majority of cases, result from a genetically determined enzyme defect with subsequent accumulation and storage of substrates within various areas of the nervous system. Another, more common example of a multifocal syndrome is progressive, diffuse myelomalacia that can develop secondary to an explosive intervertebral disk extrusion. With this disorder, an initial thoracolumbar syndrome may be followed by a lumbosacral syndrome and then by a cervicothoracic syndrome, as the lesion descends and ascends the spinal cord. In addition, multifocal syndromes are commonly encountered in animals with intoxications—e.g., in tetanus and in strychnine poisoning, tetanic spasms usually involve multiple areas of the nervous system.

The principal clinical signs of the multifocal syndrome are listed in Figure 2.13, and the diseases known to produce this syndrome are outlined in Table 2.13.

Common causes of the multifocal syndrome seen in practice: **Distemper; granulomatous meningoencephalomyelitis; feline infectious peritonitis; meningitis; mycotic diseases; progressive diffuse myelomalacia; organophosphate toxicity; lead poisoning; tetanus; strychnine poisoning.**

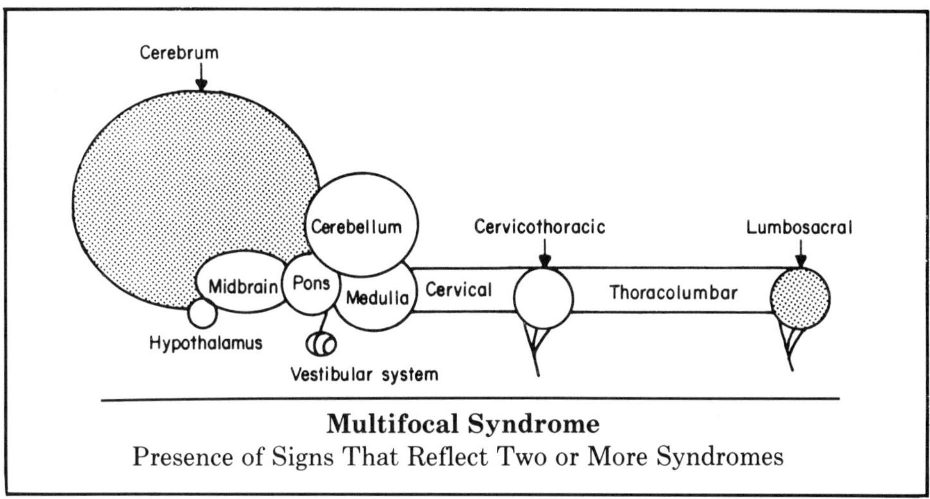

Multifocal Syndrome
Presence of Signs That Reflect Two or More Syndromes

Figure 2.13.   Multifocal syndrome.

Table 2.13. Multifocal Syndrome

Category of Disease	Acute Onset		Chronic Onset
	Progressive	Nonprogressive	
Degenerative	Progressive, diffuse myelomalacia	None	1. Fibrinoid leukodystrophy—Labrador retriever 2. Gangliosidosis (GM1)—beagle; Siamese, Korat, and domestic cats 3. Gangliosidosis (GM2)—German shorthaired pointer; domestic cat 4. Glucocerebrosidosis—Australian silky terrier 5. Sphingomyelinosis—Siamese and domestic cats; poodle 6. Globoid cell leukodystrophy* 7. Mannosidosis—Persian cat 8. Mucopolysaccharidosis—Siamese and domestic cats 9. Glycoproteinosis 10. Glycogenosis—Swedish Lapland dog; German shepherd 11. Fucosidosis—springer spaniel 12. Ceroid lipofuscinosis—English setter; dachsund; saluki; cocker spaniel; chihuahua; Siamese cat 13. Hereditary quadriplegia and amblyopia—Irish setter 14. Leukoencephalomyelopathy—rottweiler 15. Spongiform degeneration—Egyptian Mau cat; silky terrier; samoyed; Labrador retriever
Neoplastic	1. Metastatic (see Chapter 3, "Neoplastia")	None	1. Primary and secondary tumors (see Chapter 3, "Neoplasia")
Inflammatory/infectious	1. Distemper 2. Rabies 3. Postvaccinal distemper 4. Postvaccinal rabies 5. Pseudorabies 6. Granulomatous meningoencephalomyelitis 7. Herpesvirus encephalitis 8. Infectious canine hepatitis 9. Meningitis 10. Encephalitozoonosis 11. Parasitic migration 12. Toxoplasmosis 13. Mycotic diseases	None	1. Refer to Acute Onset, Progressive 2. Feline infectious peritonitis 3. Prototohecosis 4. Idiopathic feline polioencephalomyelitis
Traumatic	None	1. Cranial trauma	None

Table 2.13—*Continued*

| Category of Disease | Acute Onset | | Chronic Onset |
	Progressive	Nonprogressive	
Toxic	1. Lead 2. Hexachlorophene 3. Organophosphates and carbamates 4. Chlorinated hydrocarbons 5. Tetanus 6. Strychnine	None	1. Organophosphates and carbamates

* Cairn terrier; West Highland white terrier; beagle; blue-tick hound; poodle; bassett hound; Pomeranian; domestic cat.

Paroxysmal Syndromes

The term "paroxysmal syndromes" refers to a group of sporadically occurring disorders that usually have no structural lesions within the nervous system. Each syndrome tends to manifest distinctive clinical signs, and the animal is typically alert and responsive (i.e., without neurological deficits) between episodes. Many of these disorders cannot be accurately classified since little is known about their etiopathogenesis. The various syndromes include episodic seizures (signs may include unconscious paddling, tail biting and/or tail chasing, "fly catching," viciousness, screaming, or fear behavior), sleep (narcolepsy-cataplexy complex), syncope (fainting), cramping (e.g., "Scotty cramp"), myoclonus (e.g., familial reflex myoclonus), and weakness (e.g., congenital and acquired forms of myasthenia gravis, hypoglycemia, hyperkalemia, or hypokalemia). Rarely, a paroxysmal episode may develop into a prolonged state, e.g., status epilepticus occurring after an episodic seizural attack.

The principal clinical signs of the paroxysmal syndrome are listed in Figure 2.14, and the diseases known to produce this syndrome are outlined in Table 2.14.

Common causes of the paroxysmal syndrome seen in practice: **Seizures; myasthenia gravis; Scotty cramp.**

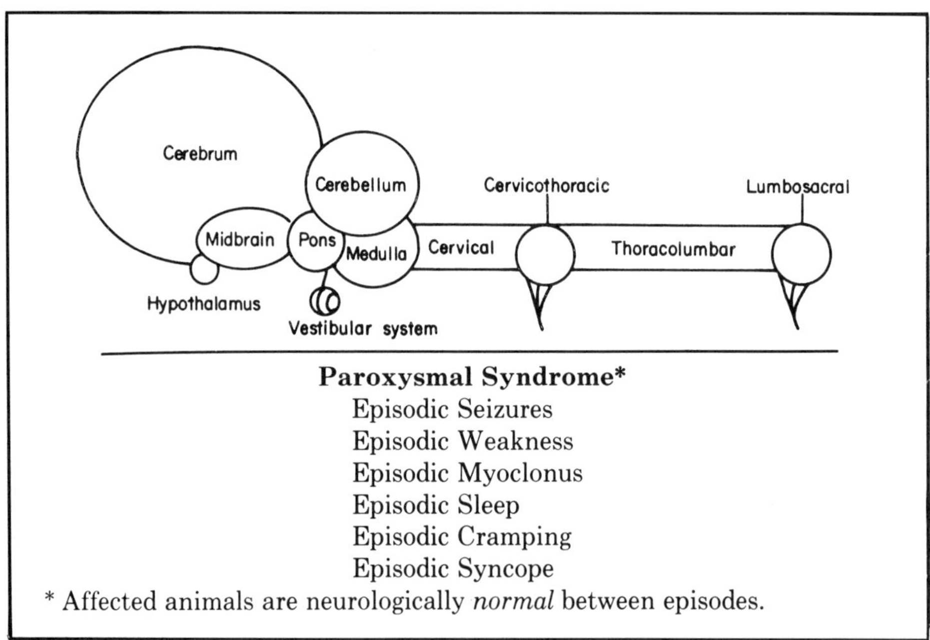

Paroxysmal Syndrome*
Episodic Seizures
Episodic Weakness
Episodic Myoclonus
Episodic Sleep
Episodic Cramping
Episodic Syncope
* Affected animals are neurologically *normal* between episodes.

Figure 2.14. Paroxysmal syndrome.

Table 2.14. Paroxysmal Syndrome

Category of Disease	Acute Onset		Chronic Onset
	Progressive	Nonprogressive	
Degenerative	None	1. Syncope 2. Hypoglycemia 3. Myasthenia gravis (congenital)—Jack Russell terrier; springer spaniel; smooth fox terrier	None
Autoimmune/ immune-mediated	None	1. Myasthenia gravis (acquired)—German shepherd	None
Metabolic	None	1. Scotty cramp—Scottish terrier; Norwich terrier; dalmation 2. Narcolepsy/cataplexy—Doberman pinscher; poodle; dachshund; Labrador retriever 3. Hypokalemia 4. Hyperkalemia	None
Idiopathic	Status epilepticus (see Chapter 3, "Seizures")—German shepherd; Saint Bernard; Irish setter	1. Idiopathic epilepsy (see Chapter 3, "Seizures") 2. Familial reflex myoclonus—Labrador retriever	None

References

1. Braund KG, Simpson ST: Localization in clinical neurology. In Slatter DH (ed): *Textbook of Small Animal Surgery*. Philadelphia, WB Saunders, 1985, vol 1, p 1256.
2. Braund KG: Localizing lesions using neurologic syndromes. 1. Brain syndromes. *Vet Med* 80:40–54, (July) 1985.
3. Braund KG: Localizing lesions using neurologic syndromes. 2. Spinal cord syndromes *Vet Med* 80:54–63, (Aug) 1985.
4. Braund KG: Localizing lesions using neurologic syndromes. 3. Neuropathic, myopathic, multifocal, and paroxysmal syndromes. *Vet Med* 80:20–34, (Sept) 1985.

3
Neurological Diseases

Abscessation

Intracranial or intraspinal abscessation may result from bacterial or fungal meningitis (1–5). Clinical signs will usually reflect a space-occupying lesion. Diagnostic and therapeutic procedures are the same as those for bacterial meningitis (see "Meningitis"). Prognosis is guarded, especially if the mass lesion is large and encapsulated, making it refractory to antibiotic therapy.

Abscesses within the CNS are uncommon in dogs and cats, but they may arise as a result of metastasis from distant foci of infection, by direct extension from sinuses, ears, and eyes, as a result of trauma (e.g., bite wound), or from contaminated surgical instruments (e.g., spinal needle). Brain abscess may also result from penetration of the cranial cavity and brain substances by an exopharyngeal foreign body (e.g., sewing needle). The common sites for direct extension are the cribriform plate and the inner ear, resulting in abscess formation in the frontal lobe and the cerebellopontine angle, respectively. Abscesses of hematogenous origin appear to have a predilection for the hypothalamus and cerebral cortex, at the junction of gray and white matter.

Three main phases in the evolution of a brain abscess have been described (6): (a) systemic and focal toxicity with early cerebritis and/or meningitis; (b) spreading cerebritis, cerebral edema, and nonencapsulated suppuration; (c) control of infection with encapsulation. Stage 3 may reactivate with rupture into the ventricle or subarachnoid space and/or formation of multiple abscesses.

Abscesses are life threatening due to systemic and local toxicity and increased intracranial pressure. During stage 1, both toxicity and intracranial pressure may cause death. In stage 2, intracranial pressure is slightly more likely to cause death. In stage 3, intracranial pressure is the predominant fatal mechanism.

When abscesses are multiple, death occurs after a short clinical course. Prolonged survival may occur when abscesses are isolated; however, with brainstem abscesses, the clinical course is usually short because of interference with vital centers.

Diagnosis is based on clinical signs correlated with history, increased cerebrospinal fluid (CSF) pressure, increased CSF cell count (particularly neutrophils), and elevated protein in CSF.

Treatment of abscesses centers around drainage and antibiotic therapy. The latter is based on culture and drug sensitivity testing of organisms isolated from the abscess. It should be noted that when an abscess becomes encapsulated there may be no evidence of infection and no systemic reaction. Accordingly, CSF examination may be of little value in excluding an abscess from the differential diagnosis.

KEY DIAGNOSTIC AIDS: **Clinical Signs, CSF Analysis**

Allergic Encephalomyelitis

A disseminated, demyelinating encephalomyelitis has been reported as a complication of rabies vaccination using phenolized brain tissue vaccines (7). This disorder is now of mainly historical interest since this vaccine has been replaced by chick embryo or tissue culture-modified live virus vaccines. The demyelination is believed to result from immunological reaction to myelin in brain origin vaccines. An ascending paralysis was observed in affected animals.

KEY DIAGNOSTIC AIDS: **Vaccination History, Clinical Signs**

Arachnoid Cysts

These rare structures have been reported in only a few dogs and are characterized as dorsal midline, intradural, extramedullary cavitational lesions that result in spinal cord compression (8, 9). The cystic cavities are reportedly separated from the compressed spinal cord by an intact pia mater. There is no evidence of inflammation within the meninges or tissues lining the cysts. Arachnoid cysts have been reported in dogs aged from 1 to 10 years and have been observed in rostral cervical and caudal thoracic sites. The pathogenesis is unknown, although congenital factors may play a role.

Clinical syndromes will reflect the lesion location. To date, cervical and thoracolumbar syndromes have been observed. Diagnosis can be made using myelography since the cysts usually fill with contrast agent. Surgical excision appears to be the treatment of choice (9).

KEY DIAGNOSTIC AIDS: **Age, Clinical Signs, Myelography**

Atlantoaxial Luxation

This is a condition of instability of the atlantoaxial articulation that produces excessive flexion of the joint and may result in severe, acute neurological deficits, thus causing the cranial aspect of the axis to rotate dorsally into the vertebral canal with subsequent spinal cord compression (10). The disorder results from separation, absence, or malformation of the dens (11–15). The pathogenesis of this developmental malformation is unknown. While hereditary factors may be involved in some lines of miniature and toy breeds of dogs in which this congenital anomaly is most common, fracture and insufficient ligamentous support of the dens may occur in any breed. Congenital atlantoaxial luxation occurs most commonly in dogs less than 1 year of age; however, older animals exposed to various stresses also may be affected. Atlantoaxial luxation has been reported in cats sporadically (16). Atlantoaxial luxation also has been reported in a dog and cat in association with bony occipitoatlantoaxial malformation (17, 18).

Clinical signs vary according to the degree of luxation. They may range from cervical rigidity and pain to spastic paraparesis, and sometimes tetraplegia. The signs may develop slowly over several months, or they may occur acutely.

When atlantoaxial luxation is suspected, survey radiographs should be made without anesthesia before manipulating the animal excessively. Lateral view radiographs will reveal widening of the space between the arch of the atlas and spinous process of the axis, angulation of the axis relative to the atlas, a fractured dens, or the rounded end of the axis indicating the absence of the dens. Oblique views may be useful in determining the presence or absence of the dens. Open mouth frontal (19) and flexed lateral views are not necessary in most cases and are likely to cause severe compression of the spinal cord (20).

The prognosis is guarded. Treatment of spinal cord trauma using glucocorticoids and/or mannitol may be indicated. Internal stabilization of the luxation generally is regarded as the therapy of choice (10, 15, 21–23). However, successful results have been reported in dogs that were managed conservatively without surgical intervention (24).

KEY DIAGNOSTIC AIDS: **Breed, Age, Clinical Signs, Spinal Radiography**

Atrophic Myopathy

This is a chronic degenerative myopathy (synonyms "atrophic myositis" and "cranial myodegeneration") (25, 26) that is characterized by atrophy of muscles of mastication. This condition, the cause of which is unknown, usually occurs in dogs of any breed without an antecedent acute phase; however, it may follow the acute phase of masticatory myositis. There is no peripheral or local eosinophilia present. The atrophy is accompanied by a state of trismus (lockjaw) which may not be reduced under general anesthesia and which may interfere with eating.

Pathological studies reveal large numbers of atrophic fibers and increased amounts of perimysial connective tissue. Focal areas of lymphoplasmacytic infiltrates may be seen occasionally in masticatory and other skeletal muscles. Degenerative changes may be seen in terminal portions of the motor trigeminal nerve.

Prognosis of this form is also guarded because of the severe trismus (27). Spontaneous regression has been observed.

KEY DIAGNOSTIC AIDS: **Clinical Signs, Muscle Biopsy**

Babesiosis

Babesiosis is caused by species of the protozoan parasite *Babesia*. Dogs may be infected with *B. canis*, *B. gibsoni*, and *B. vogeli*, while *B. felis* causes the disease in cats. Under natural conditions all babesias are transmitted by ticks. CNS involvement is rare. Piriform organisms have been observed to fill the lumen of small capillaries and small arterioles of the hippocampus and cerebrum (28). Clinical signs may be mistaken for rabies. Sudden death has been reported (29).

KEY DIAGNOSTIC AIDS: **Clinical Signs, Presence of Ticks, Histopathology**

Botulism

Botulism is a disease resulting from the ingestion of spoiled food or carrion containing a preformed exotoxin produced by *Clostridium botulinum*. The toxin associated with canine disease has been reported to be type C (30–34). Botulism is an uncommon disease in dogs. The toxin blocks release of acetylcholine from neuromuscular junctions and cholinergic autonomic synapses (35). Onset of clinical signs is from hours to several days following ingestion of toxin. Clinical signs reflect a progressive, symmetrical disorder, ranging from mild weakness to severe flaccid tetraplegia with absent spinal reflexes and evidence of weakness in muscles of the face, jaw, pharynx, and esophagus resulting in dysphonia, dysphagia, facial paralysis, and megaesophagus. Early in the course of the disease, or in mildly affected animals, the gait may be stiff and pelvic limbs may be used in a synchronous fashion ("bunny hopping").

Electrodiagnostic studies may reveal a reduction in amplitude of evoked potentials and motor unit potentials; normal or decreased nerve conduction velocities, and, sometimes, fibrillation potentials and positive sharp waves, especially in distal limb muscles (36).

The diagnosis is suggested by historical, clinical, and electrodiagnostic data. It is confirmed by identification of the toxin by neutralization with type-specific antitoxin in the material ingested or in serum, feces, or vomitus of an affected animal.

The prognosis is usually favorable in dogs. Treatment is primarily supportive. Severely affected animals should be monitored closely to avoid the potential complications of inhalation pneumonia and respiratory paralysis.

KEY DIAGNOSTIC AIDS: **History, Clinical Signs, Toxin Identification**

Boxer Neuropathy

This is a newly described neurological disease of boxer dogs (37). The etiology of the disorder is unknown, but a genetic basis is suspected.

Pathological changes in nerve roots and peripheral nerves include both axonal degeneration and demyelination/remyelination, suggesting presence of axonal and Schwann cell defects. Lesions characterized by swollen axons are widespread in the central nervous system, although there is no apparent "tract" or distal distribution of the lesions.

Onset of clinical signs is usually around 6 months of age. There is a progressive ataxia and weakness, initially in pelvic limbs, but later involving thoracic limbs. Proprioceptive function, muscle tone, and tendon reflexes are diminished or absent while pedal reflexes and pain sensation are preserved. Muscle atrophy is minimal. Electrodiagnostic studies reveal little spontaneous activity, normal or slight reduction in motor nerve conduction velocities, and smaller amplitude of evoked muscle action potentials than normal.

Diagnosis is suggested by signalment, clinical, electrophysiological, and nerve biopsy data and is confirmed by pathological evaluation of the central nervous system. Prognosis is poor. There is no treatment.

A disorder with similar clinical and pathological features has been reported in a 5-month-old Pyrenean Mountain dog (38).

KEY DIAGNOSTIC AIDS: **Breed, Age, Clinical Signs**

Brachial Plexus Avulsion

Lesions of the brachial plexus are often encountered clinically in animals, especially in dogs, following trauma. Traction of the thoracic limb or severe abduction of the scapula in dogs has been accepted as the cause of this traumatic disorder. The frequency of root avulsion is believed to be due to the lower resistance of nerve roots to stretch, probably because they lack a perineurium. The ventral roots are more susceptible to traumatic stretch than are the dorsal roots.

Avulsion is usually intradural, and the lesion in dogs is diffuse rather than circumscribed with involvement of fibers at many different levels (39, 40). Degenerative changes in dorsal and ventral nerve roots and ventral branches of spinal nerves are characterized by axonal necrosis, myelin fragmentation, and loss of myelinated fibers. Many fibers are damaged where they penetrate the leptomeninges, resulting in neuroma formation. Retrograde changes are observed in the ventral horn cells characterized by chromatolysis, cell swelling, and neuronal depletion. Retraction balls may be seen. Dorsal column degeneration occurs only with lesions central to the dorsal root ganglion.

Clinical signs reflect the distribution of damage to nerve roots, branches, and plexal cords rather than direct peripheral nerve involvement. Signs may vary from weakness of single muscle groups without sensory loss to paralysis of all thoracic limb muscle groups with accompanying sensory loss (e.g., with a lesion from C6 to T1-T2). A lesion that involves spinal cord segments C8 to T1 may produce ipsilateral loss of the panniculus reflex; while involvement of the T1 root, which contains preganglionic sympathetic fibers, frequently results in partial Horner's syndrome and anisocoria.

Sensory impairment of conscious pain is usually present to a variable degree in all dogs with brachial plexus avulsion. In general, desensitized areas of skin may be detected on lateral, medial, dorsal, and palmar surfaces of the affected thoracic limb.

Diagnosis is most commonly based on historical and clinical data. Electrodiagnostic testing is useful for detecting muscle denervation, especially minor degrees which cannot be detected from routine neurological examination. This information may be helpful in those cases where muscle-tendon transposition is being considered for surgical management. Myelography may occasionally demonstrate a contrast-outlined diverticulum at the level of the cervicothoracic junction.

The prognosis is guarded to poor. The progress of recovery is slow, requiring many months. Electrophysiological testing will detect early changes in reinnervation and recovery. Some fibers, following acute injury, may show a temporary conduction block, from which they will recover within a few days. Since the roots of the radial nerve are commonly injured in brachial plexus avulsion, an evaluation of radial nerve conduction velocity may provide early prognostic information. It has been shown that the prognosis is poor in those cases with initial, decreased radial nerve conduction velocity (41). If this situation remains unchanged after 4 weeks, with concurrent severe electromyographic changes in the triceps muscle, there is virtually no chance of spontaneous recovery. Muscle tendon transpositions have been successful in some dogs with partial avulsion. Amputation of the affected limb may be necessary if the limb is severely excoriated from dragging or self-mutilation.

KEY DIAGNOSTIC AIDS: **History, Clinical Signs, Electrodiagnostic Studies**

Brachial Plexus Neuropathy

This is a rare neurological condition involving the nerves of the brachial plexus that has been reported in dogs (42, 43). It has been suggested that this disorder may be the result of an allergic or hypersensitive reaction similar to serum neuritis in man following prophylactic inoculations, such as tetanus antiserum. The proposed pathogenesis is that the allergic condition produces spinal nerve swelling and subsequent compression at the level of the intervertebral foramina. Pathological changes described include severe axonal and myelin degeneration of peripheral nerves of the thoracic limbs. Clinical signs described in one dog were characterized by acute onset of thoracic limb paresis with depressed or absent reflexes and hypotonia, facial paresis, and neurogenic atrophy in all thoracic limb muscles. Electromyographic studies revealed denervation potentials and absence of evoked muscle action potentials in the thoracic limbs. Cerebrospinal fluid evaluation was normal.

This dog manifested two allergic episodes with facial edema and generalized urticaria over a 48-hour period prior to development of neurological signs. Immunological testing indicated that these signs were related to an all horsemeat diet. Three weeks prior to signs the dog was vaccinated with modified live rabies virus.

No improvement was noted in this dog 49 days after onset of clinical signs even with glucocorticoid therapy. In a second dog with brachial plexus neuropathy, slight improvement was reported 4 months after signs first developed.

Brachial plexus neuropathy has been reported in a cat with clinical signs similar to those in the dog (44). Conspicuous differences include absence of denervation (clinically and electrodiagnostically) and rapid recovery (3 weeks). Vaccination with modified live rabies virus was considered to be related to the neuropathy.

KEY DIAGNOSTIC AIDS: **History, Clinical Signs**

Cerebellar Degeneration

There are many degenerative disorders affecting the nervous system of domestic animals. The majority of these disorders are hereditary or are suspected of being hereditary in nature and are characterized by premature aging and by degeneration and death of various neuronal cell populations. The cause and pathogenesis are not known. The mechanism of premature degeneration of cells is termed "abiotrophy," implying an inherent lack of trophic or nutritive factor. Degenerative diseases tend to be breed related. Clinical signs frequently occur in young animals, usually within a few months after birth. Progressive signs of neurological deficits generally are present with degenerative disorders.

Antemortem diagnosis is based on clinical signs, age, breed, and by rule-out of acquired diseases. Examination of biopsy material from selected sites, such as the cerebellum, may confirm a diagnosis in some instances. In general, electrodiagnostic aids, clinical biochemistry, CSF, and radiology are of limited value in the diagnosis of degenerative disease. Prognosis is guarded to poor. There is no treatment. Cerebellar degeneration has been reported in several breeds of dogs.

Inherited Cerebellar Degeneration in the Kerry Blue Terrier

This is an autosomal recessive disease that affects Kerry blue terriers. Degenerative lesions are initially observed in the Purkinje cell (+/− granule cell) layers, followed by symmetrical, bilateral neuronal degeneration in the olivary nuclei after 3 to 4 months of clinical signs. Several months later, neurons of the substantia nigra and caudate nuclei degenerate in a symmetrical fashion (45).

Clinical signs of stiffness of pelvic limbs and head tremors reflect cerebellar disease and are seen between 8 and 16 weeks of age. Subsequent signs include dysmetria-hypermetria and, often, inability to stand by 1 year of age. The condition is progressive, and prognosis is poor. There is no treatment.

Inherited Cerebellar Degeneration in the Gordon Setter

This is believed to be an autosomal recessive, late-onset cerebellar disease affecting mature Gordon setters between 6 and 30 months of age (46–50). Lesions are restricted to the cerebellum and are characterized by profound loss of Purkinje cells throughout most of the cerebellar cortex. The molecular layer is moderately thinned, and the granule cell layer varies in thickness. It has been suggested that the degenerative process begins in Purkinje cells and that granule cells may be secondarily affected (51). Dogs appear normal during the first 6 months of life, but between 9 and 18 months, they may develop a mild thoracic limb stiffness, hypermetria, broad-based stance, and occasional stumbling. Nystagmus can occur late in the condition. These signs progress very slowly or remain static after a short period of progression.

There is no treatment. Prognosis is guarded. The disease is usually slowly and insidiously progressive over several years.

Inherited Cerebellar Degeneration in the Rough-Coated Collie

This is an autosomal recessive disease reported in rough-coated collie dogs in Australia in which there is early and rapid degeneration of Purkinje cells and granule cells of the cerebellum (52). Other changes include neuron depletion in cerebellar root nuclei, lateral vestibular nuclei, inferior olivary nuclei, and ventral horns of spinal cord.

Posterior incoordinance occurs between 1 and 2 months of age. Subsequently, animals develop a broad-based stance, hypermetria, and head tremors and, occasionally, a "bunny-hopping" gait. Affected animals frequently fall sideways or forward with their legs in extension. Severely affected dogs typically spend most of their time lying down. Clinical signs may stabilize after 12 months of age. There is no treatment.

Cerebellar Degeneration in the Border Collie

This condition appears to be very similar to that described in the rough-coated collie (53). There is a reported loss of granule and Purkinje cells from the anterior folia of the cerebellar vermis, which is flattened grossly. The disease is believed to be familial. Clinical signs are first noted at 6 to 8 weeks of age and are characterized by ataxia, hypermetria, and head tremor. Prognosis is guarded to poor since clinical signs reportedly deteriorate with time.

Cerebellar Degeneration in Bull Mastiffs

This is believed to be an autosomal recessive cerebellar disease affecting bull mastiff puppies, usually between 4 and 9 weeks of age (in one affected dog, signs were noted initially at 7 months of age) (54). Pathological findings are characterized by moderate to severe communicating hydrocephalus with dilatation of all ventricles and the cerebral aqueduct. Symmetrical lesions occur in the cerebellar nuclei, lateral vestibular nucleus, and inferior colliculus. The cerebellar lesions consist of vacuolation, gliosis, and frequent axonal spheroids. Purkinje cells appear normal. There is no cerebellar atrophy, although occasional torpedoes have been seen in the granule cell layer. A specific deficit or abiotrophy within the Purkinje system could account for degenerating axons in cerebellar and lateral vestibular nuclei, but would not explain the lesions in the inferior colliculus. The concentrations of spheroids in and adjacent to nerve cell nuclei and the paucity of degenerative changes in their nerve cell bodies may suggest that this disease is another form of neuroaxonal dystrophy.

Clinical signs include ataxia, most obvious in pelvic limbs, hypermetria, proprioceptive deficits, and head tremor which is accentuated as animals attempt to eat. To date, all affected animals have had visual deficits and slowed menace reflexes. Less constant signs include hysterical behavior, compulsive movements, circling, depression, and nystagmus.

Ancillary aids, such as hematology, blood biochemistry, and CSF analysis are within normal limits. Ventriculography can reveal enlarged lateral ventricles. The contrast passes from lateral ventricles to fourth ventricles without hindrance and into the spinal subarachnoid space, suggesting that there is no blockage and that this is a communicating form of hydrocephalus.

Prognosis is guarded. There is no treatment.

Cerebellar Degeneration in Other Breeds

Cerebellar degenerations, usually involving Purkinje cells, have been reported in families of samoyeds (with swollen axons of Purkinje neurons in the granule cell layer), Airedale terriers, Finnish harriers, and Bern running dogs. A genetic basis has been suggested. A similar disorder has been observed in single litters of Labrador retrievers, golden retrievers, beagles, cocker spaniels, cairn terriers, and Great Danes (47–50). The author has observed isolated cases of Purkinje cell degeneration and loss in German shepherd, springer spaniel, pit bull, and poodle puppies, aged between 6 and 16 weeks. Clinical signs are characterized by the typical cerebellar syndrome.

KEY DIAGNOSTIC AIDS: **Breed, Age, Clinical Signs**

Cerebellar Malformation

As with most other congenital anomalies, malformations of the cerebellum in domestic animals usually result from unknown causes. Various forms of agenesis (absence of the whole or parts), aplasia (faulty development with no tissue differentiation), and hypoplasia (faulty development with some tissue differentiation) (55) have been reported in dogs (48, 49, 56–62).

In utero infection with feline panleukopenia virus results in destruction of actively dividing cells in the external germinal layer, resulting in hypoplasia of the granular cell layer (63). Purkinje cells also may be destroyed (64). The cerebellum is frequently grossly atrophic. Postnatal infections with this virus, however, rarely involve the central nervous system.

In dogs and cats born with congenital malformations, clinical signs will be present when they first begin to ambulate. The signs of cerebellar disease are generally nonprogressive, symmetrical, and include hypermetria, head tremor, and a wide-based stance. Abnormal nystagmus can be present. Diagnosis usually is based on age, breed/species, history (e.g., of viral infection), and clinical signs. As the condition usually is nonprogressive, prognosis for longevity may be favorable. There is no treatment.

KEY DIAGNOSTIC AIDS: **Historical Data, Age, Clinical Signs**

Ceroid Lipofuscinosis

Ceroid lipofuscinosis is believed to be a lysosomal storage disease associated with accumulation of lipofuscin and its related pigment ceroid, particularly in neurons and glial cells of the CNS. The pathogenesis of this disease is unknown. However, in English setters, a deficiency of *p*-phenylenediamine-mediated peroxidase, an enzyme which presumably prevents accumulation of peroxidized lipids, may be involved (65). The presence of the pigment alone is unlikely to be the cause of the CNS disorder since the pigment is present in normal older dogs.

Neuronal ceroid-lipofuscinosis occurs as an autosomal recessive trait in English setters (66–68). There have been sporadic case reports in Chihuahuas (69, 70), dachshunds (71, 72), terrier-cross (73), saluki dogs (74), and corgis and border collies (75). A generalized form has been reported in cocker spaniels (76–78). Neuronal ceroid-lipofuscinosis has been reported also in cats (79, 80).

Neuronal ceroid-lipofuscinosis is characterized pathologically by distention of large and small neurons with fine granular storage material that stains pinkish with hematoxylin and eosin, black with Sudan Black and Luxol Fast Blue, and orange with Sudan III, is periodic acid-Schiff positive, and shows autofluorescence with ultraviolet light. Affected neurons are distributed throughout the brain and spinal cord.

Clinical signs usually occur in mature animals between 1 and 9 years of age, although most reports are of animals under 2 years of age. Signs are extremely variable and include personality changes, visual impairment, generalized ataxia, head tremors, seizures, and tetraparesis.

Hematology, blood chemistries, urinalysis, CSF, and skull/spinal radiographs are normal. Definitive diagnosis usually is made after death.

Prognosis is guarded to poor. There is no treatment.

KEY DIAGNOSTIC AIDS: **Breed, Age, Clinical Signs, Negative Ancillary Aids**

Cervical Malformation-Malarticulation

Cervical malformation-malarticulation (synonyms "wobbler syndrome," vertebral instability, vertebral subluxation, cervical spondylolisthesis, cervical stenosis, and cervical spondylopathy) (21, 81–85) is considered to represent a developmental malformation and malarticulation of cervical vertebrae in dogs. It occurs most frequently in Great Dane and Doberman pinscher dogs. The cause of this disorder is unknown but is probably multifactorial. Rapid growth rates and nutrition (86), mechanical factors (85), genetic factors (84, 87), and disk disease (88) have all been suggested as playing a role. The age of onset of clinical signs is variable, ranging from 3 months to 9 years. In general, Great Danes are affected at less than 2 years of age, while Doberman pinschers more frequently manifest signs when 2 years of age or older (81, 85, 87, 89). There is no sex predisposition in dogs.

The underlying deformity is a narrowing of the diameter of the vertebral canal that may be apparent only on flexion and/or extension of the neck (85, 90, 91). One or more of the caudal cervical vertebrae may be unstable and malarticulated so that the craniodorsal aspect of its vertebral body is displaced dorsally into the vertebral canal, or the cranial border of the vertebral orifice protrudes into the canal. If the displacement appears on both flexed and extended radiographic views, it is considered to be stable. As a result of abnormal stresses on vertebrae associated with malarticulation, the cervical vertebrae may become malformed. In dogs there may be deformity and exostoses of the cranioventral region of the ventral bodies, and degenerative changes have been observed in associated intervertebral disks, sometimes with encroachment of articular facets into the spinal canal (KG Braund and IG Mayhew, unpublished information; 85). Results of a recent study indicate that the principal lesion in the canal is redundant dorsal annulus fibrosis that produces ventral compression of the cord (88). Dorsal compression of the cord was due to the ligamentum flavum. The dorsal longitudinal ligament appeared to play a minor role. In this study, ventral flexion or linear traction of cervical vertebrae resulted in relief of cord compression, while dorsal flexion exaggerated cord compression. It has been suggested that (*a*) "hourglass" compression of the cord (as a result of dorsal annulus fibrosis ventrally, the ligamentum flavum dorsally, and the facets and fibrous joint capsules of the facets laterally) is seen principally in the Great Dane, as is compression due to ligamentum flavum redundancy; (*b*) ventral compression from a redundant dorsal annulus fibrosis occurs mainly in the older Doberman pinscher; and (*c*) the congenital bony formation can be seen in any breed but principally the Great Dane and the Doberman pinscher and usually within the first year or two of life.

In the spinal cord, degenerative changes characterized by white and gray matter necrosis are seen at the site of spinal cord compression. Wallerian-like neuronal fiber degeneration of white matter is seen above and below the compressive lesion.

Clinical signs are related to the severity of spinal cord compression and, therefore, are variable in nature and degree. The most common sign is pelvic limb ataxia and paresis, with or without thoracic limb involvement. Clinical signs usually are first noticed in pelvic limbs. Affected animals can have difficulty rising from lateral recumbency or from a sitting position and frequently have a hypermetric-like gait in thoracic limbs. The digits may knuckle when the animal walks, and nails are often worn excessively as a result of scuffing and dragging. Most dogs have a conscious proprioceptive deficit and demonstrate a wide-based stance. Sometimes pain may be elicited upon neck manipulation, especially extension. Clinical signs tend to be slowly progressive but can be abrupt in onset when external trauma is suspected as playing a major precipitating role.

Diagnosis is based on historical data, signalment, clinical data, and radiography. Many animals have more than one site of compression, which may not be apparent on survey radiography. In one study, plain films were inaccurate in 18 of 45 dogs (40%) (88). Therefore, myelography is essential to establish an accurate diagnosis and prognosis, especially if surgery is to be considered. Excessive dorsal flexion of the neck can exacerbate spinal cord compression, resulting in deterioration of clinical signs immediately following radiographic or myelographic procedures. In the older dog group, similar signs frequently are caused by a Type II disk protrusion.

Prognosis for spontaneous recovery is poor; however, marked improvement has been reported following decompressive and/or stabilizing surgery.

There have been isolated reports of a similar cervical malformation/malarticulation in other canine breeds, including Rhodesian ridgeback, Old English sheepdog, Irish setter, fox terrier, boxer, chow chow, weimaraner, golden retriever, and Pyrenian Mountain dog. A possible hereditary malformation of C2-C3 vertebrae occurs in bassett hounds less than 6 months of age (92). Spinal cord compression has been successfully relieved by surgery (93).

KEY DIAGNOSTIC AIDS: **Breed, Clinical Signs, Spinal Radiography/Myelography**

Chlorinated Hydrocarbon Toxicity

Chlorinated hydrocarbon compounds are used for prevention and control of insect infestations around farms, homes, and on animals, although regulatory agencies have banned the use of many of these insecticides because of accumulating tissue residues and environmental persistence. Dogs and cats may be poisoned by ingestion, inhalation, or absorption through the skin when the insecticide is applied topically (94). Chlorinated hydrocarbon insecticides are considered to be nonspecific stimulants of the central nervous system. Clinical signs can include anxiety, hysteria, facial muscular spasms, jaw champing, spastic gait, ataxia, mydriasis, salivation, and severe generalized seizures. External stimuli may precipitate seizures. Body temperature will usually increase significantly as a result of the seizures. Death may occur within minutes or hours, after several days, or not at all.

A presumptive diagnosis is based on historical data of recent exposure to the toxin and clinical signs. Prognosis is guarded. Signs of acute toxicosis usually abate in 1 to 2 days. Complete recovery may take weeks. Treatment is symptomatic since there is no known antidote. Seizures may be controlled using intravenous anesthetic barbiturates, given to effect. Purgatives and/or gastric lavage will help to remove residual toxin ingested, but maximum benefit is to be expected only during the initial 2 hours after exposure. Soap and water scrubs are indicated for animals exposed by the dermal route. Hyperthermic animals may be bathed in cool water. Forced diuresis with 5% mannitol in 0.9% sodium chloride can enhance urinary excretion.

KEY DIAGNOSTIC AIDS: **History of Exposure, Clinical Signs**

Chronic Relapsing Polyradiculoneuritis

A rare, chronic neurological disorder characterized by periodic remission has been reported in a dog (95). Pathological findings were of a long-standing demyelinating polyradiculoneuritis characterized by symmetrical demyelination/remyelination, prominent "onion-bulb" formation, and axonal sprouting. Inflammatory mononuclear infiltrates (including macrophages and plasma cells) were prominent.

The etiology of this disorder is not known, but the pathological changes are compatible with an autoimmune pathogenesis. Onset of signs was not related to a specific antecedent such as a raccoon bite or an urticarial reaction.

Clinical and laboratory findings include tetraparesis, diminished or absent reflexes, muscle wasting, albuminocytological dissociation (elevated protein but normal cell count in cerebrospinal fluid), muscle denervation potentials, and delayed peripheral nerve conduction velocities. The progressive course is interrupted by partial remission of signs.

A disorder has been reported in a cat in which the clinical and pathological changes resemble those in the dog with chronic relapsing polyradiculoneuritis (96).

The prognosis of animals with chronic relapsing polyradiculoneuritis appears to be poor. Treatment with glucocorticoids has not been effective.

KEY DIAGNOSTIC AIDS: **History, Clinical Signs, Clinical Course, CSF Analysis, Nerve Biopsy**

Coonhound Paralysis

Coonhound paralysis (CHP) (synonym is polyradiculoneuritis) is a rare neurological disease of dogs, occurring especially in raccoon-hunting breeds (97). However, a similar condition can occur in dogs with no possible exposure to raccoons (98, 99). The pathogenesis is unknown. A raccoon bite has been a consistent antecedent in CHP. The condition has been reproduced experimentally by injection of raccoon saliva into a dog that had recovered from two earlier spontaneous attacks (99a). Results of this work suggested that raccoon saliva contains the etiological factor for CHP and that only specifically susceptible dogs are at risk of developing CHP when exposed to this factor.

Interest has focused on CHP mainly due to its resemblance to Guillain-Barré syndrome in humans and its potential as an elucidating model. Like the human syndrome, CHP may have an immunological pathogenesis, although results of a recent study of CHP did not conform with the evidence presented in Guillain-Barré syndrome for an obligatory role of macrophages in initiating myelin damage (100). However, the observed changes do resemble those reported in immunologically mediated experimental allergic neuritis (101).

Pathological changes are associated with a polyradiculoneuritis, with both segmental demyelination and concurrent degeneration of myelin and axons. Leukocytic infiltration, consisting mostly of cells of the monocyte-macrophage series, and scattered aggregates of lymphocytes and plasma cells also are observed. Changes occur in peripheral nerves and nerve roots, especially in the latter and more consistently in ventral roots than in dorsal roots. The disease affects dogs of any breed, both sexes, and usually of adult age.

Clinical signs frequently appear 7 to 11 days after an encounter with a raccoon. Onset is marked by weakness and pelvic limb hyporeflexia. Paralysis progresses rapidly, resulting in a flaccid symmetrical tetraplegia; however, milder forms without paralysis can occur (102). Motor impairment is more pronounced than sensory changes. Many dogs appear to be hyperesthetic to sensory stimuli. Bladder and rectal paralysis usually are not observed. In severely affected animals there may be complete absence of spinal reflexes, facial weakness, and labored respiration (103). Death may occur from respiratory paralysis. The duration of paralysis varies from several weeks to 2 or 3 months. Motor nerve conduction velocities may be markedly reduced, and electromyographic studies reveal widespread denervation 6 to 7 days after the onset. Elevated protein with normal cell counts ("albuminocytologic dissociation") in cerebrospinal fluid has been reported, especially in samples obtained from lumbar puncture.

Prognosis is usually favorable; however, protection from future attacks is short-lived or nonexistent. Treatment is symptomatic. Good nursing care is essential.

KEY DIAGNOSTIC AIDS: **History, Age, Clinical Signs, Nerve Biopsy**

Cranial Trauma

Cranial trauma is a relatively common entity in dogs and cats, usually resulting from a fall or an automobile accident. Head injury frequently causes severe neurological dysfunction. It can produce shear stresses that induce transient loss of consciousness with minimal parenchymal damage, or more severe cerebral contusion, brain degeneration with or without laceration and hemorrhage, and sometimes cranial fractures, which if they involve the floor of the cranial vault, may damage cranial nerves.

An important consequence of head injury is cerebral edema. Edema of the brain can be produced by vascular leakage ("vasogenic" edema) and by cellular hypoxia which leads to accumulation of fluid within cells, especially neurons and astrocytes ("cytotoxic" edema). Vasogenic edema is prominent in white matter, whereas cytotoxic edema affects gray and white matter (104). Cerebral edema can increase intracranial pressure, which will reduce cerebral perfusion and further exacerbate cellular hypoxia. The size of the brain may increase dramatically as a result of cerebral edema, leading to possible brain herniation. The brain can herniate in several ways (105); the three most common are: (*a*) the cingulate gyrus herniates under the falx cerebri; (*b*) the occipital or temporal lobe herniates under the tentorium cerebelli (transtentorial herniation); and (*c*) the cerebellum herniates through the foramen magnum.

Hemorrhage can be an important factor in cranial trauma. Contusions may lead to subdural hemorrhage, which in animals is often diffusely distributed over the cerebral cortex (106). Hemorrhage into the brain substance from damaged vessels is commonly observed. This form of bleeding may be short-lived due to vessel spasm and microthrombi formation (107). Disruption of arachnoid vessels can lead to bleeding into the subarachnoid space. Bleeding into the inner ear is not infrequent (108).

Pathological alteration may include subdural or subarachnoid hemorrhage, bone fragments embedded within brain parenchyma, ischemic laminar necrosis of the cerebral cortex, profound hemorrhage into the substance of the brain, especially the midbrain, with associated focal or multifocal necrosis of midline structures, and edema.

Lesions may be dispersed at multiple levels of the brain. This results in a wide variation of clinical signs commensurate with a multifocal syndrome. Some animals may be completely normal after a brief period of unconsciousness that lasts a few seconds. Other animals can be comatose, confused, delirious, or depressed. Pupil size may be normal, pinpoint (suggestive of mild or moderate midbrain compression), or dilated and unresponsive to light (suggestive of severe midbrain compression, e.g., from transtentorial herniation). Normal conjugate eye movements may be depressed or absent when the head is rotated (this is suggestive of severe brainstem pathology). Other signs can include blindness, which may be transient (up to 24 hours) or permanent, various cranial nerve deficits, vestibular and/or cerebellar signs, and abnormal respiration. Limbs of recumbent animals may be rigidly extended.

Diagnosis typically is based on historical information relating to the accident, clinical evidence of cranial injury, such as abrasions or penetrating wounds, and/ or clinical signs. Skull fractures can be demonstrated using radiography.

Treatment of animals with cranial trauma can be medical, surgical, or both. Medical management is aimed at treating cerebral edema and tissue hypoxia by establishing an oxygen-rich environment, maintaining central venous blood pressure using isotonic lactated Ringer's solution, and administration of high levels of glucocorticosteroids and hypertonic agents, such as mannitol. Comatose patients should be intubated and given oxygen. Conscious animals that are depressed or delirious can be placed in an oxygen cage or supplied oxygen via a tracheostomy tube. Dexamethasone can be given using a dose of 2 to 4 mg/kg intravenously, repeated at 6- to 8-hour intervals for 24 to 36 hours, then at decreasing doses at the same intervals for a further 36 to 48 hours. Glucocorticosteroids are considered to be effective in treating vasogenic edema (105). Mannitol can be administered using a dose of 2 gm/kg intravenously given over a 10-minute period, and repeated two to three times at 3- to 4-hour intervals. Hypotonic solutions, such as mannitol, are believed to be effective in reducing cytotoxic edema (105).

Animals presenting with seizures or status epilepticus can be treated with Valium, using a dose of 5 to 10 mg intravenously or intramuscularly, which is repeated as needed every 30 minutes. Alternatively, barbiturates can be used if seizures persist. General supportive treatment includes maintaining normal body temperature, preventing decubital ulcers by placing animals on a padded surface with frequent turning, and bladder emptying.

Surgical management can be considered under the following circumstances: (*a*) animals with skull fractures and penetrating wounds; (*b*) comatose animals with miotic pupils whose condition has not improved after 24 to 36 hours of medical therapy; (*c*) animals whose signs are deteriorating despite medical treatment.

Various surgical techniques are available for cerebral decompression (109). A bilateral lateral craniotomy approach affords excellent exposure for removal of bone fragments and blood clots, for vessel ligation, and for decompression.

Prognosis is guarded. Some animals are normal after a brief period of unconsciousness. Others may have a stable condition for several days before showing signs of deterioration. Stuporous or comatose animals with dilated unresponsive pupils have a poor prognosis. A period of coma lasting 48 hours or longer is a grave prognostic sign. Deteriorating clinical signs—such as depression progressing to coma, or normal or miotic pupils becoming dilated and unresponsive—are ominous and indicative of progressive brain swelling or transtentorial herniation.

Long-term sequelae of head trauma include seizures and/or focal persistent neurological deficits.

KEY DIAGNOSTIC AIDS: **Historical Data, Clinical Signs, Radiography**

Dachshund Sensory Neuropathy

A genetic basis is suspected (110) for this neurological disease that has been reported in long-haired dachshund puppies. The pathogenesis is unknown. Pathological changes occur in distal sensory nerves, and both larger caliber myelinated fibers and unmyelinated fibers show degenerative changes. Less severe, but similar changes occur in mixed nerves. In the central nervous system, distal degeneration has been observed in the fasciculus gracilis.

Clinical signs are noted in dogs shortly after they begin to walk, and are characterized by loss of proprioception and placing reactions, especially in pelvic limbs, reduction or loss of pain sensation over the whole body in response to superficial and deep pain stimulation, and urinary incontinence. There is no evidence of paresis or muscular atrophy, and patellar reflexes are normal. Electromyographic studies and motor nerve conduction velocities are normal. Sensory nerve potentials may be reduced or absent.

Diagnosis is based on signalment, clinical, electromyographic, and pathological (nerve biopsy) data. Prognosis is poor. There is no treatment.

KEY DIAGNOSTIC AIDS: **Breed, Age, Clinical Signs**

Dalmation Leukodystrophy

A progressive neurological disorder, possibly transmitted by autosomal recessive inheritance, has been described in dalmation dogs (111). Gross pathological changes include brain atrophy, dilatation of lateral ventricles, and cavitation of the central white matter of the cerebral hemispheres. Within affected areas of white matter, there is a diffuse loss of myelin, widespread vacuolation, edema, and presence of numerous, lipid-filled macrophages.

Clinical signs are noted between 3 and 6 months of age and are characterized by visual deficiency and progressive ataxia and weakness in all limbs. Results of routine hematology, urinalysis, and cerebrospinal fluid analysis are within normal limits. Prognosis is poor. There is no treatment.

KEY DIAGNOSTIC AIDS: **Breed, Coat/Eye Color, Age, Clinical Signs**

Dancing Doberman Disease

A suspected neuromuscular disorder has been observed in mature Doberman pinscher dogs (HS Steinberg, unpublished information; 112). Preliminary studies have revealed mild degenerative changes in peripheral nerves and apparent neurogenic muscular atrophy. Clinical signs have an insidious onset and are characterized by alternating pelvic limb flexion when the animal is standing and by frequent sitting. Variable muscle atrophy can be observed in gastrocnemius, semitendinosus, and semimembranosus muscles. Patellar reflexes may be exaggerated. The clinical course is slowly progressive over several years. Positive sharp waves and fibrillation potentials have been detected on electromyographic testing. Sensory and motor nerve conduction velocities are reportedly normal. Results of hematology, blood chemistries, cerebrospinal fluid, and joint fluid examinations are within normal limits.

Prognosis for recovery appears to be guarded. The final outcome, treatment, and further characterization of this disease remain to be clarified.

KEY DIAGNOSTIC AIDS: **Breed, Age, Clinical Signs**

Deafness

Deafness as a result of disease in the receptor organ or a lesion of the auditory pathways is known as "nerve" deafness. Bony defects of the inner ear rarely are found in dogs and cats. Congenital deafness in animals is usually associated with degeneration, hypoplasia, or aplasia of the spiral organ (113–115). The etiology of congenital deafness is unclear. Maternal exposure to ototoxic drugs, such as streptomycin, or viral infection has been suggested as a cause in some instances (116). In cats, the disorder is associated with a dominant autosomal gene (117). A hereditary pattern has been suggested for dalmations, Old English sheepdogs, English setters, Australian heelers, Australian shepherds, cocker spaniels, border collies, collies, Boston terriers, Walker American foxhounds, Shropshire terriers, and bull terriers (60, 116, 118, 119).

Congenital deafness is frequently associated with pigmentation disorders, such as a white coat color and blue eyes (113, 117, 120–122). Coat color abnormalities have been linked with the "merle" color gene. In heterozygotes, this dominant gene will increase the amount of white in the animal's coat, cause dappling in the pigmented portions of the coat, and also alter the pigment in the tapetum and iris. In the homozygous state the gene commonly produces a nearly all white animal that is deaf and blind.

Pathological changes consist of total or partial agenesis of the organ of Corti, the spiral ganglion, and the cochlear nuclei (60). Additionally, in congenitally deaf collie and dalmation puppies, partial collapse of the saccule, atrophy of the saccular nerve, and obliteration of the cochlear duct have been described (115, 123). The hearing deficit is usually present from birth or within a few weeks postnatally (120, 121) and is permanent. Some animals are affected unilaterally.

Definitive diagnosis of deafness is aided by electroencephalographic audiometry. There is no treatment.

Deafness also has been reported in young dogs and cats with transient peripheral vestibular disease. It has been seen in cocker spaniels, German shepherd dogs, Doberman pinschers, Akita dogs, and Siamese and Burmese cats (81). Clinical signs, which usually begin at 3 to 12 weeks of age, include head tilt, circling, and ataxia. Nystagmus is not a feature of this disorder, but there is a deficit in normal eye movements. The few animals that have been examined histologically had no detectable lesions. The signs are generally not progressive, and improvement is usually seen over a period of weeks. This is probably due to compensation rather than resolution of the problem. There is no treatment. Genetic studies have not been done, but there have been multiple cases observed in the breeds listed.

KEY DIAGNOSTIC AIDS: **Breed, Coat/Eye Color, Age, Clinical Signs**

Degenerative Myelopathy in Dogs

This degenerative disease may have an inherited basis. It is most often observed in German shepherd dogs over 5 years of age. A similar condition has been reported in other breeds of dogs (124–126). The pathogenesis of this disease is unknown. It is unrelated to intervertebral disk degeneration, spondylosis deformans, or osseous metaplasia of dura mater. Vitamin deficiency, trauma, and vascular disease have been suggested as possible causes (127). Morphometric data (128) do not support the hypothesis that this disease represents a "dying-back" neuropathy. More recent suggestions that immunological factors (suppressor cells) may play a role (129, 130) need further clarification. The significance of reportedly abnormal activities of brush border and lysosomal enzymes in the intestine of dogs with degenerative myelopathy is unknown (131). Pathologically, the most severe lesions are found in the thoracic spinal cord and are characterized by degeneration of white matter, especially in dorsolateral and ventromedial funiculi. Dorsal root involvement and loss of neurons in dorsal gray horns of spinal cord have been observed (124, 127) in some German shepherd dogs.

The onset of the disease is insidious. Initial signs include pelvic limb ataxia and paresis. The signs progress slowly to truncal ataxia and severe pelvic limb paresis. Knuckling of paws of pelvic limbs is commonly observed. Some dogs have a depressed patellar reflex. Sphincter function remains normal. The disease usually is slowly progressive.

Diagnosis is based on clinical syndrome, breed, and age. Radiography and myelography are normal, which distinguishes degenerative myelopathy from disk protrusion and neoplasia. Prognosis is poor. There is no satisfactory treatment currently available.

A similar disorder has been reported in cats (132).

KEY DIAGNOSTIC AIDS: **Historical Data, Breed, Age, Clinical Signs**

Demyelinating Myelopathy of Miniature Poodles

A rare suspected hereditary disorder in miniature poodles has been reported (55, 133, 134). Pathologically, diffuse demyelination can occur throughout all columns of the spinal cord, but spinal cord gray matter and dorsal and ventral nerve roots are preserved. There may be loss and degeneration of axons. In some dogs, the most severe lesions occur in dorsal and ventral white columns of cervical and thoracic spinal cord segments. Focal areas of malacia also have been observed in cerebral and cerebellar peduncles, cerebellar root nuclei, and tegmentum of the midbrain. Lesions can be characterized by the presence of lipid-laden macrophages. Clinical signs first appear between 2 and 4 months of age. Initial signs of pelvic limb paresis progress to spastic paraplegia and tetraplegia. Analysis of CSF is within normal limits. Prognosis is poor. There is no treatment. There have been no additional reports of this disease during the past 20 years.

KEY DIAGNOSTIC AIDS: **Breed, Age, Clinical Signs**

Dermatomyositis

Dermatomyositis (synonym is "familial canine dermatomyositis") is a recently identified disease of collie dogs that is believed to be inherited, possibly in a dominant fashion with variable expression (135, 136). Dermatomyositis is an inflammatory disease of muscle and skin. Cutaneous lesions involving the face, lips, ears, and skin over bony prominences of the limbs, feet, sternum, and tip of the tail are noted usually between 2 and 6 months of age. The cutaneous lesions consist of vesicles, pustules, and ulcers which may progress rapidly to crusted or alopecic areas. In many cases, the lesions spontaneously regress by 6 to 8 months of age. Generalized or localized masseteric and temporalis muscle atrophy may be noted between 3 and 5 months of age. Associated signs can range from generalized weakness and exercise intolerance, to difficulty in lapping water, chewing, and swallowing. Muscle lesions consist of multifocal muscle fiber necrosis, atrophy, fibrosis, and regeneration, and mild to severe interstitial and perivascular inflammatory cell infiltrates (lymphocytes, neutrophils, plasma cells, and macrophages). It has been suggested that dermatomyositis may be immune-mediated; however, definitive evidence is lacking. Direct immunofluorescence of skin is negative, as are antinuclear antibody titers. Serum muscle enzyme levels are reportedly normal. Cerebrospinal fluid analysis and nerve conduction studies are normal. The presence of fibrillation potentials and positive sharp waves has been demonstrated electromyographically.

The clinical and pathological course and the treatment of myositis remain to be evaluated. A similar disorder has been reported in Shetland sheepdogs (shelties) (137).

KEY DIAGNOSTIC AIDS: **Breed, Age, Clinical Signs, Muscle Biopsy**

Dermoid Sinus

A dermoid sinus is a neural tube defect resulting from incomplete separation of skin and neural tube during embryonic development. Dermatoid sinus has been considered to be unique to the Rhodesian ridgeback breed or ridgeback crosses; however, the condition has been reported recently in a Shih Tzu and a boxer dog (138). It is believed that the sinus is hereditary in nature in ridgebacks, and it is assumed to be controlled by an autosomal recessive gene (139).

The dermoid sinus occurs in the dorsal midline in the cervical, cranial thoracic, and sacrococcygeal regions. One or more may occur in the same animal. The sinuses form a small external opening about 1 mm in diameter, and the hair around the orifice is concentrated in a little tuft (140–142). The sinus is lined by modified skin, incorporating hair follicles and sebaceous glands so that the lumen contains both hair and sebum. The sinus runs from the skin toward the supra-spinous ligament, to which it may or may not be attached by fibrous tissue. In some dogs, the sinus may communicate with the dura mater, especially in the sacrococcygeal region and less commonly in the thoracic region. In the cervical area, the sinus generally is attached in the area of the spinous process of the second cervical vertebra.

Clinical signs can occur in dogs at any age when the sinus communicates with the dural mater and becomes infected. Neurological signs may reflect either a cervicothoracic, thoracolumbar, or lumbosacral syndrome.

Prognosis is guarded. Surgical excision is the treatment of choice.

Incomplete segmentation between adjacent vertebrae may be detected on plain radiography. Metrizamide fistulography may help to determine the extent of the sinus, and myelography can be used to detect the presence of meningeal abnormalities.

Spinal cord myelodysplasia has been reported in one dog with a dermoid sinus (138).

KEY DIAGNOSTIC AIDS: **Breed, Clinical Signs, Fistulography**

Diabetic Neuropathy

Spontaneous diabetes mellitus is a well-recognized disorder in dogs and cats for which clinical and biochemical features have been documented. Recently, cases of clinical and subclinical polyneuropathy have been reported in adult dogs and cats with spontaneous diabetes mellitus (143–148). The author recently observed a polyneuropathy in a chow chow puppy with pancreatic islet cell hypoplasia.

The etiological factors and mechanisms by which peripheral nerve fibers degenerate in diabetic neuropathies are not known (149). It is now believed that vascular factors are unlikely to play an important role in the genesis of the symmetrical polyneuropathies associated with diabetes (150), and interest has focused on metabolic derangement of Schwann cells and on primary axonal disease (151). This metabolic dysfunction may represent another peripheral distal axonopathy/dying back disease, i.e., distal regions of peripheral nerves are first affected and subsequent degeneration occurs in the direction of the cell body located within the spinal cord (152, 153).

Pathological changes reported in dogs and cats range from active nerve fiber degeneration to demyelination/remyelination and axonal regeneration, especially in distal nerves (144, 145, 147). An associated neurogenic muscle fiber atrophy is present in skeletal muscle.

Clinical signs are extremely variable, ranging from an insidious subclinical condition to one with an acute onset of progressive paraparesis, proprioceptive deficits, muscle atrophy, and depressed spinal reflexes. Cats often assume a plantigrade posture in pelvic limbs. Diabetic cataracts may be present. Electro-diagnostic testing has revealed fibrillation potentials, positive sharp waves and fasciculation potentials in muscles, slow nerve conduction velocities, and decreased amplitudes of evoked muscle action potentials (146, 148).

Diagnosis is based on clinical pathological evidence of diabetes mellitus (hyperglycemia, glycosuria, insulin assays) and clinical, neurological, electrophysiological, and nerve biopsy data.

Prognosis is guarded; however, partial or full recovery can occur following insulin therapy (145, 147, 148).

KEY DIAGNOSTIC AIDS: **Blood Chemistries, Clinical Signs, Nerve Biopsy**

Disk Disease

Intervertebral disk disease occurs in all breeds of dogs. It is most common in dachshunds, Pekinese, beagles, miniature/toy poodles, cocker spaniels, Shih Tzus, Lhasa apsos, and Welsh corgis. Most of these breeds are characterized by varying degrees of short-limbed dwarfism and have been designated "chondrodystrophoid." Intervertebral disks in these breeds undergo an accelerated aging process (154–156).

The etiopathogenesis of disk disease is unknown; however, the most logical explanation for the prevalence of disk disease in certain breeds of dogs is a genetic one (157). The risk of occurrence of disk disease in dachshunds is stated to be 10 to 12.6 times greater than for all other breeds combined (158, 159). In some families of dachshunds, the prevalence of disk disease is greater than 60%, compared with the estimated breed prevalence of 19%. The incidence of spinal cord compression associated with disk disease in cats is very low (160, 161).

In disk "protrusion," the outer layers of the disk bulge dorsally into the vertebral canal without rupturing. This appears as a small, round to dome-shaped bulging of the dorsal surface of the disk. Disk "extrusion" is characterized by rupture of the outer dorsal layers of the disk with extrusion of disk material into the vertebral canal around the spinal canal.

Neurological signs are caused by impact injury (162) and/or mechanical compression of the spinal cord and/or nerve roots (163) following extrusion of disk material. An explosive herniation results in far more severe damage than a slow extrusion. Disk protrusion usually is not associated with clinical signs, with the possible exception of pain.

Most dogs with disk disease are between 3 and 7 years of age. Eighty-five percent of disk extrusions in dogs occur in the thoracolumbar area, and 15% are cervical. Approximately 80% of thoracolumbar extrusions occur between T11 and L3, with less than 2% occurring in the terminal lumbar region (L5-S1). Disk extrusion normally does not occur between T2 and T10, probably because of the presence of the conjugal ligament. The most common site in the cervical region is C2-C3, followed by the C3-C4 and C4-C5 segments.

The onset of clinical signs in dogs may be acute (minutes), subacute (hours), or chronic (several days or weeks). These signs may be rapidly progressive or slowly progressive, or they may remain static. Clinical signs also may undergo remission, only to recur at a later date. Clinical signs in dogs with recurrent attacks frequently are more severe than those seen at the initial episode. Recurrences usually are the result of multiple extrusions at the same disk level (164).

The two most common neurological syndromes associated with disk disease are thoracolumbar and cervical syndromes. Clinical signs of these syndromes are outlined in Tables 2.4 and 2.6, respectively. With cervical disk disease, the majority of affected animals will have a history of pain, with or without paresis. Animals may assume a posture with the nose held close to the ground and the back arched. In some dogs, one thoracic limb may be held in partial flexion, with reluctance to walk on this limb. These animals frequently show considerable pain on manipulation of the head and neck. This combination of signs is termed "root signature," since it is believed to be associated with nerve root entrapment near the intervertebral foramen as a result of lateral disk extrusion.

A lumbosacral syndrome (refer to Table 2.3) is uncommonly associated with disk disease. In a small percentage of dogs, a multifocal syndrome may develop as a result of an acute, explosive extrusion of disk material from a thoracolumbar disk that produces progressive diffuse myelomalacia. With this irreversible disorder, an initial thoracolumbar syndrome may be followed by a lumbosacral syndrome as the lesion descends the cord. As the lesion also frequently ascends the cord, signs of thoracic limb rigidity give way to flaccidity and areflexia followed by death due to respiratory paralysis.

A definitive diagnosis of disk disease requires radiographic confirmation of presence of a mass lesion or, in the absence of a mass lesion, evidence of characteristic changes in the disk-vertebral articulations. Typical radiographic features of disk disease include narrowing of the disk space, interverbral foramen, and articular facet at the site of the herniated disk, wedging of contiguous vertebral bodies so that the dorsal part of the disk space appears narrower than the ventral part, and presence of an opacified mass in the vertebral canal. In situ calcified disks in the absence of any other abnormality are a common finding in chondrodystrophoid breeds of dogs and are of little significance. In some cases, particularly in acute extrusions, plain radiographic findings may be minimal or equivocal and myelographic studies will be necessary to define the extent and location of spinal cord compression. Contrast studies also are indicated when there is evidence of more than one disk lesion. The most common myelographic change is narrowing and dorsal deviation of the ventral contrast column at the level of disk protrusion/extrusion. If the disk extrusion is acute, spinal cord swelling may result in complete blockage of contrast material at or immediately rostral to the level of the disk extrusion.

Medical management usually is directed at animals with their first signs of disk disease. Mild clinical signs often resolve after at least 3 weeks of confinement with outside activity limited to leash exercise. Recurrences of clinical signs are common in this group of animals. Severe, unremitting pain may be managed with prednisolone, 0.5 mg/kg orally twice a day for 72 hours. Muscle spasms may respond to muscle relaxants, e.g., methocarbamol (Robaxin), 20 mg/kg orally three times a day for 7 to 10 days, or diazepam, 2 to 5 mg orally three times a day for several days.

Surgical treatment is indicated in animals with clinical signs unresponsive to medical management, with recurrent and/or progressive clinical signs, or in animals that are paralyzed. The two approaches most widely used for thoracolumbar and cervical disk extrusions are dorsolateral hemilaminectomy and ventral slot-decompression, respectively.

Potential complications in some animals following high dosage and/or long-term glucocorticoid therapy are development of gastrointestinal hemorrhage, ulceration, colonic perforation, and pancreatitis (165–168). Complications may be kept to a minimum by administering glucocorticoids for as short a time as possible (or not at all). Prophylactic use of intestinal protectants, e.g., bismuth subsalicylate (Pepto-Bismol) in conjunction with frequent administration (at least four times daily) of antacids, e.g., magnesium or aluminum hydroxide, or H_2 antagonists such as cimetidine (Tagamet, 20 mg/kg orally three times a day) also may reduce the prevalence of gastrointestinal hemorrhage. When gastrointestinal complications are noted glucocorticoids should be stopped immediately.

Paralyzed patients need to be maintained in a sanitary environment, with twice daily bladder catheterization, frequent removal of soiled bedding, and use of foam rubber pads or water beds to prevent development of decubital ulcers. In addition, active physiotherapy that includes assisted standing and walking exercises and supervised swimming for 15 minutes twice daily is an integral part of the nursing care since it will delay disuse muscle atrophy.

The following statements may be used as a general guide to assess prognosis:

1. Animals that are paretic or paralyzed but have normal pain sensation have a good prognosis following medical and/or surgical management.

2. Animals that are paralyzed with loss of bladder control and that show reduced pain sensation have a guarded prognosis following surgical decompression. Early decompressive surgery will have a positive effect on the return of clinical function and on the rate of recovery.

3. Animals that are paralyzed, with loss of bladder control and loss of pain sensation, have an extremely poor prognosis regardless of the mode of treatment employed.

KEY DIAGNOSTIC AIDS: **Breed, Age, Clinical Signs, Radiography**

Diskospondylitis

Diskospondylitis is intervertebral disk infection with concurrent osteomyelitis occurring in contiguous vertebral bodies. This disorder occurs in young to middle-aged adult dogs usually of the larger breeds. Male dogs outnumber females by approximately 2:1. Juvenile large animals are more often affected than adults. Diskospondylitis has also been reported in cats (169).

Diskospondylitis may occur following iatrogenic trauma of the vertebral column (e.g., disk curettage), foreign body migration, paravertebral injection, or more commonly from blood-borne septic emboli (170–174). The source of infection is not established in most cases. Possible sites include the urinary tract, skin, gingiva, and infected heart valves. *Staphylococcus aureus* was the most common organism identified by cultures of blood, urine, or bone in two canine studies (172, 175). Other organisms identified include *Brucella canis, Nocardia, Streptococcus canis, Escherichia coli,* and *Corynebacterium diphtheroides.* Fungal organisms, including *Aspergillus terreus* and *Paecilomyces varioti,* have also been cultured from vertebrae (176–178). A cause and effect relationship between urinary tract infection and diskospondylitis remains to be established.

Clinical signs are variable, ranging from subtle spinal hyperesthesia and stiffness to severe paresis/paralysis (170, 172, 179). Affected animals may manifest depression, anorexia, and pyrexia. Heart murmurs can be detected on auscultation in some animals. The clinical neurological signs reflect the degree of bone proliferation and compression of spinal cord.

Radiographic abnormalities include a concentric area of lysis of adjacent vertebral end-plates early in the disease process. More chronic lesions are characterized by varying degrees of bone lysis and proliferation, vertebral sclerosis, shortening of vertebral bodies, and narrowed intervertebral disk spaces. Extensive destruction of a vertebra may result in its collapse. Diskospondylitis may be present in more than one disk space and commonly occurs in one or more adjacent disk spaces. Common sites of diskospondylitis are thoracic and lumbar vertebrae and the lumbosacral joint.

The severity of the radiographic changes does not necessarily correlate with the degree of clinical involvement. Radiographic signs of the disease may not appear for several weeks after the onset of clinical signs. Hence, a radiographically normal spine does not preclude the diagnosis of diskospondylosis. Blood and urine cultures should be obtained before starting antibiotic therapy. Percutaneous aspiration of the infected vertebrae using fluoroscopy shows promise. *Brucella* titers using rapid slide agglutination or tube agglutination tests should be checked because of the public health significance.

Prognosis is usually favorable with aggressive long-term antibiotic therapy if the vertebrae are stable (178, 180). Until culture results are available, the organism should be assumed to be a staphylococcus. The cephalosporins have been effective in the majority of small animal cases. Vertebral curettage may expedite clinical resolution. In animals with severe neurological signs, spinal cord decompression and vertebral immobilization are indicated (181). The resolving lesion is characterized by cessation of the lytic process and by gradual replacement with new bone, sometimes causing fusion of the adjacent vertebrae.

KEY DIAGNOSTIC AIDS: **Clinical Signs, Radiography, Culture**

Distal Denervating Disease

A degenerative neuropathy has been reported in dogs in the United Kingdom (182). In this disorder there is no breed or age predisposition. The etiology and pathogenesis of this neuropathy are unknown. Pathologically, there is degeneration of the distal intramuscular axons with collateral sprouting. Skeletal muscle changes are typical of neurogenic atrophy. Proximal and middle portions of peripheral nerves are normal, and there is no evidence of sensory nerve damage.

The rate of onset of clinical signs is variable from 1 week to greater than 1 month. The main presenting sign reported is tetraparesis. In some dogs, the head and neck cannot be supported. Mastication, swallowing, respiration, and bladder function are unimpaired. Pain sensation is preserved. Muscle atrophy may be prominent, especially involving proximal extensor muscles. There is hypotonia and depressed or absent patellar reflexes. Seventh cranial nerve dysfunction has been observed. Moderate to marked spontaneous potentials (fibrillations and positive sharp waves) are present in limb, paraspinal, and masticatory muscles, and in the tongue. Motor nerve conduction velocities are in the low-normal range. The amplitude of evoked potentials is reduced. Sensory nerve potentials are normal.

The prognosis for full recovery is good, with appropriate nursing care. Most dogs recover spontaneously within 1 to 5 months of onset of clinical signs.

KEY DIAGNOSTIC AIDS: **Clinical Signs, Clinical Course, Nerve Muscle Biopsy**

Distal Symmetrical Polyneuropathy

A distal symmetrical sensorimotor polyneuropathy has been reported in young adult dogs (1.5 to 3 years) (183, 184; BR Farrow, unpublished information). This condition is clinically and pathologically different from other reported peripheral neuropathies in dogs. The cause and pathogenesis are not known; however, a dying-back process of peripheral axonopathy has been suggested. In one dog, the condition was noted after canine heartworm disease therapy (thiacetarsamide), which was complicated by disseminated intravascular coagulation.

Pathological changes characterized by fiber degeneration and loss, especially of larger caliber myelinated fibers, are present in distal parts of appendicular and laryngeal nerves. Sensory and autonomic nerves appear to be affected to a lesser degree. No lesions are found in the central nervous system. There is evidence of neurogenic atrophy in distal skeletal muscles.

Clinical signs include chronic pelvic limb paresis that progresses to involve thoracic limbs, and bilateral atrophy of bulbar and distal appendicular musculature. A reduced response to painful stimuli has been observed.

Electrodiagnostic studies indicate fibrillation potentials, positive sharp waves in distal limb muscles (below stifle and elbow), and absence of evoked muscle action potentials.

Diagnosis is based on clinical, electrodiagnostic, and nerve biopsy data. Prognosis is poor. There is no known effective treatment.

KEY DIAGNOSTIC AIDS: **Clinical Signs, Clinical Course, Electromyography, Nerve Biopsy**

Distemper

Canine distemper encephalomyelitis (CDE) is caused by a paramyxovirus closely related to measles virus of man and to rinderpest virus of cattle (185, 186). Although the incidence is decreasing, CDE is still one of the most common central nervous system disorders in the dog. The virus initially invades and multiplies in lymphatic tissue and then spreads to epithelial and nervous tissue (187, 188). Results of experimental studies suggest that central nervous system infection may be initiated by migrating virus-infected lymphocytes (189). This pantropic/neurotropic virus usually affects both white and gray matter. The distemper virus has been incriminated as a cause of polioencephalomalacia in dogs (189a, 190–192).

Several clinical syndromes have been recognized in dogs (193, 194).

Canine Distemper Encephalitis in Immature Animals

Microscopic lesions are generally found in many of the visceral organs, including the bladder, kidney, gastrointestinal tract, bronchioles, and tonsils. Lesions in the central nervous system are characterized by mononuclear perivascular cuffing, gliosis, microglial proliferation, and inflammatory cell infiltration of the pia-arachnoid (55, 60). Adventitial cell proliferation and endothelial swelling are commonly seen. Neuronal changes, including nuclear pyknosis and shrunken cells, chromatolysis, and neuronophagia, are found in the cerebral cortex, pontomedullary nuclei, Purkinje cells, and gray matter of the spinal cord. In some dogs, hippocampal cells can be selectively involved (195). Intranuclear and intracytoplasmic inclusion bodies may be present in neuronal cells, astrocytes, histiocytes, meningeal cells, and ependymal cells. The distribution of inclusion bodies in distemper virus encephalitis is erratic, and their presence is not an indication of the severity of the disease process.

Changes in the white matter vary according to the duration and intensity of the infection. There is an apparent predilection for change in the central white matter of the cerebellum, the cerebellar peduncles, the optic nerves and tracts, and the spinal cord. Demyelinating lesions can be focal or disseminated, isolated or confluent. Nerve fibers may undergo degeneration, resulting in the formation of swollen axonal ovoids. Pronounced gliosis may be evident in association with these changes. In many severe lesions, there is evidence of tissue necrosis, edema, and macrophage infiltration. These lesions are often situated in the cerebellar peduncles or central white matter.

This is the most common form of distemper virus infection and is frequently characterized by systemic evidence of gastrointestinal and respiratory disturbances: vomiting, diarrhea, coughing, and seromucopurulent oculonasal discharges. Hyperkeratosis of the foot pad may be seen. Additionally, many animals have conjunctivitis and chorioretinitis. Neurological signs are quite varied and usually suggest a multifocal distribution of lesions. Cortical and subcortical signs include generalized seizures and sometimes personality changes, such as depression and disorientation. Signs of localization in the brainstem include incoordination, hypermetria, falling, head tilt, and nystagmus. Occasionally, monoplegia and paraplegia are observed. A sign that is characteristic of distemper encephalitis is myoclonus, or more correctly, flexor spasm (196). Appendicular flexor muscles, abdominal muscles, and the cervical musculature are the most frequently involved. Sometimes the masseteric, temporalis, and periorbital muscles are affected. These rhythmic contractions are not necessarily associated with limb paresis or paralysis and usually persist during sleep. The movements are temporarily abolished by intravenous injection of local anesthetic agents. The muscle contractions are caused by an abnormality in the motor neuron-interneuron pool in the spinal cord. It is not dependent on sensory nerves or descending pathways from the brain. Visual impairment is frequently reported and is generally associated with abnormal pupillary reflexes. Canine distemper virus is probably the most common cause of convulsions in dogs less than 6 months of age.

Multifocal Encephalitis Secondary to Canine Distemper Virus in Mature Animals

In mature dogs between the ages of 4 and 8 years, canine distemper virus can produce a type of encephalitis that is characterized by a chronic course (193, 194). It is not unusual for an animal to be presented for care with a history of neurological signs that have been present for 12 months. The incidence of this disease is relatively low and does not appear to be related to breed or sex. Animals that have received vaccinations against distemper virus may be affected. This disease is not preceded by, nor is it coincident with, the systemic signs that are seen in younger dogs. Furthermore, it is not unusual for this slowly progressive disease to remain clinically and pathologically static.

The pathological changes that occur in mature dogs with this disease are usually restricted to the central nervous system. The lesions tend to be multifocal and necrotizing and are frequently found in the cerebellopontine angle adjacent to the fourth ventricle, in the cerebellar and cerebral peduncles, in the central cerebellar white matter, in the optic tracts, and in spinal cord white matter. Cystic lesions may be noted along with a loss of the original architecture of the tissues and strong fibrillary astrogliosis. The focal lesions may be associated with thick, perivascular, mononuclear cuffs. Small, plaque-like demyelinative lesions may be found in the capsula interna and corona radiata. Inclusion bodies are rarely found and, when present, are usually located within astrocytic nuclei. Lesions generally are not found in the cerebral cortex.

The initial neurological signs that are commonly seen in mature dogs with distemper virus encephalitis include weakness of the pelvic limbs, generalized incoordination, and occasional falling. These signs frequently progress to tetraplegia. Generalized seizures or personality changes are not features of this disease, and affected animals maintain a normal mental state. Many dogs will have unilateral or bilateral menace deficits, with normal or abnormal pupillary reflexes. Some animals will have signs of facial paralysis, head tilt, and nystagmus. Although head tremors may be seen, myoclonic movements or flexor spasms are not present.

Old Dog Encephalitis

Old dog encephalitis (ODE) (synonyms "disseminated encephalomyelitis in mature dogs," "subacute diffuse sclerosing encephalitis," and "chronic dementional distemper"), in which canine distemper virus has been incriminated as the etiological agent, is a subacute or chronic progressive panencephalitis that occurs rarely in mature dogs.

Affected animals are usually over 6 years of age; however, younger dogs may be affected. There are no related systemic signs, nor is there any apparent predisposition according to breed or sex. There is some speculation that this form of distemper no longer exists since no cases have been reported in several institutions over the past 6 to 8 years.

Pathological changes associated with the disorder are restricted to the central nervous system and are characterized by disseminated perivascular infiltration with lymphocytes and plasma cells, diffuse microglial proliferation, astrogliosis, neuronal degeneration, and neuronophagia. The lesions have a diffuse distribution throughout all divisions of the cerebral cortex. Similar lesions are usually found throughout the basal nuclei, thalamus, hypothalamus, and midbrain. The perivascular mononuclear cuffs often extend beyond the Virchow-Robin space and infiltrate the nervous parenchyma. Diffuse demyelination is seen in subcortical areas, internal capsule, and cerebral peduncles, and often is observed in the pontine area and middle cerebellar peduncles. Large eosinophilic inclusion bodies are seen in the nuclei and cytoplasm of neuronal and glial cells. Necrotizing lesions may be present in the cerebral cortex, characterized by diffuse loss of neuronal cells with replacement of the parenchyma by fibrillary astrocytes.

The most common initial neurological sign is visual impairment. Old dog encephalitis is an invariably progressive disorder and is accompanied by the development of increasing mental depression, compulsive circling, hyperkinesia, and head-pressing against objects (obstinate progression (197). A bilateral menace deficit of a central or peripheral nature is also a common sign. An affected animal may manifest a personality change and fail to recognize its owners. Signs of involvement of the brainstem are rare.

Old dog encephalitis is clinically and pathologically different from multifocal distemper encephalitis in mature dogs. The nature of the lesions (diffuse sclerosis versus multifocal necrosis) and their topographic localization (cerebral cortex and upper brainstem versus lower brainstem and spinal cord) are quite distinct in old dog encephalitis and multifocal distemper encephalitis, respectively. In contrast to multifocal distemper encephalitis, the cerebellum is mostly spared in old dog encephalitis. Clinical differentiation between the two diseases is facilitated by the development of progressive cortical and subcortical signs (mental depression, unresponsiveness, obstinate progression) in old dog encephalitis.

The interest generated by ODE is related to its clinical, pathological, and immunological similarities with subacute sclerosing panencephalitis in man (198–201), even though there appear to be different mechanisms operating in the maintenance of persistent infection and pathogenesis of these two chronic viral diseases (202).

The diagnosis of canine distemper encephalomyelitis (in young dogs especially) is usually based on history and clinical signs. The index of suspicion is higher in affected dogs that are not vaccinated. Positive diagnosis is assured by isolating the virus, usually by inoculation of tissues into ferrets or dogs, and by demonstrating a rise in antibody titers of paired sera samples. Hematological and biochemical data are nonspecific, and electroencephalographic traces may indicate presence of inflammatory disease only. Cerebrospinal fluid analysis may reveal a moderate pleocytosis (15 to 60 white blood cells/mm^3) of mononuclear (lymphocytes and macrophages) cells, and elevated γ-globulins (203). Increased β-glucuronidase levels have been reported in serum and CSF (204). Specific neutralizing antibody in CSF occurs 2 to 3 weeks after onset of disease and is the most definite evidence for canine distemper. It is normally not present in the CSF of vaccinated dogs, dogs that develop circulating antibody quickly and remain asymptomatic after exposure, or dogs that die from acute canine distemper infection (187). Fluorescent antibody (FA) testing for viral antigen in smears made from conjunctival or tracheal washes (or from a footpad biopsy) may be positive (187), especially in young dogs; however, the FA test can be positive in recently vaccinated animals (205).

Ophthalmoscopic examinations may detect a chorioretinitis (206) characterized by areas of hyperreflectivity and bright-colored "medallion" lesions, indicative of past or latent infection (207). Examination of buffy coat smears may demonstrate inclusion bodies in lymphocytes, particularly in the early phase of the disease. Immunofluorescent techniques to detect canine distemper viral antigen in brain sections and other tissues (e.g., mononuclear cells in blood smears) from dogs of all ages have been described (187, 208, 209).

Experimental transmission of distemper encephalitis from young dogs and from dogs with multifocal distemper encephalitis has been relatively easy (194, 210); however, it is only recently that CDV has been isolated from dogs with ODE (211).

The suggested link between dog ownership with the associated possible exposure to canine distemper virus and multiple sclerosis (212, 213) has not been substantiated (186, 214–216).

There is no treatment for CDE, and dogs with progressive neurological signs leading to incapacitation need to be euthanatized. The prognosis is better in dogs with nonprogressive neurological sequelae, such as intermittent seizures, myoclonus, and visual impairment, although only seizures may respond to medication.

KEY DIAGNOSTIC AIDS: **Historical (Vaccination) Data, Clinical Signs, CSF Analysis, Ophthalmoscopy, Fluorescent Antibody Testing, Conjunctival Smears/Tracheal Washes**

Drug Toxicities

Prolonged administration of high doses of aminoglycoside antibiotics (streptomycin, dihydrostreptomycin, kanamycin, gentamycin, neomycin) may cause degeneration of labyrinthine receptors of the auditory and/or vestibular systems (217–220). Vestibular signs of loss of balance, head tilt, falling/rolling, and nystagmus may be reversible following withdrawal of the drug (streptomycin in cats is often incriminated); however, hearing loss is usually permanent.

Chronic experimental intoxication with lead, organophosphates, and toxic hexanes may produce peripheral neuropathies in dogs and cats. Such neuropathic toxicities are rarely encountered in clinical practice.

Aminoglycoside antibiotics also may interfere with neuromuscular transmission, producing neuromuscular weakness. The effects are considered to be due to pre- and postsynaptic blocks. Infusion of calcium gluconate may overcome the presynaptic component, and the use of parenteral neostigmine will antagonize the curare-like effects of these drugs.

Tetracyclines may also have a neuromuscular blocking effect, via a curare-like postsynaptic action.

KEY DIAGNOSTIC AIDS: **History, Clinical Signs**

Dural Ossification

Dural ossification (synonyms "osseous metaplasia of the dura mater" and "ossifying pachymeningitis") is a degenerative disorder of dogs characterized by deposition of bone plaques on the inner surface of the dura mater. These plaques occur in over 60% of both large and small breeds over 2 years of age and occur most often in cervical and lumbar areas of the spine (221, 222). The etiology of this condition is unknown.

At necropsy, gross plaques of bony tissue are found. In extreme cases, the dura may be transformed into a solid bony tube (55; M Vandevelde, unpublished information). The plaques often contain marrow cavities. In general, dural ossification rarely causes clinical disease, but spinal cord compression with secondary degenerative changes in white and gray matter have been reported in dogs (55, 223). Degenerative changes also may occur in nerve roots closely associated with plaques. Affected animals may be presented with a history of chronic (months) paresis, sometimes with atrophy of limb musculature (55, 223). Dural ossification is detected radiographically, usually as an incidental finding, and is characterized by thin radiopaque linear shadows in cervical and lumbar areas, especially at the site of intervertebral foramina.

If a definitive diagnosis is made in a dog with neurological signs, decompressive surgery may be attempted. More common disorders should be given priority in the differential diagnosis of chronic spinal cord compression.

KEY DIAGNOSTIC AIDS: **Clinical Signs, Spinal Radiography/Myelography**

Encephalitozoonosis

Encephalitozoonosis is a rare disease caused by the obligate intracellular protozoal parasite *Encephalitozoon caniculi*. This protozoan disease has been reported in many mammals, including man, dogs, cats, foxes, and laboratory animals. It has been reported in Africa, England, and more recently in the United States (224–232).

The pathogenesis of canine encephalitozoonosis is uncertain; however, it is probably transmitted transplacentally or neonatally. It is shed in urine of affected animals. The condition has been reported only in young dogs, especially in those 4 to 8 weeks of age. Vasculitis is considered to be the basic lesion in canine encephalitozoonosis (231). Pathologically, severe necrotizing nonsuppurative to granulomatous meningoencephalitis and nephritis have been seen in affected puppies (226). Vasculitis and fibrinoid necrosis of small to medium arteries are present in brain and viscera (228–231).

Clinical signs of disease in young dogs with *Encephalitozoon* infection vary considerably and range from none to severe CNS disturbance, coma, and death. Poor growth, ataxia, tremor, blindness, and seizures are characteristic features of the disease in acute and subacute forms (231). Organisms have been identified in urine sediment. In chronic stages, affected animals may have palpably enlarged kidneys, renal anemia, and mild to severe increases in blood urea nitrogen. Results of CSF analysis from affected animals are unremarkable. The clinical signs may be identical to those seen with distemper encephalitis in young dogs. Clinical diagnosis can be suggested by a combination of neurological and renal disease in young dogs. Similar neurological signs have been observed in kittens with encephalitozoonosis.

Definitive diagnosis of this rare disease may be based on renal biopsy, routine histopathology, or culturing and electron microscopy (225). Prognosis is poor. Insufficient data are available concerning treatment.

Similar neurological signs have been observed in kittens with encephalitozoonosis.

KEY DIAGNOSTIC AIDS: **Age, Clinical Signs, Urinalysis, Renal Biopsy, Hematology/ Blood Chemistry**

Esophageal Hypomotility

This condition has been termed "esophageal achalasia," "megaesophagus," and "esophageal neuromuscular disease." Both congenital and acquired esophageal dysphagias have been seen in the dog and cat (233–236). The congenital form is common in Great Dane, German shepherd, and Irish setter dogs. The condition occurs as an inherited disease in wirehaired fox terriers and miniature schnauzers (237–239). In cats, Siamese and Siamese-related breeds may be predisposed to esophageal hypomotility (240). The congenital form is usually apparent in animals around the time of weaning and has been attributed to immaturity of esophageal innervation at birth.

Acquired esophageal hypomotility may occur in any dog or cat at any age. In most cases, the cause is unknown; however, the condition has been observed in association with certain systemic neuromuscular disorders, such as myasthenia gravis, hypothyroidism, hypoadrenocorticism, polymyositis, myotonic myopathy, polyradiculoneuritis, distemper, and giant axonal neuropathy (241–247).

The pathogenesis is unknown, but neural rather than muscular mechanisms are considered to be involved. In the dog, the striated muscle of the esophagus is innervated by fibers that pass from the nucleus ambiguus to the esophagus in the vagus nerves. Electrolytic lesions of the nucleus ambiguus in dogs and of the parasympathetic nucleus of the vagus in cats produce esophageal dysfunction similar to the clinical syndrome (248). A reduction of the normal number of neuronal cell bodies in the nucleus ambiguus has been recorded in an affected dog but not in affected cats.

Clinical features are postprandial regurgitation of undigested food, with radiographic evidence of megaesophagus to the level of the diaphragm. Abnormal esophageal motility with failure of the gastroesophageal junction to dilate when swallowing is initiated may be demonstrated by contrast radiography. In most animals, there is no true achalasia or primary failure of the gastroesophageal junction to relax. In some dogs, respiratory signs, such as cough, dyspnea, and/or abnormal secretions, may be the only signs observed.

Prognosis is generally good in young dogs by feeding in an elevated position in order to enhance gravity flow of the ingesta through the esophagus into the stomach (249). These animals, by the time they mature, appear normal by radiographic, manometric, and clinical examination. However, in a recent report of 18 dogs with congenital esophageal hypomotility, none showed clinical improvement with time (250).

Acquired idiopathic esophageal hypomotility has a poor prognosis for recovery, although clinical improvement has been reported. Cachexia becomes an important complication, and death is a common consequence of aspiration pneumonia. Clinical improvement has been noted in dogs following treatment of the primary disease process, e.g., myasthenia gravis or polyradiculoneuritis.

KEY DIAGNOSTIC AIDS: **Breed, Age, Clinical Signs, Plain/Contrast Radiography**

Exertional Myopathy

Exertional myopathy (synonym "exertional rhabdomyolysis") is a disease that affects many animal species, including man (251). It is an important complication commonly arising in newly captured wild animals. Exertional myopathy occurs most frequently in racing greyhound dogs. It has also been reported in a dog as a secondary complication of prolonged convulsive seizures (252). The pathogenesis is poorly understood. In racing greyhounds severe acidosis leading to muscle cell swelling, local ischemia, muscle cell necrosis, and myoglobinuria with nephropathy has been proposed as a likely sequence of events (253–255).

Pathological findings in muscle include multifocal hemorrhage and myonecrosis.

Clinical signs generally occur during a race or trial and are characterized by extreme distress, hyperpnea, and generalized muscle pain, especially over back and hindquarters. Myoglobinuria and death within 48 hours are common in severe, acute cases.

Prognosis depends on the severity of clinical signs. Dogs with hyperacute signs usually die within 48 hours from renal failure. Mortality rate is low in less severe cases that are treated with intravenous fluids, bicarbonate, anabolic steroids, antibiotics, cooling, and rest.

KEY DIAGNOSTIC AIDS: **History, Breed, Clinical Signs**

Familial Reflex Myoclonus

This is a recently reported, possibly inherited disease reported in Labrador retriever puppies (256). The pathogenesis is unknown. Clinical signs develop in puppies at about 3 weeks of age and are characterized by intermittent muscle spasms and progressive muscle stiffness to the point where affected animals are unable to walk or rise without assistance. Animals lay in lateral recumbency and develop generalized extensor rigidity and opisthotonus in response to handling, voluntary activity, and auditory stimuli. During severe episodes, respiratory distress can be observed. Animals tend to relax in a quiet environment. There is no evidence of muscle pain or percussion dimpling. Neurological deficits are not detected. Electromyograms have increased motor unit amplitude (up to 5000 mV) with polyphasic action potentials. There are no myotonic discharges, and motor nerve conduction velocities are normal. Results of urinalysis, hematology, blood chemistries, and muscle biopsies are within normal limits. Prognosis is guarded to poor. Therapeutic trials with diazepam and clonazepam have little effect on the muscle contractions.

KEY DIAGNOSTIC AIDS: **Breed, Age, Clinical Signs**

Feline Dysautonomia

This new disease (synonyms are "Key-Gaskell syndrome" and "feline autonomic polyganglionopathy") was reported by Key and Gaskell (257) in the United Kingdom. The etiopathogenesis of this disease is unknown. To date, no organisms have been isolated, and there is no evidence of antibodies to *Aspergillus fumigatus* or Epstein-Barr or feline leukemia viruses. In one study, there was no consistent factor identified when management, vaccinal status, and drug therapy were examined (258). Pathology primarily involves neuronal perikarya, especially autonomic ganglia, both sympathetic and parasympathetic (259–261). Lesions are characterized by neuronal degeneration and loss, neuronophagia, and occasionally mild mononuclear perivascular cuffing. Degeneration has been found in many autonomic nerves. Changes are also frequently present in the dorsal nucleus of the vagus and motor nuclei of cranial nerves 3, 5, 7, and 12, ventral horn cells, and intermediolateral gray matter of the spinal cord. Sensory ganglia (e.g., dorsal root ganglia and ganglia of cranial nerves) are affected to a much lesser degree. Clinical signs suggest involvement of the parasympathetic nervous system. The pathology has features in common with grass sickness of horses.

In one series of 40 cats (258), age at the onset of clinical disease ranged from 4 months to 8.5 years, with an average of 2.25 years. In the majority of cases, clinical signs developed in less than 48 hours, but may take up to 7 days. Historically, cats begin vomiting/retching and become depressed and anorexic. The third eyelid protrudes, and pupils are dilated and poorly responsive to light stimulation. Cats may be febrile, emaciated, constipated, and dehydrated. Urinary and fecal incontinence may develop. Sneezing may occur and the nose is often dry. Dried exudate may block the external nares. Occasionally, very mild posterior ataxia or more generalized paresis, depressed proprioception, and absent anal reflex have been detected. Megaesophagus is often present and is usually associated with regurgitation. Many cats have bradycardia of less than 120 beats/minute. Heinz bodies have been demonstrated in up to 50% of the red blood cells; however, their significance is uncertain.

No specific treatment is available but supportive therapy is indicated. Prognosis is guarded, especially in cats which suffer from persistent regurgitation/vomiting. In one study, 28 of 40 cats did not survive the illness (258). Cats which begin to produce secretions and to eat and drink have the best prognosis. Clinical recovery may take up to 12 months.

A single case of canine dysautonomia has been reported in which the clinical and pathological features are identical to those described in the cat (262).

KEY DIAGNOSTIC AIDS: **History, Clinical Signs**

Feline Infectious Peritonitis

This immunopathological disease is caused by a coronavirus (263). Two forms of feline infectious peritonitis (FIP) have been reported: an effusive ("wet") form resulting from diffuse fibrinous peritonitis accompanied by excessive abdominal fluid (264, 265) and a noneffusive ("dry") form characterized by perivascular granulomas around small blood vessels in various sites, especially meninges, brain, and uvea (266).

Coronavirus infection is common in cats, but the majority of infections are subclinical. Approximately 50% of cats with clinical coronavirus disease also test positive for feline leukemia virus (267, 268). The prevalence of coronavirus infection is highest in cats 1 to 2 years of age; however, the disease has been reported in animals as young as 12 weeks of age (269). There is no breed or sex predisposition. The route of infection and the incubation period are uncertain. The CNS lesions appear to result from an immune complex-mediated vasculitis. Neurological signs accompanying FIP are more often observed in the dry form. Similarly, central nervous system pathology is more often observed in the dry form of FIP (266, 267, 270) compared with the effusive form (264, 265); however, cats without neurological deficits still may have microscopic CNS involvement (271). The pathological lesions typical of feline coronavirus disease in the CNS include a pyogranulomatous inflammatory cell infiltration of leptomeninges, choroid plexus, ependyma, and brain parenchyma. Perivascular cuffing and fibrin deposition are prominent. Subependymal periventricular necrosis is commonly observed, as is the infiltration of macrophages, lymphocytes, neutrophils, and plasma cells. Inflammatory or degenerative vascular changes and thrombosis are sometimes present, and many animals have associated panophthalmitis. Several cases of FIP-associated hydrocephalus have been reported (266, 270–273).

The clinical and neurological vagaries of FIP were recognized in earlier reports (266, 270, 271, 273) and include pelvic limb paresis, generalized ataxia, dorsal thoracolumbar hyperesthesia, nystagmus, anisocoria, seizures, tetraparesis, and intention tremors. Multifocal or diffuse CNS involvement is typical of feline coronavirus disease.

Premortem diagnosis, especially in noneffusive FIP, is often difficult. It is suggested by clinical signs, including ocular changes (anterior uveitis), laboratory evidence of increase in CSF protein and neutrophils, and plasma hypergammaglobulinemia. High serial titers for virus antibody level may support the diagnosis. Confirmation generally is made by neuropathological examination.

The prognosis for clinically affected cats is very poor since most animals die within a few weeks or months. There is no satisfactory treatment.

KEY DIAGNOSTIC AIDS: **Age, Clinical Signs, Serum Proteins, CSF Analysis, Serum Antibody Titers**

Fibrinoid Leukodystrophy

A rare fibrinoid leukodystrophy (synonym is "Alexander's disease") characterized by diffuse pallor and rarefaction of CNS white matter and by the presence of irregularly shaped eosinophilic structures designated as Rosenthal fibers has been reported in two Labrador retriever dogs and in a Scottish terrier (274, 275;

NR Cox, unpublished information). The fibers are arranged most densely around blood vessels, subependymal, and subpial areas. Affected white matter can be characterized by increased vascularity. Astrocytic proliferation is commonly seen. Neuronal loss may be evident in the cerebral cortex and subcortical gray structures. The cause of this disease is not known; however, an astrocytic dysfunction is suspected. Clinical signs are noted at about 6 months of age and include pelvic limb paresis, progressive ataxia, generalized weakness, and personality changes. Prognosis is poor. There is no treatment.

KEY DIAGNOSTIC AIDS: **Breed, Age, Clinical Signs**

Fibrotic Myopathy

A chronic progressive disorder has been reported in German shepherd dogs, usually male, with an age range from 2 to 7 years (276, 277). The cause of the condition is unknown. Excessive exercise over a long period resulting in tearing and stretching of muscle fibers has been proposed.

The condition is associated with a palpable thin fibrous band that extends from the tuber ischii to the tibia within the belly of the semitendinosus muscle. Lameness is observed in the affected limb resulting from failure to extend the limb fully. Histologically the band consists of an abundance of dense collagenous connective tissue, with a distinct interface between connective tissue and muscle bundles.

Prognosis is poor since the condition tends to recur within 3 to 8 months following surgical resection of the fibrous band. Similar fibrous bands have been observed in gracilis and quadriceps muscles in dogs.

KEY DIAGNOSTIC AIDS: **Breed, Age, Clinical Signs**

Fucosidosis

Fucosidosis is a lysosomal storage disease resulting from a deficiency of the enzyme α-L-fucosidase in various tissues including central and peripheral nervous systems, kidney, pancreas, lymph nodes, and lung. As a consequence of this enzyme deficiency, there is an intralysosomal accumulation of a substrate, probably α-L-fucose. This disease has been reported in English springer spaniels (75, 278–280), in which the disease is believed to be inherited as an autosomal recessive trait.

A notable gross autopsy finding is the pronounced enlargement of various nerves including optic, vagus, trigeminal, glossopharyngeal, and spinal nerve roots, especially those supplying the brachial plexus. Dorsal root ganglia can be enlarged. The lesions in the CNS are characterized by extensive cytoplasmic vacuolations and swelling of many neurons and supporting glia throughout the brain and spinal cord. Occasional axonal spheroids are present in the cerebellar white matter. Many phagocyte-like cells with a foamy, vacuolated, periodic acid Schiff-positive cytoplasm are present either free in the parenchyma or as pronounced cuffs about larger vessels. Peripheral nerves are infiltrated by foamy macrophages, and fibers are separated by edematous, finely fibrillar ground substance. There is minimal degenerative change in peripheral nerves.

Clinical signs develop in English springer spaniels 1.5 to 3 years of age. Signs are characterized by progressive change in temperament, loss of learned behavior, seizures, visual deficits, loss of balance, and apparent deafness. Additional signs can include head tremor, nystagmus, dysphonia, dysphagia, anisocoria, circling, head pressing, and spasms of jaw champing.

Hematological studies indicate that 3 to 40% of lymphocytes have marked cytoplasmic vacuolation. CSF analysis can reveal low glucose levels and elevated cell count, up to $500/mm^3$, comprising macrophages and lymphocytes.

A premortem diagnosis can be established by enzyme assay of cultured fibroblasts or blood leukocytes. Prognosis for longevity may be favorable. There is no treatment.

KEY DIAGNOSTIC AIDS: **Breed, Age, Clinical Signs, Enzyme Assays**

Gangliosidosis

Ganglioside storage diseases are inherited (autosomal recessive) defects of lysosomal hydrolase enzymes that result in accumulation of gangliosides and complex metabolites within lysosomes of most neurons throughout the nervous system (70, 281–283). The storage material produces widespread neuronal degeneration.

In dogs and cats, several gangliosidoses have been identified and categorized according to the enzyme deficit and degree of visceral involvement. GM1 gangliosidosis, due to a deficiency of β-galactosidase, has been reported in the dog and cat. GM1 gangliosidosis with visceral involvement has been termed GM1 type 1, and the form has occurred in a 5-month-old beagle-cross dog (284) and a 3-month-old cross-bred cat (285). GM1 gangliosidosis without visceral involvement is termed GM1 type 2. This is the more common form and has been reported in Siamese, Korat, and domestic cats (286–290). Signs first appear when cats are 2 to 5 months of age.

GM2 gangliosidosis also has been reported in dogs and cats. GM2 type 1 is caused by a deficiency of hexosaminidase A and has been reported in German shorthaired pointers and Japanese spaniels (291–294). There is no visceral involvement. Signs are severe in animals 12 to 18 months of age. A second form of the disease, termed GM2 type 2, has been reported in domestic cats. Storage material occurs in visceral organs as well as in neurons, and it results from a deficiency of both A and B isoenzymes of hexosaminidase (295, 296). Clinical signs are observed in kittens approximately 3 months of age.

Clinical signs of gangliosidoses are very similar in dogs and cats and are highlighted by their relentlessly progressive nature. Ataxia, discrete head tremor, and dysmetria typically are the first signs observed, followed by spastic paraplegia or tetraplegia, visual impairment, depression, sometimes dementia, seizures, and death. Corneal clouding has been seen in feline gangliosidoses.

Definitive diagnosis requires biochemical identification of the accumulated or storage product and absence or marked reduction in activity of specific lysosomal enzymes required for hydrolysis of accumulated compounds.

Antemortem diagnosis can be made by enzyme assay of whole skin, cultured skin fibroblasts, and purified leukocytes. Postmortem diagnosis is made most reliably by enzyme assay of brain.

Prognosis is grave. There is no treatment.

A suspected lysosomal storage disease has been reported in Abyssinian kittens, in which the clinical signs are very similar to those reported above (297, 298).

KEY DIAGNOSTIC AIDS: **Breed, Age, Clinical Signs, Clinical Course, Enzyme Assays**

Giant Axonal Neuropathy

Giant axonal neuropathy is a rare neurological disease of German shepherd dogs which is inherited as an autosomal recessive trait (299–302). The pathogenesis is unknown, but a slowing or blocking of slow axonal transport in nerves has been suggested. Pathologically the disease is characterized by the loss of myelinated nerve fibers and the presence of giant axons in myelinated and unmyelinated fibers (303, 304). The swollen axons contain masses of neurofilaments. Similar changes are found in the central nervous system. In both peripheral and central nervous systems, lesions predominate at the end of large nerve fibers; thus, the disease exemplifies a "central-peripheral, distal axonopathy" (152).

Clinical neurological signs, which are noted around 14 to 16 months of age, are more obvious in pelvic limbs and are progressive. They are characterized by paresis, proprioceptive loss, diminished patellar reflexes, and pelvic limb hypotonia with atrophy of muscles below the stifles. Conscious perception of pain is gradually reduced in pelvic limbs. Bark may be lost or diminished, and there may be fecal incontinence. Megaesophagus develops around 18 months, resulting in regurgitation and occasional inhalation pneumonia. Electrophysiologically, amplitude of evoked compound muscle action potentials are decreased several months prior to clinical evidence of neuropathy. This decrease is progressive. Denervation potentials are demonstrated by electromyography in distal muscles of pelvic limbs and thoracic limbs by 18 months.

Diagnosis is based on signalment, clinical, electrophysiological, and pathological (nerve biopsy) data. Prognosis is poor. There is no treatment.

KEY DIAGNOSTIC AIDS: **Breed, Age, Clinical Signs, Nerve Biopsy**

Globoid Cell Leukodystrophy

Globoid cell leukodystrophy (synonyms are "Krabbe's disease" and "galactocerebrosidase") is a rare lysosomal storage disease that results in progressive degeneration of white matter of the central and peripheral nervous systems. The disease is caused by an accumulation of galactocerebroside, possible within oligodendrocytes and Schwann cells, as a result of a deficiency of the enzyme β-galactosidase.

Significant lesions are confined to the nervous system where any level of the brain and spinal cord may be affected. The disease is characterized by destruction of white matter and replacement by aggregates (often in a perivascular fashion) of nonsudanophilic, nonmetachromatic, periodic acid-Schiff (PAS)-positive macrophages called "globoid cells." In the peripheral nervous system, lesions are typified by segmental demyelination, axonal degeneration, and endoneurial globoid cell accumulation.

Globoid cell leukodystrophy is inherited as an autosomal recessive trait in young (3- to 6-month-old) cairn and West Highland white terriers (305–313). The disease also has been reported in a 4-month-old beagle (314), a 2-year-old poodle (315), a 4-year-old bassett hound (316), 4-month-old blue tick hounds (317), two Pomeranians ranging in age from 5½ months to 14 years (316, 318), and domestic shorthaired kittens (319).

The clinical signs associated with this disease are variable. Animals often present with signs of either an ascending posterior paralysis or a cerebellar syndrome or both. Signs of a neuropathic syndrome are rarely observed but may include depressed spinal reflexes, reduced muscle tone, and muscle atrophy.

Results of ancillary aids usually are nonspecific. Hematology, blood chemistry, ophthalmology, and spinal/skull radiography are normal. Analysis of cerebrospinal fluid (CSF) can reveal an elevated protein level, but cell counts usually fall within normal limits (albuminocytological dissociation). PAS-positive cells are rarely identified in CSF (320). Electroencephalographic traces may indicate diffuse cerebral involvement, and fibrillation potentials, positive sharp waves, and slow nerve conduction velocities may be found using electrodiagnostic techniques.

Antemortem diagnosis may be established by enzyme activity in leukocytes. In dogs with globoid cell leukodystrophy, the mean enzyme activity is reportedly 18% of the activity in normal dogs, whereas heterozygous carriers have a mean enzyme activity of about 50% of normal activity. Postmortem diagnosis is made most reliably by enzyme assay of brain and/or spinal cord.

KEY DIAGNOSTIC AIDS: **Breed, Age, Clinical Signs, Leukocyte Enzyme Assays**

Glucocerebrosidosis

Glucocerebrosidosis (synonym is "canine Gaucher disease") is a rare lysosomal storage disease caused by a deficiency of glucocerebrosidase (β-glucosidase). The disorder has been reported in Australian silky terriers (321, 322). Glucocerebroside accumulates in neurons throughout the brain. The cytoplasm of these cells is foamy, finely vacuolated, and often contains weakly eosinophilic granules. Severe degenerative changes can occur in the cerebellum. Glucocerebroside storage occurs also in visceral cells of the mononuclear-phagocytic system.

Clinical signs reportedly occur around 6 months of age and are characterized by severe incoordination, wide-based stance, stiff gait, generalized tremors, and hypermetria.

Premortem diagnosis can be established by determining enzyme activity in white blood cells (lymphocytes and granulocytes) preparations. Postmortem diagnosis is made most reliably by enzyme assay of brain.

Prognosis is poor. There is no treatment.

KEY DIAGNOSTIC AIDS: **Breed, Age, Clinical Signs, Enzyme Assays**

Glycogenosis

Glycogen storage diseases, (glycogenosis) are rare myopathic disorders in dogs and cats. These diseases represent inborn errors of metabolism which lead to accumulations of glycogen due to the deficient activity of one of the enzymes involved in glycogen degradation or synthesis. The enzyme defects result in inadequate glycogen utilization, glycogen accumulation within muscle cells, and, often, fasting hypoglycemia. Clinical signs of weakness, exercise intolerance, vomiting, collapse, and seizures may be observed.

A glycogen storage disease (glycogenesis type II) due to acid α-glucosidase enzyme deficiency, has been reported recently in related Lapland dogs (323). Clinical signs developed in animals after 6 months of age and were characterized by progressive muscle weakness, frequent vomiting and regurgitation, megaesophagus, dysphonia, persistent panting, and cardiac abnormalities. Death occurred before the age of 2 years. Electromyographic studies revealed prolonged insertion activity, bizarre high frequency discharges, and occasional fibrillation potentials and positive sharp wave activity. The main lesions consisted of massive glycogen accumulation in most organs and tissues, especially in skeletal muscle. An autosomal recessive mode of inheritance is suggested. Attempts are being made to identify heterozygous animals by their partial deficiency of acid α-glucosidase (324).

Prognosis is poor. There is no treatment.

A glycogenosis similar to Cori's disease (glycogenosis type III) of man, and associated with a deficiency of the debranching enzyme amylo-1,6-glucosidase, has been reported in German shepherd dogs (325, 326). Muscular weakness was noted as early as 2 months of age. Other clinical signs included progressive abdominal distention as a result of hepatomegaly. Glycogen-like material occurred in liver, smooth and skeletal muscle, nerve, and glial cells of the CNS.

A suspected glycogen storage disease which was accompanied by growth retardation, progressive muscular weakness, and atrophy of pelvic limbs and death between 1 and 4 months of age has been reported in cats (327). There was hepatomegaly, splenomegaly, and focal necrosis of muscle and elevated creatine phosphokinase and aldolase activity. Glycogen-like material occurred in reticuloendothelial cells, liver, and muscle cells.

KEY DIAGNOSTIC AIDS: **Breed, Age, Clinical Signs, Muscle Biopsy**

Glycoproteinosis

It has been suggested that neuronal inclusion bodies found in beagles with epilepsy, and rarely in other breeds, are similar to Lafora bodies in human myoclonic epilepsy (328–331). These basophilic inclusions contain polysaccharide, are periodic acid-Schiff positive, and occur also in peripheral nerve, liver, spleen, and lymph nodes.

However, the relationship between seizures and these inclusion bodies remains to be proven, since similar inclusions have been observed in older dogs of various breeds with no signs of clinical disease (332, 333). Furthermore, in a recent study of epilepsy-prone beagles only 6 of 68 dogs (8.8%) had Lafora-like inclusion bodies (334).

Granulomatous Meningoencephalomyelitis

Granulomatous meningoencephalomyelitis (GME) is a worldwide, sporadic, nonsuppurative inflammatory disease of the central nervous system of dogs (and, rarely, of cats) (335–346). Lesions of GME may be disseminated or focal. The disseminated form has been previously described as "inflammatory reticulosis" and "histiocytic encephalitis." The focal form of GME has been described as "neoplastic reticulosis."

Lesions are confined to the central nervous system and are characterized by dense aggregations of mesenchymal cells arranged in a whorling, perivascular pattern. Perivascular cuffs are usually composed of histiocytes (macrophages) and varying numbers of lymphocytes, monocytes, and plasma cells set in nests of reticular fibers. Neutrophils and multinucleate giant cells are sometimes present in small numbers.

In the disseminated form of GME, lesions usually are distributed widely throughout the central nervous system, especially in the white matter of the cerebrum, lower brainstem, cerebellum, and cervical spinal cord. Comparable lesions can occur in gray matter and in leptomeningeal and choroid plexus vasculature. Coalescence of granulomatous lesions from many adjacent blood vessels can produce a true space-occupying mass, which represents the focal form of GME. The cells of this mass can have neoplastic features, such as variable mitotic index and varying degrees of pleomorphism. Focal lesions are usually single and most commonly occur in the brainstem (especially in the pontomedullary region) and cerebral white matter. Animals with focal GME usually have accompanying disseminated lesions. In some dogs, an ocular form occurs with granulomatous cuffs initially involving the optic nerves, optic disk, or retina. In these dogs, disseminated or focal lesions of GME can develop subsequently.

The cause of GME is unknown. The lesions resemble experimental allergic encephalomyelitis, suggesting a possible immunological basis for the disease. Immunohistological studies indicate that many of the lymphocyte cells present in GME are immunoglobulin bearing (347). It is possible that GME represents an altered host response to an infectious agent; distemper and rabies-like inclusion bodies and toxoplasma-like organisms have been reported in some dogs (343, 348, 349).

Disseminated and focal forms of GME are more common than the ocular form. GME appears to occur more commonly in small (toy) breed dogs, particularly in poodles and terriers. The majority of confirmed cases occur in young to middle-aged dogs (1 to 8 years of age). The disease occurs in both sexes; however, there may be a higher prevalence in females.

The onset of disseminated GME usually is acute with a progressive course over a 1- to 8-week period. In approximately 25% of affected dogs, there is rapid deterioration of clinical signs leading to death within 1 week. In more than 50% of the cases, the clinical course is from 2 to 6 weeks. The ocular form also tends to have a sudden onset and may remain static or may be progressive, especially if disseminated lesions coexist. The focal form of GME has a more insidious onset and can slowly progress over a 3- to 6-month period.

Clinical signs are variable and reflect lesion localization. The ocular form of GME is characterized by acute onset of blindness and dilated pupils that are unresponsive to light stimulation, as a result of unilateral or bilateral optic neuritis. Ophthalmic examination may reveal a hyperemic and edematous disk. Vessels may be dilated, and focal hemorrhage may be present (350–353).

Focal GME usually produces clinical signs suggestive of a single, space-occupying lesion, e.g., cerebral, midbrain, pontomedullary, vestibular, cerebellar, or cervical syndrome. In animals with disseminated GME, clinical signs usually reflect a multifocal syndrome. Common signs include incoordination, ataxia and falling, cervical pain, head tilt, nystagmus, facial and/or trigeminal nerve paralysis, circling, seizures, and depression. Occasionally, fever will accompany the clinical signs.

Hematological, serum chemical, and radiographic studies are usually normal, while electroencephalographic tracings are frequently nonspecific. Computerized tomography may detect a mass lesion in those dogs with the focal form of GME. The most useful diagnostic aid is cerebrospinal fluid (CSF) analysis. In most dogs, CSF is abnormal with mild to pronounced pleocytosis ranging from 50 to 600 white blood cells/mm^3, consisting of lymphocytes, monocytes, and variable presence of large anaplastic mononuclear cells with abundant lacy cytoplasm. Corticosteroid therapy can dramatically decrease CSF cellularity. Protein in CSF usually is elevated mildly, ranging from 40 to 100 mg/dl. Occasionally, protein can be elevated without pleocytosis.

Prognosis for permanent recovery is poor. Shortest survival periods, ranging from several days to weeks, are seen with the disseminated and ocular forms. Dogs with the focal form can survive for 3 to 6 months or longer. Long-term therapy is generally unsatisfactory, although temporary remission is often achieved with corticosteroid medication (e.g., oral prednisolone, 1 to 2 mg/kg/day initially, before reducing the dose to 2.5 to 5 mg, given on alternate days). Most dogs require continued therapy to prevent recurrences of clinical signs. Improvement may last for several months in some dogs, although nearly all eventually succumb to the disease. Cessation of corticosteroid therapy is invariably associated with rapid and dramatic clinical deterioration. The ocular form of GME can be treated initially with repository retrobulbar corticosteroids, e.g., 2.5 mg of betamethasone in conjunction with oral prednisolone therapy.

KEY DIAGNOSTIC AIDS: **Age, Breed, Clinical Signs, CSF Analysis**

Hemivertebra

A wide variety of congenital developmental abnormalities of the spinal column can occur in animals, but the majority, at least in dogs, are minor and cause no clinical signs (354).

Vertebral anomalies often result from disruption of normal development and regression of the embryonic notochord, segmentation of mesoderm into somites, or vascularization and ossification of the vertebrae (355).

Hemivertebra is a malformation that may be the result of hemimetameric displacement of somites resulting in right and left hemivertebrae and scoliosis, or it may result from altered vascularization and ossification of vertebrae (356).

While the majority of cases do not produce any obvious clinical signs, hemivertebra is more often associated with neurological deficits than any other congenital vertebral anomaly. Affected animals are usually less than 1 year of age (357, 358). Neurological signs may result from progressive kyphosis, ultimately producing cord compression, or may follow vertebral luxation or fracture at the site of hemivertebra following a sudden jump, fall, or trauma. The breeds of dogs that have been reported to be most commonly affected are the "screw-tailed" breeds, the English bulldog, French bulldog, and Boston terrier (the kinked tail is due to hemivertebrae in the coccygeal region). Vertebrae most commonly affected are in the region T7 to T9. Clinical signs are varying degrees of pelvic limb paresis and paralysis, muscular atrophy, pain on palpation of the spinal column, and, often, fecal and urinary incontinence. In addition, abnormal spinal conformation, including scoliosis and kyphosis, may be present. Radiographs show an obvious abnormality of the spinal column affecting a single or in some cases several vertebrae. There is usually a marked dorsal deviation of the thoracic vertebral column with one or more wedge-shaped vertebral bodies. Disk spaces are usually well preserved. The vertebral end-plates are smooth and of normal thickness. Myelography will often outline compression of the subarachnoid space over one or more of the anomalous vertebrae.

A relationship between abnormal congenital vertebral development and neonatal mortality has been suggested in English bulldogs (358).

Diagnosis of clinically significant hemivertebrae is based on age, breed, clinical history, clinical signs, and radiography. Dogs may be treated with surgical decompression and stabilization.

Other vertebral anomalies that may occur in animals include block vertebrae and butterfly vertebrae.

Block vertebrae result from disturbed somite segmentation. This anomaly may involve vertebral bodies, arches, or the entire vertebra. Block vertebrae are generally stable and are rarely clinically significant.

Butterfly vertebra is an anomaly that results from persistance of the notochord or sagittal cleavage of notochord producing a sagittal cleft of the vertebra body. Butterfly vertebrae are most often detected in brachycephalic, screw-tailed breeds (French and English bulldogs, pugs, Boston terriers and Pekinese). This anomaly is rarely clinically significant.

KEY DIAGNOSTIC AIDS: **Breed, Clinical Signs, Radiography**

Hemorrhage

In contrast to the high incidence in man, massive intracerebral hemorrhage resulting from spontaneous rupture of vessels and/or saccular aneurysms rarely occurs in animals (359). Intracranial and intraspinal hemorrhage has been occasionally reported in dogs in association with arteriovenous vascular malformations—telangiectatic hamartomas and angiomas (360–363). Small ring-like hemorrhages reportedly increase in frequency in dogs over 11 years of age (359). The hemorrhages were associated with an amyloid angiopathy and occurred mainly in the upper layers of the cerebral cortex. Cerebellar cortex, white matter, subcortical and brainstem gray matter were rarely involved. Clinical signs compatible with a cerebral syndrome were observed.

Hemorrhage can often be present in the CNS of animals with (*a*) migrating parasitic disorders, e.g., cuterebriasis in dogs; (*b*) protozoan infections, e.g., toxoplasmosis in dogs; (*c*) bacterial meningitis; (*d*) viral diseases, e.g., canine hepatitis; (*e*) degenerative disorders, e.g., thiamine deficiency in cats; (*f*) toxins, e.g., warfarin poisoning; (*g*) systemic metabolic disorders, e.g., disseminated intravascular coagulopathies, platelet dysfunction (thrombocytopenia), and coagulation factor deficiencies; and (*h*) cranial or spinal trauma.

Hemorrhage into primary and secondary brain tumors is also frequently observed in dogs, especially oligodendrogliomas, glioblastomas, ependymonas, and hemangioendotheliomas.

Onset of clinical signs in animals with sudden hemorrhage is usually acute. Presence of macrophages in cerebrospinal fluid containing red blood cells or hemosiderin ("siderophages") may suggest a recent hemorrhagic episode. Prognosis of animals with hemorrhage is guarded.

KEY DIAGNOSTIC AIDS: **Clinical Onset, CSF Analysis, Pathology**

Hepatic Encephalopathy

Hepatic encephalopathy in dogs and cats is a complex metabolic disturbance of the central nervous system that results from diminished hepatic function, urea cycle enzyme deficiency, or shunting of portal blood around the liver (364–372). As a result, the metabolic and detoxification functions of the liver are impaired and/or bypassed, and the unaltered constituents of the portal blood go directly to the systemic circulation. Many "toxic" substances derived from intestinal degradation, including ammonia, amino acids, short-chain fatty acids, mercaptan, and various biogenic amines, indoles, and skatoles have been incriminated in causing hepatic encephalopathy. Ammonia has been the most studied and is considered to be a leading cause of the pathogenesis of hepatic encephalopathy.

Hepatic encephalopathy can occur with (*a*) acute liver failure; (*b*) chronic liver disease and acquired portal systemic shunting; and (*c*) congenital portosystemic anomalies that shunt portal blood around the liver.

Irrespective of the cause, the neurological signs of hepatic encephalopathy are similar. Mild cases can be characterized by subtle alterations in behavior or personality. More severe changes can induce ataxia, circling, aimless wandering, head pressing, and blindness. Advanced neurological alterations can cause depression, stupor, coma, or seizures. Intermittent salivation may be an additional sign in cats.

Acute hepatic failure may occur in animals of any age. The onset of signs is rapid with a fulminant course. Nonspecific signs may include depression, anorexia, and vomiting. Dogs with encephalopathy associated with chronic liver disease are typically middle-aged or older. Weight loss, depression, anorexia, gastrointestinal signs, polydipsia, and polyuria may be observed.

Congenital portosystemic anomalies and/or enzyme defects usually occur in young dogs and cats. Affected animals are often stunted. Clinical signs are intermittent and are frequently seen a few hours after eating a high protein meal. Signs can include intolerance to certain drugs, such as tranquilizers or anesthetics, anorexia, depression, weight loss, and polydipsia. Jaundice and ascites may be observed in animals with hepatic encephalopathy. The liver tends to be small in affected animals.

Acute hepatic failure is characterized by marked elevations in the serum glutamic pyruvic transaminase (SGPT) and total bilirubin with variable levels of serum alkaline phosphatase. Chronic liver disease or cirrhosis is typified by variable levels of SGPT and total bilirubin with marked elevations in serum alkaline phosphatase. Liver enzyme levels can be normal or mildly elevated in animals with congenital shunts. Albumin levels drop, and clotting times can be prolonged in animals with impaired hepatic function, regardless of etiology.

In hepatic encephalopathy, sulfobromophthalein (BSP) retention is often increased, blood urea nitrogen may be abnormally low (due to the inability of the liver to convert ammonia to urea), and blood ammonia levels are often increased, which may result in the presence of ammonium biurate crystals in the urine sediment. Another clinically useful diagnostic aid is the ammonia tolerance test (373). Serum bile acid values reportedly are sensitive indicators of hepatic dysfunction in the diagnosis of portosystemic venous anomalies (374). The most definitive procedure to confirm the presence of portal vein anomalies is contrast radiography. Several angiographic procedures are available, including injection of a contrast agent into the body of the spleen and catheterization of an exteriorized mesenteric or splenic vein.

The principal objectives in the specific therapy of hepatic encephalopathy are removal of toxic agents (e.g., fasting, especially with respect to dietary protein, bowel cleansing using enemas and/or cathartics, and intestinal antibiotics), supportive therapy (maintaining fluid, electrolyte, and acid-base balance), and prevention of precipitating factors. Lactulose, a nonabsorbable synthetic disaccharide, can be useful in the treatment of hepatic encephalopathic crises. A recommended dose is 10.0 ml of a 3.35 gm/5 ml solution by gastric tube twice daily for 7 days. Lactulose results in a marked reduction in the pH of the colonic contents. This in turn significantly reduces the formation and absorption of ammonium ions and other nitrogenous toxins into the portal circulation.

Some congenital shunts can be surgically corrected. Correction of a shunt by partial ligation rather than by complete occlusion is recommended. The prognosis for animals with hepatic encephalopathy is guarded because of the potential for progressive deterioration of liver function; however, surgical correction can result in complete recovery.

KEY DIAGNOSTIC AIDS: **Historical Data, Age, Clinical Signs, BSP, Blood Ammonia**

Hereditary Ataxia in Smooth-Haired Fox Terriers and Jack Russell Terriers

Hereditary ataxia is an autosomal recessive disorder in smooth-haired fox terriers in Sweden that has been reported as a clinical entity since 1941 (375, 376). A similar condition has been described in Britain in Jack Russell terriers, a type of short-legged, smooth-haired terrier developed within the smooth-haired fox terrier breed. Pathologically, a focal, wallerian degeneration is found in the dorsolateral and ventromedial white matter of cervical and thoracic spinal cord. In the Jack Russell terriers, degenerative changes also are found in central auditory pathways and peripheral nerves.

Clinical signs in both breeds occur between 2 and 6 months of age when weakness and pelvic limb incoordination are observed (375, 377). The incoordination progresses to involve all limbs, and a prancing or dancing type of gait is observed. Animals appear to be unable to gauge the extent of a movement, which is unpredictable in direction (93). Severely affected animals frequently fall and are unable to rise to their feet again.

Clinical signs may stabilize after several months, and some affected animals are able to carry on a relatively normal life in spite of the abnormal movements. In no case has the disease, per se, proved to be fatal. Routine hematological, radiographic, urine, and CSF tests are within normal limits.

Breeding trials will help to eliminate the disease.

KEY DIAGNOSTIC AIDS: **Breed, Age, Clinical Signs**

Hereditary Myelopathy of Afghan Hounds

This disease in Afghan hounds of either sex has an autosomal recessive mode of inheritance (378–380). Histological lesions are limited to the CNS. Cavitation and necrosis occur in white matter extending from caudal cervical regions to midlumbar segments but especially in midthoracic cord segments where all funiculi are affected. Lesions are symmetrical bilaterally. Funicular axons remain intact. Gray matter involvement, when present, is confined to the dorsal nucleus of the trapezoid body and to the periphery of the spinal ventral gray columns. The cause of these lesions has not been determined.

Clinical signs occur between 3 and 13 months of age. Pelvic limb paresis and ataxia often are the first signs observed, and affected animals may have a "bunny-hopping" gait. Within 1 to 3 weeks, these signs progress to paraplegia, thoracic limb paresis, and/or tetraplegia. Spinal reflexes may be depressed, and breathing may be abdominal. Death frequently results from respiratory failure. Pelvic limbs and caudal thorax may be analgesic.

CSF examination may reveal slight elevations in protein level (40 to 80 mg/dl) but no increase in cell count. Blood chemistry values, routine spinal radiography, and myelography are usually normal. Prognosis is poor to grave. There is no treatment.

KEY DIAGNOSTIC AIDS: **Breed, Age, Clinical Signs, Clinical Course**

Hereditary Myopathy of Labrador Retriever Dogs

A severe degenerative myopathy that is inherited as an autosomal recessive trait has been reported in Labrador retriever dogs in the United States and United Kingdom (381–386). The pathogenesis of this condition is unknown. Pathological findings include increased central nucleus counts (sometimes involving 40% of fibers) and pronounced fiber size variation associated with atrophic and hypertrophic fibers. Atrophic fibers are angular, round, or polygonal, often form small groups, and are represented by type I and type II fibers. Hypertrophic fibers, often with splits and a whorling myofibrillar pattern, also can be a feature. A deficiency of type II fibers has been reported in some muscle groups. Intramuscular and peripheral nerves appear to be normal.

Clinical signs, observed between 2 and 6 months of age, are characterized by exercise and cold intolerance, symmetrical wasting of proximal limb and masticatory muscles, stiff-stilted gait, and difficulty in maintaining the head in an erect position. A "bunny-hopping" pelvic limb gait is frequently seen. Spinal reflexes, especially patellar, are often depressed. Signs improve with rest. Clinical signs tend to stabilize in animals after 6 to 12 months of age; however sporadic exacerbations of clinical signs may occur, often as a result of stress, such as exposure to cold, exercise, or excitement, during which time creatine phosphokinase levels are often elevated.

Variable occurrence of fibrillation potentials, positive sharp waves, and high frequency bizarre waves of short duration (myotonic potentials) have been recorded with electrodiagnostic testing.

Diagnosis is based on signalment, clinical, and muscle biopsy data. Prognosis is poor for recovery but is generally good for longevity. There is no treatment.

KEY DIAGNOSTIC AIDS: **Breed, Age, Clinical Signs, Muscle Biopsy**

Hereditary Quadriplegia and Amblyopia in the Irish Setter

This is an autosomal recessive, lethal disease of Irish setters. All animals are affected at birth. Although they make coordinated walking or paddling movements, they are unable to stand or walk unaided, and they propel themselves on their bellies with a swimming type of action (93, 387). Signs progress to visual impairment, nystagmus, head tremor, and seizures. No convincing neuropathological changes have been found to account for the clinical signs (93, 387).

Results of routine hematological, radiographic, urine, and CSF tests are within normal limits. Prognosis is poor. There is no treatment.

KEY DIAGNOSTIC AIDS: **Breed, Age, Clinical Signs**

Herpesvirus Encephalitis

Sporadic outbreaks of neonatal death in puppies caused by an infection with a herpesvirus have been reported (388). Transmission occurs in utero, by direct contact with diseased littermates, or by inhalation or ingestion of infected material. The virus is believed to spread to the CNS via the hematogenous route, after initial replication in the oronasopharynx (389). The high susceptibility of newborn puppies to disseminated canine herpesvirus (CHV) infection is related to their relatively low body temperature (390). Older puppies appear to be resistant to the virus (391) and can serve as asymptomatic carriers of CHV.

At necropsy, ecchymoses and foci of necrosis in lung, liver, and kidney, diffuse pulmonary congestion, and splenomegaly are noted (392). In the CNS, an acute encephalitis is a feature of this disease. The main lesions are focal or laminar areas of necrosis involving mainly the Purkinje cell and granular layers of the gray matter of the cerebellum. Focal gliosis and perivascular cuffing by lymphocytes and macrophages are often seen in cerebrum, thalamus, and pons. Intranuclear inclusions may be observed occasionally in neurons and glial cells adjacent to the malacic areas. Meningitis with necrosis of capillary walls may be found. Perivascular edema and hemorrhages occur in many visceral organs (391).

The syndrome is characterized by acute onset of signs, including crying, diarrhea, dyspnea, and abdominal tenderness (388). Terminal depression and death usually occur 1 to 3 days after the onset of clinical signs.

Diagnosis is based on age, clinical signs, and pathological findings. Although ara-A, a nucleoside analogue, has been used with some success in people with herpes encephalitis, and acyclovir has reduced mortality from herpes encephalitis in mice, results of clinical therapeutic trials are not currently available in dogs and cats.

KEY DIAGNOSTIC AIDS: **History, Age, Clinical Signs**

Hexachlorophene Toxicity

Hexachlorophene is used as a germicide in soaps, shampoos, and disinfectant solutions. Dogs and cats may be exposed by percutaneous absorption of hexachlorophene following skin application, or dogs may eat soap containing hexachlorophene (393, 394). Nursing puppies have been poisoned following application to the mammary glands of the bitch (395). The toxin produces spongiform changes in the white matter of the brain and spinal cord. The vacuoles are associated with intramyelinic edema (396). Significant elevations in cerebrospinal fluid pressure have been recorded in cats with experimental hexachlorophene toxicity (397).

Clinical signs in dogs are usually characterized by acute onset of tremors, especially of the head, that can increase with excitement. Tremors may disappear during inactivity or sleep. Neuromuscular twitchings, spasms, opisthotonus, severe seizures, and death have been reported in some affected animals. In cats, vomiting, weakness, ataxia, and spastic paralysis have been reported (397).

Prognosis is guarded. Some animals recover spontaneously. Gastric lavage or saline cathartic treatment may help animals that have ingested the toxin. In experimental cats, hexachlorophene toxicosis has been reversed by slow intravenous injection of 30% urea (2 gm/kg) in a 10% aqueous glucose solution (397). Barbiturates reportedly are ineffective in controlling seizures in dogs with experimental hexachlorophene toxicity (394).

KEY DIAGNOSTIC AIDS: **History, Clinical Signs**

Hound Ataxia

A degenerative myelopathy has been recognized in Britain in adult foxhounds, harrier hounds, and beagles (93, 398). Histologically, severe wallerian degeneration is found in the spinal cord involving all tracts except dorsal columns. Lateral columns are also unaffected in the cervical cord region. Tract degeneration extends into the brainstem, and occasional, degenerative changes are present in sciatic nerves. Changes are most severe in the midthoracic region of the cord, frequently associated with neuronal degeneration in gray matter. The etiology of this condition remains unknown, although a dietary factor may be involved.

Age of onset varies from 2 to 7 years. Initial signs are pelvic limb weakness, ataxia, and exaggerated elevation of these limbs when retracted at a gallop. Occasionally the pelvic limbs are dragged. The panniculus reflex is usually absent at levels caudal to the thirteenth thoracic to the second lumbar segments. Muscle atrophy is not observed, and spinal reflexes are normal. Affected animals usually become unworkable due to increasing pelvic limb incoordination within 6 to 18 months from the onset of symptoms. Thoracic limb function is normal. To date, there is no specific treatment.

Results of hematological, radiographic, and CSF tests are within normal limits.

KEY DIAGNOSTIC AIDS: **Breed, Age, Clinical Signs, Negative Laboratory Tests**

Hydranencephaly

This rare malformation is characterized by virtual absence of the cerebral hemispheres and basal ganglia with remnants of mesencephalic structures. The cerebral hemispheres are replaced by CSF-filled sacs lined by leptomeninges, a glial membrane, and ependymal remnants. The pathogenesis of this anomaly is not always certain. A fetal cerebrovascular accident may result in massive necrosis and resorption of tissue (399). In utero viral infections with destruction of large portions of CNS tissue occur with certain viruses in other species and may result in hydranencephaly (400, 401). Hydranencephaly believed to be associated with feline panleukopenia virus has been reported in a cat (402).

Affected animals may have dummy-like characteristics and are blind, ataxic, unable to suckle, and indifferent to their environment. Unilateral hydranencephaly has been observed in an 8-month-old miniature poodle whose only clinical sign was a visual defect (81).

KEY DIAGNOSTIC AIDS: **Age, Clinical Signs, Radiography/Ventriculography**

Hydrocephalus

Congenital hydrocephalus has been reported in most species of domestic animals and is one of the most common congenital malformations of the canine nervous system (55). It has multiple causes and usually is divided into communicating (nonobstructive) and noncommunicating (obtructive) forms. The latter type results from a block within the ventricular system and represents the most common cause of hydrocephalus (403). Congenital stenosis, forking, gliosis, and septum formation of mesencephalic aqueduct have been described in animals and persons (399, 404, 405). In communicating hydrocephalus, cerebrospinal fluid passes through the ventricular system into the subarachnoid space, where absorption is impaired. This form of hydrocephalus is considered to be uncommon in animals but has been reported in cats in association with feline infectious peritonitis (270) and in bull mastiff pups in familial cerebellar ataxia (54).

In a recent epizootiological study of canine hydrocephalus (403), small, "toy," and brachycephalic breeds (Maltese, Yorkshire terrier, English bulldog, Chihuahua, Lhasa apso, Pomeranian, toy poodle, etc) were identified as being at high risk. These findings support results of previous studies (60, 361). The smaller the adult dog (whether dwarf or miniature in size, or brachycephalic), the higher the risk of hydrocephalus. In this study, 53% of 564 hydrocephalic dogs manifested clinical signs by 1 year of age. A distinction between congenital and acquired forms of hydrocephalus may be very difficult from a clinical viewpoint, especially since infectious agents are believed to cause hydrocephalus postnatally in young puppies (406). Furthermore, the confusion in terminology is reflected in the results of a recent epizootological study from 14 veterinary schools in United States in which 30% of 564 dogs classified as having "hydrocephalus due to congenital origin" were over 2 years of age (403).

The pathophysiology of hydrocephalus remains unclear. Autoradiographic studies in dogs (407) demonstrated transependymal flow of albumin and fluid. A reversal of CSF flow has been documented in experimental communicating hydrocephalus in the dog (408). Cranial trauma, infections, agents causing encephalitis and meningitis, and neoplasia have all been incriminated in acquired hydrocephalus in animals (60). In Siamese cats, hereditary hydrocephalus is transmitted as an autosomal recessive trait (409). In obstructive hydrocephalus pressure from ventricular enlargement may result in disruption of septum pellucidum and atrophy of associated structures, including subcortical white matter, optic radiation, internal capsule, and auditory radiation. In severe cases the cerebral hemispheres contain extremely large, fluid-filled lateral ventricles, with the cerebral cortex often being reduced to 3 to 4 mm in thickness. On gross inspection the brain may be enlarged with loss of gyral pattern and decreased depth of sulci. Due to increased intracranial pressure, herniated portions of the cerebellum and terminal medulla oblongata may be found (55). The entire ventricular system may be dilated in communicating hydrocephalus. The mesencephalic aqueduct is often stenotic in obstructive hydrocephalus. The ependymal lining is frequently disrupted, and false diverticula may be observed. A pronounced subependymal edema is usually present.

Clinical examination of newborn and immature hydrocephalic animals often will indicate an enlarged, dome-shaped cranium and open sutures and/or fontanelles in an animal that continuously cries out and has visual and auditory impairment and altered mental status (ranging from hyperexcitability to severe depression). Seizures can occur sporadically. Gait is often incoordinated, spastic, and clumsy, and affected animals may circle and press their heads into objects. Pupils may be dilated and fixed. Ventrolateral strabismus may be evident (410). The strabismus is frequently caused by the encroachment on the orbit from the expanding frontal bones, in which case eye movements are normal.

Hydrocephalus may be confirmed by radiographic demonstration of enlarged lateral ventricles by ventriculography. Plain radiography will often reveal a ground glass appearance throughout the cranial vault. Cranial sutures and/or open fontanelles may be evident after the normal age for closure and skull ossification.

Electroencephalographic traces usually have a characteristic pattern of high amplitude (25 to 200 mV), slow wave (1 to 5 Hz) activity, often with a superimposed fast frequency of 10 to 12 Hz. Electroencephalography has proved useful in substantiating a clinical diagnosis of occult hydrocephalus in absence of radiographic abnormalities (411). CSF pressure usually is in the low-normal range in animals with noncommunicating hydrocephalus. It may be elevated in cases of communicating hydrocephalus.

Prognosis is poor. Treatment of animals with severe congenital hydrocephalus is futile due to the large amount of tissue destruction and atrophy. Indeed, the efficacy of glucocorticosteroids and surgical shunt procedures in animals with "acquired" hydrocephalus remains uncertain due to the lack of well-controlled clinical trials and to incomplete knowledge of the underlying pathogenesis of hydrocephalus. Successful shunting procedures have been reported in "acquired" hydrocephalus in older dogs (109, 412, 413).

Dexamethasone, administered at an oral dose of 1 mg divided four times daily for 3- to 5-lb dogs, has been used empirically. This dose is gradually reduced over a 2- to 3-week course of therapy. Some animals may be maintained on alternate-day dosage schedules. Glucocorticosteroids are believed primarily to affect brain bulk and CSF production, but not CSF absorption (414).

KEY DIAGNOSTIC AIDS: **Breed, Age, Clinical Signs, Skull Radiography/
Ventriculography**

Hyperadrenocortical (Cushing's) Myopathy

An acquired degenerative myopathy has been reported in dogs in association with hyperadrenocorticism (HAC) (241, 415–417). Hyperadrenocorticism may be idiopathic or secondary to anterior pituitary gland adenoma or to an adrenal gland adenoma. The pathophysiological basis for hyperadrenocortical myopathy is unknown, although the changes probably result from excessive circulating glucocorticoids, since identical muscle changes are observed in dogs receiving glucocorticosteroids (417, 418). Histological findings are mild degenerative changes of fiber size variation, focal necrosis and fiber splitting, and fiber atrophy, especially of type II fibers. Fiber grouping may be present, and evidence of demyelination/remyelination has been noted in appendicular nerves.

Clinical signs of HAC include polydypsia, polyuria, alopecia, and pendulous abdomen. Myopathic signs are characterized by gradual development of a stiff-stilted gait, weakness, and muscular atrophy. Pelvic limb rigidity, especially in poodles, is not unusual.

Electromyographic studies reveal evidence of bizarre high frequency discharges, often producing a "dive-bomber" sound. Myotonic dimpling may also be elicited in some patients.

Diagnosis is based on clinicopathological evidence of HAC (plasma cortisol levels, adrenocorticotropic hormone (ACTH) response testing, and dexamethasone suppression), signalment (mature female poodles may be predisposed), clinical, and electrophysiological findings.

Prognosis is guarded. Myopathic signs may abate following surgical or medical management of the hyperadrenocorticism.

KEY DIAGNOSTIC AIDS: **Clinical Signs, ACTH Response Testing, Plasma Cortisol Levels, Muscle Biopsy**

Hyperkalemia

Episodic weakness, collapse, and paralysis may occur in dogs with hyperkalemia precipitated by exercise and/or excitement (419). Attacks may last 10 to 15 seconds, after which the dog may appear drowsy but will soon resume normal behavior. The pathogenesis of this disorder (synonym is "hyperkalemic periodic paralysis") is unknown but is thought to involve increased permeability to sodium in muscle cells. Attacks are usually associated with increased plasma potassium levels.

Treatment with acetazolamide, 2 mg/kg orally twice a day, can be beneficial. It has been suggested that acetazolamide stimulates release of insulin and glucagon, thereby increasing potassium movement into muscle.

Increased serum potassium values also may occur in association with adrenocortical insufficiency, diabetes mellitus, acute renal failure, or severe acidosis. In conjunction with the characteristic signs of these diseases, animals may manifest episodic weakness. Diagnostic aids include serum potassium and sodium, plasma cortisol, ACTH response testing, blood glucose, blood urea nitrogen, urinalysis, creatinine, and blood pH values.

KEY DIAGNOSTIC AIDS: **History of Episodic Exercise Intolerance, Clinical Signs, Hyperkalemia**

Hypertrophic Neuropathy

An autosomal recessive neurological disease has been reported recently in Tibetan mastiff dogs (420). This disease results in a reduced density of myelinated fibers, widespread demyelination, and primitive onion-bulb formation with relatively little axonal degeneration in peripheral nerves and roots. Results of initial studies suggest an inborn defect in the Schwann cell's ability to form or maintain a stable myelin sheath.

Clinical signs appear in animals from 7 to 12 weeks of age and consist of generalized weakness, hyporeflexia, and muscle hypotonia. Severely affected pups may become totally recumbent within 3 weeks of onset with subsequent development of sternal compression and limb contractures. Some pups may regain the ability to stand and walk. Mild muscle wasting occurs, and ambulatory pups have a shuffling, plantigrade gait. Pain perception is normal.

Electrodiagnostic studies reveal moderate to severe reduction in nerve conduction velocities and infrequent denervation potentials. There is inconstant elevation in cerebrospinal fluid protein.

Diagnosis is based on signalment, clinical, electrophysiological, and nerve biopsy data. Prognosis is poor. There is no treatment.

KEY DIAGNOSTIC AIDS: **Breed, Age, Clinical Signs**

Hypervitaminosis A

Hypervitaminosis A (synonym is "cervical spondylosis") is a crippling degenerative and proliferative bony disorder affecting the cervical and thoracic vertebral column and various long bones in cats fed whole liver diets (421–425). The disorder is caused by high levels of vitamin A. Clinical signs typically occur when cats of either sex are from 2 to 4 years of age. Affected animals assume a rabbit- or kangaroo-like sitting posture, walk with pelvic limbs flexed, and may show lameness of one or both thoracic limbs. The head may be held in a ventroflexed position, and there may be scoliosis of the cervical spine, which is palpably rigid. Radiographic studies reveal extensive new bone formation and autolysis of cervical and rostral thoracic vertebrae. Periosteal exostoses can be seen involving multiple long bone articulations, especially in elbow and shoulder joints. Ribs, sternebrae, pelvic girdle, and hip joints also can show exostoses. Neurogenic muscle atrophy can result from spinal roots compromised by the bony proliferation.

A high intake of vitamin A is necessary for several weeks before cervical exostoses develop, and trauma may be a contributing factor in the pathogenesis due to constant movement of the neck in coat cleaning. Prognosis is poor. A change in diet may halt the development of the disease but is unlikely to result in resolution.

KEY DIAGNOSTIC AIDS: **Dietary History, Clinical Signs, Radiography**

Hypocalcemia

As a result of reduction in extracellular fluid concentration of calcium ions, the nervous system becomes increasingly excitable due to increased neuronal membrane permeability. Nerve fibers discharge spontaneously, resulting in skeletal muscle contraction and tetany.

In dogs and cats, hypocalcemic tetany (serum calcium levels <6 mg/dl) may result from hypoparathyroidism, postparturient eclampsia, terminal renal failure, protein-losing enteropathy, and severe alkalosis.

Clinical signs of hypocalcemia include nervousness, panting, pacing, muscle spasm, ataxia, tonic-clonic spasms, and sometimes seizures and status epilepticus. Animals are frequently febrile.

Diagnosis is based on clinical signs and serum-ionized calcium levels. Eclampsia in dogs may be treated using a slow intravenous injection of 5 to 10 ml of 10% calcium gluconate, followed by oral calcium gluconate, 0.5 to 2.0 gm/day.

KEY DIAGNOSTIC AIDS: **History, Sex, Clinical Signs, Serum Calcium Levels**

Hypoglycemia

Glucose is the major nutritive carbohydrate substrate used by the brain. The brain uses approximately 66% of the total hepatic glucose production. Since the brain does not store glucose, a sudden drop in blood glucose values can produce neuronal dysfunction. A common cause of hypoglycemia in dogs is a functional islet cell tumor (synonyms are "hyperinsulinism," "beta cell tumor," and "insulinoma") (426–431). These tumors occur in middle-aged to older dogs and are associated with increased insulin secretion by functional, neoplastic β cells ("islet" cells) of the pancreas. Certain breeds—including German shepherds, Irish setters, standard poodles, boxers, and fox terriers—appear to have a higher incidence than other breeds. Clinical signs are characterized by weakness and generalized seizures. Less common signs include ataxia, muscle tremors or fasciculations, posterior paresis, depression, and abnormal behavior. Signs are often intermittent initially but become more frequent as the disease progresses. Polyneuropathy may be a rare complication (432, 433).

Tentative diagnosis is commonly based on demonstration of Whipple's triad (neurological disturbances associated with hypoglycemia, fasting plasma glucose concentration <40 mg/dl, and relief of neurological disturbances by feeding or administration of glucose). The diagnosis can be supported by the amended insulin:glucose ratio which is calculated as follows:

$$\frac{\text{Serum insulin (mU/ml)} \times 100}{\text{Serum glucose (mg/100 ml)} - 30}$$

Amended insulin:glucose ratio levels higher than 30 are considered diagnostic of insulinoma (426, 431). Elevation of serum insulin concentrations in hypoglycemic patients is also highly suggestive of islet cell neoplasia. However, some beta cell tumors secrete predominantly proinsulin, which has only 10 to 15% of the biological activity of insulin. In such cases, insulin serum levels may be within normal limits.

Provocative testing, such as the glucagon tolerance test, can be useful in determining the cause of the resting hypoglycemia. Definitive diagnosis is obtained by biopsy and histopathological examination of the tumor. Most islet cell tumors in dogs are malignant, and metastatis to regional lymph nodes, liver, or spleen is common and occurs early in the course of the disease.

Surgical removal is the treatment of choice. In inoperable cases (e.g., extensive local tumor or metastatic disease), prednisolone, 0.25 to 0.5 mg/kg orally/day, in two divided doses, and diazoxide, 3 to 5 mg/kg orally three times a day, can be used singly or in combination to provide long-term medical management of functional islet cell tumors by virtue of their anti-insulin effects (434). Prednisolone promotes gluconogenesis, while diazoxide inhibits the release of insulin, enhances epinephrine-induced glycogenolysis, and increases the rate of mobilization of free fatty acids. Neither drug has any effect on tumor growth or metastasis.

A 50% dextrose solution, at a dose of 0.5 to 1.0 ml/kg given slowly intravenously, may be given for temporary control of seizures in animals with a hypoglycemic crisis.

The long-term prognosis for animals with islet cell tumors is poor. In surgical cases, a mean postoperative survival time is reported to be 12 to 14 months (430, 431). Temporary postoperative complications can include acute pancreatitis and diabetes mellitus (possibly from chronic beta cell suppression by the excessive insulin levels). Sometimes the diabetes persists, necessitating a low carbohydrate diet and/or insulin administration.

Hypoglycemia also has been reported in association with non-islet cell tumors in dogs, especially hepatocellular carcinomas (435). Transient hypoglycemia may occur in neonatal pups and in toy and miniature-breed puppies less than 3 months of age as a result of cold, starvation, or gastrointestinal disease. These disorders usually respond to a dietary carbohydrate source. Another cause of juvenile hypoglycemia is glycogen storage disease.

In adult dogs, hypoglycemia may occur with severe hypoadrenocorticism, liver disease, and sepsis. It can be a complication of excessive insulin administration to animals with diabetes mellitus. Hypoglycemia in highly nervous hunting dogs is well recognized. Attacks are characterized by apparent disorientation, weakness, and generalized seizures. Recovery is rapid, but the animal's hunting ability is compromised. Frequent feedings with protein-rich foods and/or candy bars may prevent the attacks. The cause has not been determined.

KEY DIAGNOSTIC AIDS: **Clinical Signs, Amended Insulin:Glucose Ratio, Pancreatic Biopsy**

Hypokalemia

Decreased serum potassium levels uncommonly may result from severe vomiting, diarrhea, urinary loss, excessive fluid therapy, or insulin administration. Clinical signs are characterized by episodic weakness.

KEY DIAGNOSTIC AIDS: **History, Clinical Signs, Hypokalemia**

Hypomyelinogenesis

Abnormal myelination of the nervous system has been reported in a variety of animal species (60, 361, 436, 437). The hereditary nature of this disorder has been established in the pig (438). Hypomyelination of the CNS in chow chow dogs is believed to be hereditary (439, 440). In these dogs, a severe myelin deficiency is found throughout the central nervous system, especially in subcortical white matter and foliated white matter of the cerebellum. Axons have thin or uncompacted myelin sheaths, separated from each other by massive astrocytosis, and bizarre myelin formations. Peripheral and cranial nerves are myelinated normally. The myelin deficiency in absence of degenerative changes indicates a disorder of myelin formation rather than breakdown. Retarded myelination may be due to a dysfunction of delay in glial maturation. Animals show clinical signs at 2 to 4 weeks of age. Clinical signs are characterized by wide-based stance, hypermetria, head and body intention tremors, and, often, a bunny-hopping gait. Tremors decrease or cease completely when affected animals lie quietly or are asleep. Clinical signs plateau from 6 to 12 months, followed by gradual improvement. A similar tremor syndrome and hypomyelinogenesis have been reported in two 4-week-old, male, crossbred lurcher puppies (441). Signs regressed completely in one puppy over a 12-week period.

Another similar myelin disorder has been reported shortly after birth in male springer spaniels that is suggestive of an intrinsic defect of oligodendrocyte metabolism. A sex-linked recessive inheritance has been proposed for this condition (442). Hypomyelination occurs throughout the CNS; it is more marked in the cerebrum and optic nerves than in the spinal cord. Myelination appears to increase with age. Peripheral cranial and autonomic nerves are myelinated normally. Tremors in springer spaniels are much more severe than those in chow chows. Animals have great difficulty standing or performing useful coordinated movements, and they cannot feed without assistance. Affected dogs are approximately half the size and weight of normal littermates. Most animals are euthanatized as a result of progressive morbidity.

Cerebrospinal hypomyelinogenesis has been observed in a 5-week-old dalmation puppy (443). On pathological examination, myelin was not found anywhere in the CNS. There was no evidence of active white matter degeneration. The peripheral neuron system was normally myelinated. Generalized body tremors were present at birth. The puppy could not walk voluntarily, and horizontal pendular nystagmus was observed.

KEY DIAGNOSTIC AIDS: **Breed, Age, Clinical Signs**

Hypothyroid Myopathy

A subclinical myopathy has been reported in mature dogs with primary hypothyroidism (444). The etiopathogenesis of this endocrine myopathy is unknown. A disturbance in carbohydrate metabolism has been proposed to explain the preferential type II fiber atrophy which occurs in human and canine muscle. Atrophic type II fibers are oval or angular in outline and are distributed throughout all muscle fascicles. A deficiency of type II fibers has been noted in some dogs. Nemaline rod inclusions may be observed in some muscle fibers, especially in type I fibers (445). No cellular response or myodegeneration is seen, and intramuscular and peripheral nerves are normal. Myopathic changes are considerably more pronounced in muscles of hypothyroid dogs with a concomitant endocrinopathy, namely, diabetes mellitus and hyperadrenocorticism (446). Nerve degeneration reportedly occurs in some affected dogs (445).

Clinical signs of bilaterally symmetrical flank alopecia and obesity are often associated with the hypothyroidism. Presence of weakness and reduced exercise tolerance in some dogs with chronic hypothyroidism may reflect an underlying myopathy. Electrodiagnostic findings may reveal the presence of myotonic potentials. Reversal of the myopathy following thyroid hormone replacement has not been determined by clinical trials.

KEY DIAGNOSTIC AIDS: **Age, Clinical Signs, Thyroid-Stimulating Hormone Response Test, Muscle Biopsy**

Hypotrophic Myopathy

A subclinical myopathy has been reported in pectineus muscles of German shepherd dogs (447, 448). Hypotrophy of the pectineus muscle is characterized by a retardation in muscle fiber growth, particularly of type II fibers. It has been suggested that hypotrophy of the pectineus muscle may potentially influence the development of the coxofemoral joint; however, additional studies have not substantiated the relationship between pectineal myopathy and subsequent development of hip dysplasia (449). Indeed, hip dysplasia can still develop in dogs in which the pectineus muscle has been exercised.

Idiopathic Facial Paralysis

Facial nerve paralysis of acute onset has been reported in mature dogs with an apparent predisposition for cocker spaniels (450). The cause of this condition is unknown. The facial paralysis is unrelated to otitis media.

Pathological studies of facial nerve biopsies reveal active degeneration of myelinated fibers, especially those of larger diameter. Clinical signs are characterized by ear drooping, lip commissural paralysis, sialosis, and collection of food on the paralyzed side of the mouth. Menace response testing and palpebral reflexes are absent. Bilateral facial paralysis may be observed. There is no evidence of Horner's syndrome.

Electrodiagnostic testing may reveal spontaneous denervation potentials in superficial facial muscles. Stimulation of the facial nerve external to the stylomastoid foramen may fail to evoke muscle action potentials. Skull radiographic studies are noncontributory.

Prognosis is guarded. Improvement may take place in a few weeks or months or may never occur. Chronic lip paralysis may result in permanent contracture, and inability to close the eyelids often leads to corneal lesions due to lack of lacrimal lubrication. Treatment is empirical. The efficacy of steroid therapy is unknown. Artificial tears may assist with corneal dryness.

Unilateral or bilateral facial paresis or paralysis in dogs has also been seen in association with hypothyroid neuropathy or pituitary neoplasia or both, sometimes accompanied by peripheral vestibular signs (81). Results of thyroid hormone replacement in such animals have been variable.

Facial nerve paralysis following anesthesia in lateral recumbency has been documented in the dog, resulting from compression of the superficial branches of the facial nerve outside the stylomastoid foramen (451).

KEY DIAGNOSTIC AIDS: **History, Breed, Age, Clinical Signs**

Idiopathic Feline Polioencephalomyelitis

This is a chronic, slowly progressive neurological disease that has been described in immature and mature cats (452). In this report five of six cats were female and of different breeds. The cause of feline polioencephalomyelitis is unknown. Pathological changes suggest a viral infection; however, viral isolation attempts have been unsuccessful. The pathogenesis of this disease may be associated with panleukopenia or feline leukemia virus.

Pathological changes consist of severe neuronal degeneration and loss, especially in segments of the thoracic spinal cord and, to a lesser extent, in the cerebral cortex, basal and diencephalic nuclei, midbrain, periaqueductal gray matter, and oculomotor and pontomedullary nuclei. Diffuse degeneration of white matter (demyelination and axonal necrosis) is usually present in ventral and lateral columns of the spinal cord.

Clinical signs include incoordination, paresis, and hypermetria. Intention tremors may be seen involving the head. Affected cats are usually mentally alert. Cranial nerve function is normal except for depressed direct and consensual pupillary reflexes in some animals. Postural reactions and segmental reflexes of the spine may be noticeably depressed in affected limbs. Occasionally, a localized area of apparent hyperesthesia is evident. In some cases, a psychomotor-like pattern of seizures that is characterized by hallucinations, wild stares, clawing, and hissing and biting at imaginary objects has been reported in sleeping animals.

Some cats have leukopenia, myeloid hypoplasia, and nonregenerative anemia. Electroencephalographic traces may be abnormal. Prognosis is guarded. Data on treatment are lacking.

KEY DIAGNOSTIC AIDS: **Historical Data, Clinical Signs**

Idiopathic Feline Polymyopathy

A polymyopathy of unknown cause has been observed in cats usually over 1 year of age, without breed or sex predisposition. Histological findings include myonecrosis, lymphocytic cellular infiltrates, internal nuclei, and fiber regeneration (453). Clinical signs are characterized by a persistent ventroflexion of the neck, appendicular weakness, especially in the thoracic limbs, painful muscles, and exercise intolerance. Serum levels of creatine phosphokinase and aldolase are elevated. Electromyography reveals fibrillation potentials, positive sharp waves, and bizarre high frequency waves.

Prognosis is guarded. Some cats may recover spontaneously, and others appear to respond to glucocorticosteroids. Recurrences have been observed.

KEY DIAGNOSTIC AIDS: **Age, Clinical Signs, Serum Enzymes, Muscle Biopsy**

Idiopathic Feline Polyneuritis

A severe, acute polyneuritis associated with anemia and transient icterus and fever has recently been reported in a 4-year-old neutered female cat (454). Pathological findings were largely restricted to peripheral nerves and axons and consisted of extensive destruction of myelin and axons and macrophage infiltration. The variable presence of perivascular cuffs of lymphocytes and plasma cells was commensurate with an inflammatory disease and suggests a possible viral and/or immune-mediated etiology. Clinical signs included tetraparesis progressing to tetraplegia, lack of placing and tendon reflexes, depressed flexor reflexes, and hyperesthesia. Cranial nerves, perineal reflex, and tail are normal. Mental status was normal. Severe muscle wasting was present in all limbs after 2 weeks. Electrodiagnostic data were not available. The prognosis appears to be poor. Treatment remains to be established.

KEY DIAGNOSTIC AIDS: **Age, Clinical Onset, Clinical Signs, Nerve Biopsy**

Idiopathic Vestibular Disease

An acute vestibular syndrome without evidence of inflammatory lesions is seen in cats of all ages and in older dogs. Both have signs of peripheral vestibular involvement, including head tilt, asymmetrical ataxia, and horizontal or rotatory nystagmus. More severe signs of falling, rolling, and vomiting (especially in the dog) are seen occasionally. The signs appear suddenly, often causing severe incapacitation. In a few days, the animal tends to stabilize and gradually improves for several weeks. Residual deficits, such as a mild head tilt, may be seen.

It is important to exclude an infection as the cause since the idiopathic syndrome and acute labyrinthitis have identical clinical signs. In the idiopathic disease, the external, middle, and inner ear are grossly normal. Otoscopic and radiographic examinations are normal. The canine disease must also be differentiated from brainstem disease. The syndrome has been mistaken for an acute vascular accident (i.e., infarction or hemorrhage) of the brainstem. The signs of the idiopathic syndrome are only those of peripheral vestibular dysfunction. Postural reactions and other cranial nerves are not affected. In the early stages, postural reactions may be very difficult to test, and the peripheral nature of the syndrome may not be obvious until the second or third day.

The peracute onset of clinical signs and absence of otitis media/interna based on otoscopic and/or radiographic examinations suggest a diagnosis of idiopathic vestibular disease.

Prognosis for spontaneous remission is good; however, recovery may take 2 or 3 weeks. Recurrences may be noted. A variety of treatments have been tried, including antibiotics, anti-inflammatory agents, anti-motion sickness drugs, and others. There is no evidence that any treatment changes the course of the disease. If infection cannot be absolutely excluded, antibiotics are recommended, but aminoglycosides should be avoided.

Signs of peripheral vestibular disease have been observed in several breeds of puppies and kittens (81, 455–457) including cocker spaniels, German shepherds, Doberman pinschers, and Siamese and Burmese cats. Signs may be noted from birth to 3 or 4 months of age, and typically include a pronounced head tilt, circling, and often falling and/or rolling. Nystagmus is not a feature in these young animals. Some animals may be deaf. The cause of this disorder is unknown. Pathological studies have failed to produce any evidence of inflammation, degeneration, or malformation. Prognosis is guarded since clinical signs may regress completely, recur, or remain static. There is no treatment.

KEY DIAGNOSTIC AIDS: **Breed, Age, Clinical Signs, Negative Laboratory Findings**

Immobilization Myopathy

A myopathy in the quadriceps muscle has been reported in dogs following treatment of femoral fractures by limb immobilization in hyperextension for 3 to 7 weeks (458). The pathogenesis is not well understood. It has been proposed that joint stiffness occurs as a result of fibrous adhesions in and around the stifle while it is maintained in an extended position. Immobilization of muscle induces muscle atrophy. This change is especially influenced by the degree of stretch in which the muscle is held. In animals with limb immobilization in extension, the quadriceps muscle group, held in a shortened state, undergoes selective and progressive atrophy.

Pathological findings in vastus lateralis muscle include fiber size variability, increased perimysial fibrosis and focal necrosis, and pronounced type I fiber atrophy.

The clinical syndrome is characterized by limb hyperextension, generalized muscle atrophy of the affected limb, abducted gait, and limited range of joint motion.

Prognosis is guarded. Breakdown and removal of adhesions by surgical management may result in a return of function of the femorotibial joint and reversibility of the type I fiber atrophy (459).

Similar clinical signs are seen in dogs with congenital limb contractures.

KEY DIAGNOSTIC AIDS: **History, Clinical Signs, Muscle Biopsy**

Infarction

Infarction or necrosis (synonym is "malacia") of CNS parenchyma results from cerebrospinal vascular occlusion. Infarction most commonly occurs in association with fibrocartilaginous emboli in dogs and with ischemic encephalopathy in cats. Rare causes of infarction in dogs and cats include cerebrovascular abscessation (sometimes associated with hypothyroidism), atherosclerosis, arteriosclerosis, and thrombosus (460, 461). Aortoiliac thrombosus in cats results in a neuromuscular pelvic limb ischemia, rather than spinal cord infarction (refer to **"Ischemic Neuromyopathy"**).

Fibrocartilaginous Embolization

This disease process is an ischemic necrosis of spinal cord parenchyma that has been associated with fibrocartilaginous emboli in arteries and veins (462–467). Any level of the spinal cord may be involved. The disorder has been reported mainly in dogs, immature and adult, small and large breeds. It may also occur in cats. Infarction at the level of the cervicothoracic or lumbosacral spinal cord may result in a neuropathic syndrome as a result of necrosis of ventral horn cells within the spinal cord gray matter.

The pathogenesis is not clear. Intervertebral disk material is considered to be the source of the fibrocartilage. The fact that this disorder occurs in young adult nonchondrodystrophoid breeds of dogs that are not prone to disk disease at this age is enigmatic. The condition has not been reported in chondrodystrophoid breeds of dogs, which are at high risk of disk disease; however, fibrocartilaginous emboli have been demonstrated recently in pulmonary vessels of chondrodystrophoid breeds of dogs with signs of clinical disk disease.

Pathologically, malacia and necrosis of spinal cord gray and white matter are present. Infarcted areas are usually ischemic but may be hemorrhagic. Neutrophils and phagocytic mononuclear cells are often abundant within the lesions. Onset of signs is typically hyperacute. Clinical signs will reflect location of the lesion within the spinal cord. While any level of the spinal cord may be affected, cervical or lumbar cord segments are commonly involved. If areas of the cord that supply the limb muscles are involved, clinical signs will be characterized by depressed reflexes, reduced muscle tone, and muscle atrophy after 5 to 7 days. If the lumbosacral cord is involved, there may be paralysis and analgesia of the tail, anal sphincter, bladder, and rectum. Affected animals do not typically show evidence of pain.

Plain radiographs are normal. Myelography is usually normal, but if performed early, it may suggest slight cord swelling at or rostral to the level of the lesion. Cerebrospinal fluid analysis may reveal an elevated neutrophil count within a few hours of clinical onset, and protein levels in CSF may be slightly elevated.

Prognosis is guarded and depends on the location and extent of infarction. Animals with extensive gray matter involvement of the cervicothoracic and/or lumbosacral spinal cord have a poor prognosis. Any improvement should be apparent in 10 to 14 days. Residual effects are common. Treatment with dexamethasone (1 to 2 mg/kg body weight, repeated at 6-hour intervals) may be beneficial in reducing cord swelling, but only if given within 24 hours of the onset of signs. The dosage is then reduced to 0.1 mg/kg every 12 hours for 2 to 3 days.

KEY DIAGNOSTIC AIDS: **Clinical Onset, Clinical Signs, Negative Ancillary Tests**

Feline Ischemic Encephalopathy

This is an ischemic necrosis of cerebral tissue that occurs sporadically in adult male and female cats of all ages, especially in summer months (468, 469). Lesions may be unilateral or bilateral and may involve up to 75% of one cerebral hemisphere. The major area of infarction is frequently in the distribution of the middle cerebral artery. Vascular occlusive lesions including thrombosis and vasculitis have been found only occasionally. Affected animals do not have cardiomyopathy.

Clinical signs are nonprogressive and variable but acute in onset. Clinical signs include depression, circling to seizures and change in attitude, often to the point of aggression. Mydriasis and visual impairment may be present. Clinical signs may be modified or disappear with time (several days to weeks). Hematology, skull radiographs, and CSF analysis usually are normal. Abnormal brain trace pattern may be detected with electroencephalography.

Prognosis is usually favorable since many of the signs seen initially will ameliorate; however, behavioral changes and uncontrollable seizures may persist.

KEY DIAGNOSTIC AIDS: **Historical Data, Age, Clinical Signs**

Infectious Canine Hepatitis

Infectious canine hepatitis is an adenovirus (CAV-1) infection that is a highly contagious systemic disease of younger dogs and foxes. The virus is transmitted by direct contact with infected animals (saliva, respiratory secretions, urine, or feces) or by contact with contaminated objects. The virus spreads to local lymph nodes via the oropharynx and is disseminated throughout the body by the hematogenous route (470). It has special predilection for vascular endothelium and liver, kidney, and lymph nodes (471). Signs of encephalitis related to damage of vascular endothelium are rare in the dog; but may include rapidly progressive tetraparesis, coma, seizures, and death. These signs may be accompanied by vomiting, abdominal pain, fever, and jaundice.

Diagnosis is substantiated by demonstration of the virus in blood or biopsy material (e.g., observing characteristic cytopathic effects in dog-kidney cell monolayer cultures), and confirmed by histological examination of tissues. Large intranuclear inclusion bodies are found in hepatic cells.

Treatment is usually futile.

KEY DIAGNOSTIC AIDS: **Age, Clinical Signs, Clinical Course**

Ischemic Neuromyopathy in the Cat

This is a disorder that occurs not infrequently in cats and is associated with cardiomyopathy (472, 473). The cause of the disease and emboli formation in the heart are uncertain. The emboli may be carried to any site within the arterial circulation. The most common site of occlusion is the aortic trifurcation. Thrombi which extend into the iliac arteries are termed "saddle thrombi." Vasoactive substances released from the thrombus may be involved in the pathogenesis (474, 475). Cats of all ages may be affected. There is a predilection for male cats and cats of the Persian breed (476).

Pathologically, changes occur in skeletal muscle and peripheral nerve (477). Lesions in peripheral nerves begin in the midthigh region, with the central fibers in a fascicle being more susceptible than the peripheral. The majority of fibers show changes of wallerian type degeneration, while others have evidence of paranodal/segmental demyelination. In skeletal muscle, ischemic myopathy characterized by focal necrosis, myophagia, internal nuclei hypertrophy, and occasional infiltrates contributes to the clinical signs.

Clinical signs are acute in onset and usually include pelvic limb pain, plantigrade stance, and paraparesis or paralysis. Femoral pulse may be weak or absent, the gastrocnemius muscle is firm and often painful, and the limbs are cool. Distal limb muscles below the stifle are particularly affected. Flexion and extension of both hip and stifle joints and the patellar reflex are usually present. Pain sensation typically is absent in the distal limbs. The nail bed of pelvic limbs is cyanotic.

Electrodiagnostic studies reveal an absence of or a much reduced evoked potential from interosseous and cranial tibial muscles. Nerve conduction velocities may be either normal or reduced (477). Chest radiography may indicate cardiopulmonary disease. Diagnosis of occlusive vascular disease can be confirmed from an aortogram.

Although the collateral circulation does return in the majority of cases with return of function to varying degrees within 6 weeks to 6 months, the long-term prognosis is guarded because of the potential of further thromboembolism. Femoral pulses frequently return within 1 to 2 weeks. At present there are no results which show that any therapy produces a significantly better recovery than no therapy. The effectiveness of embolectomy is uncertain.

KEY DIAGNOSTIC AIDS: **Clinical Onset, Clinical Signs**

Labyrinthitis

Labyrinthitis or otitis interna refers to an inflammation of the inner ear resulting in dysfunction of the membranous labyrinth. This disorder is usually associated with otitis media, which, in turn, is most commonly associated with otitis externa (478). The nasopharynx is also a source of retrograde infection by way of the eustachian tubes. A third source of infection of the middle-inner ear structures is hematogenous spread. Extension of infection from middle-inner ear areas to the meninges is a potential untoward sequela and occurs more often in cats.

Most infections are caused by bacteria, including staphylococci, α-streptococcus, *Proteus* species, *Pseudomonas* species, and *Escherichia coli*. Foreign bodies, such as grass awns, may initiate inflammation and predispose to secondary microbial infection. Animals predisposed to chronic otitis externa and chronic ear mite infestations would appear to have an increased risk of developing otitis media-interna; however, in a recent survey, no breed was disproportionately represented, compared to the hospital population examined (478).

Varying degrees of vestibular disturbance will reflect labyrinthine disease. Signs may range from head tilt, nystagmus (frequently rotatory), and ataxia to torticollis, circling, falling, and rolling. Attendant middle ear inflammation may disturb function of the facial and sympathetic nerves that course through the middle ear, resulting in facial paresis/paralysis and Horner's syndrome, respectively. Hemifacial spasms have been reported in dogs with otitis media (479). Signs, probably due to facial nerve irritation, are characterized by blepharospasm, elevation of the ear, and deviation of the nose—all on the same side as the otitis media. Similar signs have been reported in a dog without otitis media but with a brainstem lesion in the area of the facial nucleus (480). Another structure commonly involved in labyrinthitis is the cochlear nerve, dysfunction of which results in deafness. Occasionally, labyrinthitis is bilateral. In the event the infection spreads to the brain, signs of meningitis, pyrexia, depression, brainstem involvement, and seizures may be observed.

The diagnosis of labyrinthitis is suggested by clinical signs and confirmed by otoscopic examination and skull radiography (481). Otoscopy may reveal an otitis externa and evidence of erosion, rupture, or bulging of the tympanic membrane. Fluid in the middle ear produces bulging of the tympanic membrane, which may appear opaque and hyperemic. Fluid and/or inflammatory exudate should be cultivated from the external and middle ear by aspiration if the tympanic membrane has ruptured, or by myringotomy (surgical incision of the typanic membrane). Radiographic examination of the petrous temporal bones using ventrodorsal, lateral-oblique, and open mouth projections may reveal middle ear inflammation as suggested by fluid density, osteitis, sclerosis, or erosion of the bulla. Normal detail of the bony labyrinth may be lost.

Prognosis is usually favorable with prolonged oral and topical antibiotics chosen from positive culture and sensitivity studies. In more chronic cases, surgical debridement and drainage of the middle ear may be required. In some animals neurological signs may persist or recur.

KEY DIAGNOSTIC AIDS: **Clinical Signs, Otoscopy, Skull Radiography**

Laryngeal Paralysis

Spontaneous laryngeal paralysis has been reported sporadically in dogs and is rare in cats. A hereditary form (autosomal dominant) has been documented in Siberian huskies and Bouvier des Flandres either as unilateral or bilateral disease (482–484). About 74% of affected Bouvier des Flandres are males. The acquired disease has been reported mostly in middle-aged and old large and giant breed dogs, such as St. Bernard, Chesapeake Bay retriever, and irish setter (485), but medium and small/toy breeds also may be affected. Male dogs, particularly if castrated, were more frequently affected than females in a recently reported survey (486). Of the four reported cases of laryngeal paralysis in cats, all have been male and three had been castrated (487, 488).

The etiology of laryngeal paralysis is unknown. The motor innervation to the muscles of the larynx is derived largely from branches of the recurrent laryngeal nerves, dysfunction of which results in impaired abduction of the dorsal crico-arytenoid muscle and, hence, the vocal cords. Histological evidence of neurogenic atrophy is found in intrinsic laryngeal muscles. Axonal degeneration, with increase in endoneurial connective tissue and the number of Schwann cells, is present in right and left recurrent laryngeal nerves. Changes occur along the entire length of these nerves, suggesting that the primary lesion is in the neurons of origin. Degenerative changes have been documented in the nucleus ambiguus in Bouvier des Flandres. Degenerative changes also have been described occasionally in vagus and sciatic nerve, raising the question of associated neuromuscular disease (e.g., hypothyroidism) in some dogs with laryngeal paralysis.

Onset of clinical signs in the hereditary form in dogs is from 4 to 6 months of age. The acquired form may develop in animals from 1.5 to 13 years of age. Clinical signs reflect respiratory (inspiratory) distress and are characterized by increasing loss of endurance, increasing laryngeal stridor, voice changes, absence of purring, dyspnea, cyanosis (during episodes of severe dyspnea) and collapse with complete airway obstruction. Clinical signs are usually of several months' duration. Pelvic limb weakness and "foot drop" associated with bilateral cranial tibial muscle denervation have also been observed in dogs with hereditary and acquired forms of laryngeal paralysis.

Diagnosis of larnygeal abductor dysfunction is made by laryngoscopy. Recurrent laryngeal paralysis is confirmed by detection of denervation potentials in individual intrinsic laryngeal muscles using electromyography, and by evidence of neurogenic atrophy in biopsy specimens of the cricoarytenoid muscle.

Prognosis is usually favorable with surgical management, such as arytenoidectomy and vocal fold removal, arytenoid lateralization, and castellated laryngofissure in acquired paralysis, but it has been variable in hereditary paralysis (489, 490). Prevention of the inherited form by breeding control is indicated; however, it has been reported that clinically silent carriers can transmit hereditary laryngeal paralysis in Huskie crosses (491).

KEY DIAGNOSTIC AIDS: **Breed, Age, Clinical Signs, Laryngoscopy**

Lead Poisoning

Accidental lead poisoning is one of the more common intoxications of dogs and cats (492–497). It may occur from many sources, including linoleum, putty, roofing felt, golf balls, and old car batteries; however, lead-based paints are the most frequent source of poisoning. Lead is believed to inhibit sulfhydryl groups of essential enzymes of cellular metabolism. One important consequence of this is inhibition of heme synthesis. Lead can disrupt the blood-brain barrier by damaging capillary endothelial cells with resultant cerebral edema and hemorrhage. In the brain, histological changes range from diffuse capillary proliferation to status spongiosus and cerebral cortical necrosis (498). Peripheral neuropathy may occur sporadically with spontaneous lead poisoning.

Lead poisoning is more commonly reported in dogs than in cats. Affected animals usually are less than 1 year of age. The incidence is reportedly higher in summer and early fall. Clinical signs of central nervous system dysfunction usually are preceded or accompanied by gastrointestinal malfunction. Signs may be acute or chronic. The most common gastrointestinal signs are vomiting, abdominal pain, and anorexia. Common neurological signs include seizures, hysteria (barking and/or whining continuously, aimless running, and snapping at objects), ataxia, blindness, and jaw champing.

Diagnosis is suggested by finding numerous nucleated erythrocytes in a stained blood smear. The presence of basophilic stippling in red blood cells, elevated urinary levels of aminolevulinic acid, presence of diffuse radiopaque material in the gastrointestinal tract, and radiopaque bands in long bone metaphyses of young dogs also support the diagnosis. Levels of 60 μg or more of lead/100 ml of whole blood are considered definitively diagnostic of lead poisoning (496). There is no direct correlation between severity of clinical signs and blood level content.

Treatment with the chelating agent calcium ethylenediaminetetraacetic acid (EDTA) using a dose of 25 mg/kg intravenously four times a day for 2 to 5 days, often results in rapid recovery within 36 to 48 hours. Alternatively, oral penicillamine may be given in a dose of 100 mg/kg daily for 1 to 2 weeks. Treatment is repeated over another 5-day period if signs persist.

The prognosis is favorable in the majority of lead poisoning cases treated with chelating agents.

KEY DIAGNOSTIC AIDS: **Historical Data, Clinical Signs, Blood Lead Levels**

Leukoencephalomyelopathy of Rottweiler Dogs

A degenerative disorder of the spinal cord and lower brainstem has been reported recently in two rottweiler dogs (499). A 3-year-old female and a 4-year-old male had a slowly progressive course for 7 to 9 months. Demyelinating lesions were found in the brainstem, deep cerebellar white matter, and spinal cord. Axons are preserved. Lesions tended to be bilaterally symmetrical. The cause and pathogenesis are unknown. Clinical signs included ataxia, tetraparesis, dysmetria, delayed proprioceptive positioning, and exaggerated spinal reflexes. All diagnostic studies—including CSF analysis, electromyography, plain radiography, and myelography—were normal. One dog was treated with corticosteroids for 2 months without improvement. The clinical and pathological course and treatment remain to be evaluated.

KEY DIAGNOSTIC AIDS: **Breed, Age, Clinical Signs**

Lissencephaly

This rare defect is characterized by a small, smooth-appearing brain with few or no gyri present and derangement of cells of the cerebral cortex. It results from disturbance of neuronal migration and proliferation during development. This anomaly has been reported in Lhasa apso dogs (500, 501), wirehaired fox terriers, Irish setters (49), and in a cat associated with cerebellar hypoplasia (58).

Clinical signs usually are detected in the first year of life and are characterized by erratic behavior patterns (episodes of aggressivness, growling at imaginary objects, confusion, hyperactivity), visual deficits, and seizures. Apart from abnormal wave tracings detected electroencephalographically, results of all other ancillary aids are normal.

Prognosis is guarded. Treatment is symptomatic. Seizures may be controlled with anticonvulsant therapy.

KEY DIAGNOSTIC AIDS: **Breed, Age, Clinical Signs, Negative Laboratory Tests**

Lumbosacral Stenosis

Stenosis or narrowing of the vertebral canal or intervertebral foramina or both (synonyms are "cauda equina syndrome," "spondylolisthesis," and "lumbosacral malarticulation and malformation") in the lumbosacral area with compression of the lumbosacral cord segments or nerve roots that form the cauda equina is an entity recently reported in dogs (502–504) and also in a cat (504a). Acquired or degenerative stenosis may develop in association with tumors or infectious processes, intervertebral disk prolapse, degenerative spondylosis deformans, or vertebral luxation (502, 504, 505–507). Thickened lamina, pedicles, facets, and ligaments often accompany acquired lumbar stenosis. A form of congenital ("idiopathic") stenosis in dogs has been reported and is characterized by shortening of the pedicles, thickened and sclerotic apposition of the lamina and articular processes, infolding and hypertrophy of the ligamentum flavum, and sclerotic and bulbous articular facets that bulge into the dorsal half of the canal. Lumbosacral instability is considered to be a factor in lumbosacral stenosis, leading to chronic inflammatory changes in soft tissues and bony structures.

Large breed dogs, the German shepherd in particular, were most commonly affected in one study of dogs with acquired stenosis. Smaller breed dogs were more often affected with the congenital form. In both forms, clinical signs are noted usually in mature to middle-aged dogs.

Irrespective of etiology, dogs with lumbosacral vertebral stenosis usually manifest a syndrome complex that reflects varying degrees of cauda equina involvement depending on the level and extent of the lesion. Commonly reported clinical signs include pain on palpation of the lumbosacral area, difficulty rising, slight pelvic limb paresis or lameness in one pelvic limb, tail paresis, hypotonia of anal sphincter with fecal incontinence, and urinary incontinence. In some animals self-mutilation of pelvic limbs, tail, perineum, anal area, and genitalia may be noted.

Radiographic findings may include spondylosis and/or subluxation of L7-S1 vertebrae and stenosis of the vertebral canal. In some dogs, there may be evidence of degenerative disk disease, tumor, or infection, such as diskospondylitis. Myelographic studies may not provide useful information because of the lumbosacral location of the lesion. Electromyographic studies can demonstrate fibrillation potentials in lumbosacral paraspinal muscles, pelvic limbs, coccygeal muscles, and anal sphincter. In those cases where results of ancillary aids are equivocal, exploratory dorsal laminectomy may be the only means available for diagnosis and treatment.

Prognosis is usually favorable with surgical decompression alone for congenital stenosis, and in combination with mass removal or vertebral stabilization for acquired stenosis. Medical treatment has usually been ineffective.

KEY DIAGNOSTIC AIDS: **Age, Clinical Signs, Radiography, Exploratory Dorsal Laminectomy**

Malignant Hyperthermia

Malignant hyperthermia is characterized by peracute development of hypercatabolism and contracture in skeletal muscle. The pathogenesis of this disorder is believed to be associated with abnormal regulation of myoplasmic calcium leading to overstimulation of glycogenolysis and contractile protein activity. This, in turn, results in depletion of glycogen stores, hypoxia, and accumulation of heat, CO_2, and lactic acid.

In man and swine, malignant hyperthermia may develop in response to certain inhalation anesthesia and quarternary amide muscle relaxants or to severe psychological stress. Anesthesia-induced malignant hyperthermia has been reported sporadically in dogs (508–512) and in a cat (513). More recently, a colony of malignant hyperthermia-susceptible dogs has been reported (514). The disorder has been reported in various breeds: greyhound, St. Bernard, border collie, pointers, spaniels, and crossbred animals with Doberman pinscher, German shepherd, and hound features. There is no apparent sex predisposition. The disease is considered to be inherited, possibly with a polygenic mode of transmission. Dogs susceptible to malignant hyperthermia may be nervous and difficult to handle. Their muscles may be hypertrophic with greater than normal muscle tone and strength. Resting body temperature may be high-normal or slightly above, and serum creatine kinase and aspartate transaminase may be mildly elevated. There is recent evidence that stress alone may induce malignant hyperthermia in dogs (515, 516).

In dogs, malignant hyperthermia is most commonly induced using halothane anesthesia. It should be noted that this disorder does not always occur during the first exposure to halothane anesthesia. Clinical signs can include hyperthermia, tachycardia, tachypnea, severe limb rigidity, and trismus, followed by respiratory and cardiac arrest. In some animals, extreme trismus and generalized muscle rigidity occur immediately after death.

Histopathological features in skeletal muscle include fiber size variation, fiber hypertrophy, and increased numbers of internal nuclei in muscle cells.

Halothane, succinylcholine, and enflurane have been implicated as triggers of malignant hyperthermia in the dog. To date, methoxyflurane has not been reported as an inducer of this syndrome in dogs.

Diagnosis of fulminating malignant hyperthermia can be suggested by historical data relating to breed or colony susceptibility, and by development of characteristic clinical signs while under anesthesia. Signs may occur after 30 to 300 minutes of halothane exposure.

Prognosis is guarded. Removal of triggering agents and symptomatic treatment (total body cooling, corticosteroids, sodium bicarbonate, intravenous fluids) usually are ineffectual in reversing malignant hyperthermia episodes. Administration of dantrolene is usually necessary for survival (517). A recommended dosage is 5 mg/kg intravenously (518).

In instances where malignant hyperthermia is suspected, susceptible animals can safely undergo anesthesia if triggering agents are avoided. An in vitro caffeine contracture screening test is now available in some institutions for detecting malignant hyperthermia-susceptible animals. Another potential screening test is erythrocyte osmotic fragility (519).

KEY DIAGNOSTIC AIDS: **Historical Data, Breed, Clinical Signs, Caffeine Contracture Test**

Mannosidosis

Mannosidosis is a lysosomal storage disease resulting from a deficiency of the enzyme acidic α-D-mannosidase in various organs, including brain, kidney, and liver. As a consequence of this enzyme deficiency, there is accumulation of mannose-rich material in the tissues and excretion in the urine of mannose-rich oligosaccharides (520, 521). This rare disease has been reported in a 7-month-old domestic shorthaired cat presenting with multiple skeletal anomalies, diminutive size, and neurological disturbances characterized by progressive generalized ataxia and intention tremors. More recently, a hereditary form of mannosidosis has been reported in Persian kittens in which similar neurological signs, but no skeletal abnormalities, appeared at 2 months of age (522). Microscopic lesions are characterized by extensive vacuolation of lymphocytes, visceral organs, and neurons and glial cells of the nervous system. Poor myelination of the cerebral white matter and axonal spheroid formation in cerebral and cerebellar white matter have been observed in 2- and 3-month-old Persian kittens. Diagnosis is based on demonstrating a deficiency of acidic α-D-mannosidase in brain, liver, or kidney or the detection of mannose-rich oligosaccharides in urine.

Prognosis is poor. There is no treatment.

KEY DIAGNOSTIC AIDS: **Age, Clinical Signs, Clinical Course, Enzyme Assays, Urinalysis**

Masticatory Myositis

This inflammatory myopathy (synonym "eosinophilic myositis") is one of the most commonly recognized myositides in dogs and is observed most commonly in adult German shepherd dogs (523, 523a). This disease is characterized by recurrent inflammation of muscles, especially those of mastication (masseteric, temporalis, and pterygoid muscles), often in association with peripheral blood eosinophilia and the presence of eosinophils in muscle lesions. The etiopathogenesis is unknown. The suggestion that it represents an autoimmune disease remains unconfirmed.

Lesions consist of myonecrosis, hemorrhage, edema, and cellular infiltrates (macrophages, lymphocytes, plasma cells, occasionally neutrophils, and sometimes eosinophils). Clinical signs are characterized by acute onset of painful, swollen masticatory muscles. The jaw is held partially open ("pseudotrismus"), and passive manipulation is painful. Dogs are often febrile, and tonsils and mandibular lymph nodes may be swollen. The acute phase may last 2 to 3 weeks, with signs reaching a peak by 10 to 14 days. Serum creatine phosphokinase (CPK) levels are elevated early in the disease, and γ-globulin levels may be increased.

Diagnosis is based on signalment, clinical, and muscle biopsy data. Prognosis is guarded. The acute disease is usually responsive to glucocorticosteroids, e.g., prednisone 0.5 to 1.0 mg/kg orally twice a day. The dose is reduced after remission and gradually withdrawn using alternate-day therapy. Repeated clinical episodes are not uncommon, resulting in muscle atrophy.

KEY DIAGNOSTIC AIDS: **Age, Breed, Clinical Signs, Muscle Biopsy**

Meningitis

In contrast with domestic large animals, meningitis is not a common disease of the dog and cat. Bacterial invasion of the CNS usually results in both encephalomyelitis and meningitis. Bacterial infections of the CNS occur via hematogenous spread from distant foci within the body, by direct extension from sinuses, ears, and eyes, as a result of trauma (e.g., bite wound), or from contaminated surgical instruments (e.g., spinal needle). Organisms usually disseminate via CSF pathways and produce cerebrospinal meningitis, often associated with microabscess formation of brain and spinal cord. One important source of bacterial infection of meninges and CNS parenchyma in dogs is bacterial endocarditis.

Bacteria are probably the most common cause of purulent meningitis. Organisms that have been cultured from dogs with bacterial meningitis include *Pasteurella* sp., *Pasteurella multocida*, *Staphylococcus aureus*, *Staphylococcus epidermidis*, *Staphylococcus albus*, *Actinomyces* sp., and *Nocardia* sp.

Pathological changes that are characteristic of bacterial meningitis include diffuse infiltration of inflammatory cells into the leptomeninges by both polymorphonuclear and mononuclear cells. Frequently, inflammation is found throughout the entire subarachnoid space of the brain and spinal cord. Vasculitis is often pronounced. Bacterial invasion of CNS parenchyma is characterized by mononuclear and polymorphonuclear inflammatory infiltration and large perivascular cuffing. Necrosis of gray and white matter may be observed with infiltrations of macrophages, neutrophils, and plasma cells. Irrespective of the etiological agent, bacterial meningitis usually is acute in onset and tends to be characterized by a group of clinical signs that include hyperesthesia, pyrexia, and cervical rigidity. Pyrexia is believed to be secondary to bacterial invasion of the blood stream and cerebrospinal fluid, accompanied by the release of leukocytic pyrogen and hypothalamic stimulation. In humans, inflammation of the subarachnoid space activates protective reflexes, resulting in nuchal rigidity and hyperextension of the neck and vertebral column. A similar mechanism probably exists in the dog and serves as an explanation of the signs of cervical rigidity and the occasionally seen opisthotonus with thoracic limb hyperextension. In addition, emesis, anorexia, occasional cranial nerve deficits, and seizures may be observed (193, 481, 524–526).

The clinical diagnosis of bacterial meningitis is supported by the finding of highly pleocytic cerebrospinal fluid (500 to 1000 or more white blood cells/mm^3) with a high proportion of polymorphonuclear cells. The protein content of the cerebrospinal fluid is usually increased as well (100 to 1000+ mg/dl). Low CSF glucose, relative to plasma glucose values, is typical. Electroencephalographic traces may demonstrate high voltage (30 to 70 μV), fast (20 to 35 Hz) or slow (5 to 10 Hz) wave activity. Definitive diagnosis is made by bacterial culture of CSF. Blood cultures may incriminate a pathogenic organism when CSF cultures are negative. Rickettsial infections (Rocky Mountain spotted fever or ehrlichia) should be considered in dogs with evidence of meningitis and negative cultures (rickettsial meningoencephalitis). Also, parasitic migration through the CNS can result in aseptic, suppurative meningitis. Trypanosomiasis occasionally may involve the central nervous system, producing a severe chronic meningoencephalitis in dogs (527).

Prognosis is guarded. Appropriate use of antibiotics, according to the culture results, is basic to successful therapy of bacterial meningitis (encephalomyelitis). Chloramphenicol has the highest penetrability of the central nervous system, followed by sulfonamides and trimethoprim. Ampicillin and penicillin enter the nervous system only with meningeal irritation. Aminoglycosides and cephalosporins reportedly do not adequately penetrate the CNS, even when inflammation exists (528). Intrathecal administration of antibiotics should only be considered in refractory cases. Glucocorticoids, in general, are contraindicated in the treatment of bacterial or fungal meningitis; however, a suppurative meningitis of unknown etiology has been observed in some dogs with clinical and laboratory evidence of bacterial meningitis (encephalomyelitis), and in whom abatement of signs occurs only following glucocorticoid therapy (81, 529). An immunological pathogenesis is suspected.

KEY DIAGNOSTIC AIDS: Historical Data, Clinical Signs, Cerebrospinal Fluid Analysis, Culture of Blood/CSF

Meningitis and Vasculitis

A severe form of meningitis and polyarteritis has been reported in beagles (530, 531). Lesions are characterized by periarteritis involving vessels in the meninges and heart. Partial and complete vessel occlusion may be present. There is extensive perivascular and leptomeningeal infiltration by mainly mononuclear cells, some of which contain IgG. Amyloidosis and lymphocytic thyroiditis are present in some dogs.

Affected animals usually are 4 to 6 months old. The first sign is altered gait and posture. The head, neck, and spine are held in a straight line, sometimes with the nose elevated and sometimes with it directed toward the ground. Pain is seldom elicited on manipulation of the head and neck. Affected animals have a recurring fever. Hematological studies typically reveal a neutrophilic pleocytosis (in some dogs as high as 10,000 cells/mm^3).

An autoimmune disorder has been proposed for this disorder. The prognosis is guarded due to the recurrences. Chloramphenicol, corticosteroids, and aspirin can produce temporary improvement.

A similar form of necrotizing vasculitis has been observed in a 10-month-old boxer dog and in a 4-month-old Labrador retriever (532).

KEY DIAGNOSTIC AIDS: Breed, Age, Clinical Signs, CSF Analysis

Mucopolysaccharidosis

The mucopolysaccharidoses are a group of generic lysosomal diseases that result from deficits in the metabolism of glycosaminoglycans which accumulate in various connective tissues and/or are excessively excreted in urine. There are two mucopolysaccharidoses described in cats, both considered to be recessively inherited. Mucopolysaccharidosis I (synonym is "Hurler's syndrome"), caused by a deficiency of α-L-iduronidase, has been reported in a 10-month-old domestic shorthaired cat (533). This cat was presented because of progressive lameness, a broad face with depressed nasal bridge, small ears, corneal clouding, and multiple bone dysplasia, including fusion of vertebrae over the cervicothoracic junction, pectus excavatum, and bilateral coxofemoral subluxation. The cat excreted excessive amounts of glycosaminoglycans in its urine, and glycosaminoglycan storage was evident in fibroblasts and neurons. Gross postmortem fndings included hepatosplenomegaly. Swollen, vacuolated neurons may be seen in the central nervous system. Activity of α-L-iduronidase was deficient in cultured fibroblasts and leukocytes.

Mucopolysaccharidosis VI (synonym is "Maroteaux-Lamy syndrome") has been reported in 2- to 3-month-old Siamese cats (534, 535). This disorder is caused by a deficiency of the enzyme arylsulfatase B. The clinical features of affected animals are almost identical to cats with mucopolysaccharidosis I; however, Siamese cats have toluidine blue-positive granules in circulating neutrophils. It has been estimated that approximately 25% of cats 4 to 7 months of age with mucopolysaccharidosis VI develop clinical signs of thoracolumbar spinal cord dysfunction secondary to cord compression from focal bony protrusions into the vertebral canal (536). Clinical signs are characterized by varying degrees of pelvic limb paresis that may progress to paraplegia, incontinence, and depressed pain sensation caudal to the level of the thoracolumbar lesion. Seizures have been reported in an affected 2-year-old Siamese cat (537).

Leukocyte assay of arylsulfatase B activity is the diagnostic method of choice. Enzyme activity is less than 10% of normal in affected homozygotic cats; it is 50% lower than normal in asymptomatic obligate heterozygote cats.

Prognosis can be favorable with surgical decompression early in the course of the disease; however, the long-term prognosis for cats with mucopolysaccharidosis I or VI remains to be determined.

KEY DIAGNOSTIC AIDS: **Breed, Age, Clinical Signs, Leukocyte Enzyme Assays**

Multiple Cartilaginous Exostosis

Multiple cartilaginous exostosis (MCE) is a benign proliferative disease of cartilage and bone (538, 539). Any bone may be affected that is formed by enchondral ossification; however, vertebrae, ribs, and long bones are the most frequent location of exostoses. The condition has been reported in dogs and cats. There is no apparent sex or breed predisposition, although a familial tendency is probable. The condition is related to abnormal differentiation of cartilage cells that give rise to exostoses.

Neurological signs in animals relate to spinal cord compression secondary to vertebral exostosis, which are most common in thoracic and lumbar regions. Signs progress from pelvic limb paresis to paraplegia. Onset of neurological signs typically occurs prior to 1 year of age. Diagnosis is based on radiography and/or myelography, and microscopic examination of a biopsy specimen. Surgical excision is necessary in animals with evidence of progressive spinal cord compression. Prognosis is guarded.

KEY DIAGNOSTIC AIDS: **Age, Clinical Signs, Radiography**

Mutilating Neuropathy

This rare disease, believed to be inherited, has been reported recently in English pointer dogs (540, 541).

Pathologically, changes affecting the primary sensory neurons are observed, including small spinal ganglia with reduced numbers of cell bodies, degeneration of unmyelinated and myelinated fibers in the dorsal roots and peripheral nerves, and reduced fiber density in the dorsolateral fasciculus of the spinal cord.

The pathogenesis of this disease is presently unclear; however, a deficiency in growth and/or differentiation of primary sensory neurons may be involved. Fiber degeneration may progress slowly with age to include sensory systems not affected in early postnatal life. The loss of primary sensory neurons is associated with a notable reduction in staining of substance P, an excitatory agent that mediates nociception (i.e., pain sensation) (542).

Clinical signs are characterized by nociceptive loss and acral mutilation. This nociceptive loss is more apparent in distal parts of limbs, so that acral analgesia is replaced by hypalgesia proximal to the carpus and tarsus. No nociceptive loss is detected about the face. Although blunting of digital pain has been detected prior to weaning, clinical signs usually become apparent at 3 to 8 months when affected dogs suddenly begin to lick and bite their paws. Acral changes include swollen reddened paws, ulcerations, lacerations, paronychia, painless fractures, and autoamputations.

There is no evidence of proprioceptive loss, ataxia, or depressed tendon reflexes. Electromyographic studies and sensory and motor nerve conduction studies are normal.

Diagnosis is based on signalment, clinical, and normal electrophysiological data. Pathological evaluation of nerve or spinal ganglia biopsy samples may support the clinical diagnosis.

Prognosis is poor because of high potential for osteomyelitis secondary to autoamputation. There is no treatment for the underlying sensory neuropathy.

An apparently similar, recessively inherited entity has been reported in shorthaired pointer dogs and has been called "toe necrosis," "hereditary neurotrophic osteopathy," and "ulceromutilating acropathy" (543–545).

KEY DIAGNOSTIC AIDS: **Breed, Age, Clinical Signs**

Myasthenia Gravis

In animals, two forms of myasthenia gravis (MG) occur—an acquired and a congenital form. Acquired MG is an uncommon disorder characterized by failure of neuromuscular transmission that has been frequently observed in large breeds of dogs, especially German shepherds, with an average age of onset of 5 years (247, 546, 547). The condition has also been reported in cats (548, 549). There is no sex predominance. Acquired canine MG is an immune-mediated disease caused by production of antibodies directed against acetylcholine receptors of the neuromuscular junction. Reactive antibodies are demonstrable in the sera of 90% of dogs with acquired MG (550), and immune complexes have been localized at the neuromuscular junction (NMJ) (550a, 551). A deficiency of functional acetylcholine receptors at the NMJ reduces the sensitivity of the postsynaptic membrane to the transmitter, acetylcholine.

Acquired MG in dogs has also been seen in association with mediastinal tumors, such as thymomas (247, 552), and antibodies reactive with muscle striations may coexist with a high titer of autoantibodies to acetylcholine receptor.

Clinical signs are characterized by excessive muscular weakness and reduced tolerance to exercise. The thoracic limbs are predominantly affected, and the stride becomes progressively shorter. Facial features may droop. The animal may have difficulty in closing its mouth and holding up its head, and the bark may have a high pitch. Dysphagia and regurgitation are common. Most affected dogs have intrathoracic megaesophagus which can be detected by radiography. Clinical signs are exacerbated by exposure to cold.

Diagnosis is based on clinical signs, electrodiagnostic evidence of decremental response of muscle action potentials after repeated nerve stimulation, serological testing for autoantibodies, and amelioration of signs following administration of the short-acting anticholinesterase edrophonium (Tensilon), using a dosage of 0.1 to 1.0 mg intravenously, depending on the size of the animal. An animal that has been previously recumbent can be restored immediately to normal activity, which will last for a few minutes before muscle weakness gradually recurs.

Prognosis is guarded. One potential complication is inhalation pneumonia. Long-acting anticholinesterase drugs, such as pyridostigmine (Mestinon), may result in clinical control. Dosages range from 30 to 60 mg orally, two or three times a day. Dosage depends on the severity of signs and on the size of the dog. In smaller breeds, such as the Jack Russell terrier, a dose of 7.5 mg of Mestinon is adequate. Overdosage will produce a cholinergic crisis with signs similar to those of undertreatment. Some dogs may recover spontaneously while others become refractory to anticholinesterase therapy after a period of successful treatment. In such instances, administration of corticosteroids (e.g., 2 mg/kg of prednisolone every second day) in conjunction with the anticholinesterase therapy may be beneficial in some dogs (553, 554).

Congenital MG occurs in young dogs, usually appearing between the ages of 6 and 9 weeks, with multiple cases in a single litter. Congenital MG has been described in three breeds: Jack Russell terrier (555), springer spaniel (556), and smooth fox terrier (557, 558). Breeding studies suggest that congenital myasthenia gravis is inherited as an autosomal recessive trait.

The physiological basis of congenital MG is the same as that of acquired MG; however anti-acetylcholine receptor antibodies are not demonstrable in serum or muscle in congenital MG. There appears to be an absolute deficiency of acetylcholine receptors in the postsynaptic membrane.

With the exception that pelvic limbs show weakness before the thoracic limbs and megaesophagus is uncommon, clinical signs, electrophysiological findings, and prognosis of animals with congenital MG are similar to those described for acquired MG. Diagnosis is based on response to Tensilon, using a dosage of 0.1 to 0.5 mg intravenously. Mestinon is used for treatment at a dosage of 7.5 to 30 mg orally once daily. Clinical response to this drug is often erratic.

KEY DIAGNOSTIC AIDS: Breed, Age, Clinical Signs, Tensilon Response Test

Mycotic Diseases of the CNS

Mycotic agents sporadically produce a granulomatous meningoencephalomyelitis in dogs and cats. The more common mycotic infections of the CNS are caused by *Cryptococcus neoformans*, *Blastomyces dermatitidis*, *Histoplasma capsulatum*, and *Coccidioides immitis* (559–568). Each agent has a particular geographic distribution in the United States (Table 3.1). The pathogenesis is similar for blastomycosis, histoplasmosis, and coccidioidomycosis. The organism is present in the soil, producing mycelia and airborne spores. The coccidia of spores are probably inhaled, deposited in the alveoli, phagocytized, and converted into the spherical parasitic, budding yeast form. This form is disseminated via lymphatics producing local hilar lymphadenopathy, and there is hematogenous spread to other organs. The fate of the infected host is believed to be dependent upon time and ability to develop cellular immunity to fungal antigens.

Unlike other mycotic diseases, *C. neoformans* exists only in the yeast form and has a worldwide distribution. Endemic areas have not been identified. Crypto-

Table 3.1. Mycotic Diseases of the Central Nervous System

Disease	Etiology	Regional Distribution	CNS Involvement	Predilection Sites	Clinical Signs
Cryptococcosis	*Cryptococcus neoformans*	Throughout US	Fairly common	Respiratory tract, brain	Mucopurulent, watery/hemorrhagic, chronic nasal discharge; firm swelling over bridge of nose. Peripheral lymphadenopathy; multiple skin lesions of head (ulcerated/draining). Depression, circling ataxia, posterior paresis, anisocoria, seizures, blindness, anosmia.
Blatomycosis	*Blastomyces dermatitidis*	Eastern seaboard of US	Uncommon	Lungs, lymph nodes, eyes, skin, bone, brain	Weight loss, emaciation, dyspnea, harsh bronchial sounds, fever, lymphadenopathy, ulcerated/draining skin lesions, epiphora, ocular redness and pain, corneal/lenticular opacification, blindness, lameness. Variable (usually multifocal) neurological signs (refer to Cryptococcosis).
Histoplasmosis	*Histoplasma capsulatum*	Eastern seaboard of US	Uncommon	Reticuloendothelial cells in liver, spleen, bone marrow, and lymph nodes	Coughing, dyspnea, hepatomegaly, splenomegaly, anemia, ocular lesions, ulcerated/draining skin nodules. Variable (usually multifocal) neurological signs (refer to Cryptococcosis).
Coccidioidomycosis	*Coccidioides immitis*	Southwestern US	Uncommon	Lungs, lymph nodes, bone	Fever, cough, malaise, depression, peripheral lymphadenopathy/abscessation, lameness. Variable (usually multifocal) neurological signs (refer to Cryptococcosis).

coccosis frequently causes disease usually in mature dogs and cats that are immunodepressed (569). Cats contract the disease more frequently than dogs (570). The natural route of infection is generally believed to be the respiratory tract, with subsequent hematogenous and lymphogenous dissemination to other areas of the body. Approximately 5% of cats with cryptococcosis have concurrent feline leukemia infection.

As with bacteria, mycotic infections also may reach brain and spinal cord by direct spread from an adjacent infection, e.g., from the nasal chambers, tooth alveolus and sinuses, outer ear, eustachian tube, middle/inner ear, petrous temporal bone, and basilar bone.

While the incidence of CNS involvement by mycotic diseases is low, *C. neoformans* may be more likely to be incriminated than the other organisms. A striking feature of mycotic lesions, particularly in the CNS, is the relative lack of a tissue response on the part of the host. Neurological signs will vary according to lesion location and severity. The signs may reflect either a focal mass lesion or a diffuse multifocal disease process. Variable neurological signs may include seizures, depression, disorientation, circling, ataxia, falling, pelvic limb paresis, paraplegia, anisocoria, pupillary dilatation, and blindness.

Diagnosis of mycotic infection is based on demonstration of the organisms in tissue sections or in material taken from aspirates or impression smears, culture, and serology. Commercial kits for intradermal skin testing or for fluorescent antibody testing are not available for cats or dogs. *Histoplasma* organisms may be found in neutrophils or monocytes of buffy coat or bone marrow smears.

Organisms may be observed in CSF which usually will be pleocytic (increase in numbers of mononuclear and polymorphonuclear cells) and will have elevated protein levels. Eosinophils may be present with cryptococcosis.

Prognosis of mycotic infection is always guarded, especially in the disseminated form. Most of the organisms are sensitive to treatment with amphotericin B, e.g., using a dosage of 0.3 mg/kg body weight intravenously three times weekly. The treatment of choice for cryptococcosis is amphotericin B and flucytosine (571). A recommended dosage for flucytosine is 100 mg/kg body weight, divided into four equal doses daily. For the management of coccidioidal meningitis, intrathecal administration of amphotericin is recommended.

Other mycotic agents have been reported to produce CNS infection sporadically. These include *Cladosporidium trichoides*—brain abscessation (572–574); *Paecilomycosis*—brain abscess/granulomas, diskospondylitis (575–577); *Flavobacterium meningosepticum*—meningitis (578); *Geotrichum candidum*—cerebral granulomas, choriomeningitis (579); and *Aspergillus* sp.—cerebral granulomas (580).

KEY DIAGNOSTIC AIDS: **Clincal Signs, CSF Analysis, Hematology, Impression Smears**

Myotonic Myopathy

"Myotonia" refers to a state in which active contraction of a muscle persists after cessation of voluntary effort or stimulation. This condition is characterized by muscle spasm (stiffness) and by temporary inability to initiate movement. Congenital and acquired forms of myotonia have been reported in dogs.

Congenital myotonic myopathy occurs in several breeds, including chow chows, Staffordshire terriers, Irish terriers, and golden retrievers (243, 581–587).

A severe myotonic myopathy affecting almost all skeletal muscles occurs in immature chow chow and Staffordshire terrier puppies, often soon after they become ambulatory. An autosomal recessive inheritance is suspected for this disease in chow chows. The pathogenesis of this disorder may be associated with a decrease in resting chloride conductance of the muscle membrane, similar to myotonia congenita in man. The possibility of a multisystem membrane defect associated with low serum cholesterol has also been considered.

Myopathic changes are mild and consist of occasional angular atrophic fibers, internal nuclei, and marked size variation of type I and type II fibers. A relative increase in number of type II fibers has been reported.

Clinical signs are characterized by stiffness in the first movements after a period of rest, splaying of thoracic limbs, "bunny hopping" pelvic limb gait, and occasional falling over and remaining rigid in lateral recumbency for up to 30 seconds. Some affected dogs may manifest respiratory difficulty from impaired abduction of vocal cords, and regurgitation of food. Stiffness and weakness largely disappear with exercise. Proximal limb and neck muscles and tongue are hypertrophied. Signs are worse in cold weather. In older animals, an increasing period of exercise is necessary for muscle relaxation to occur. Percussion of muscles results in formation of dimples. This reaction is elicited in conscious and anesthetized dogs and in those administered neuromuscular blocking agents.

Serum creatine phosphokinase levels may be slightly elevated. Electromyographic studies are characterized by the presence of trains of high frequency bizarre myotonic potentials producing an audible "dive-bomber" sound.

Diagnosis is based on signalment, clinical, and electrodiagnostic data. Prognosis is guarded. Membrane stabilizing agents (procainamide, quinidine, and phenytoin) have been shown to be beneficial in the treatment of myotonia. Results of long-term therapeutic trials are lacking.

Myotonic myopathy in Irish terrier puppies is believed to be an autosomal recessive, sex-linked, hereditary condition. The pathogenesis is unknown, although mitochondrial changes suggested a defect in oxidative phosphorylation. At necropsy, muscles are pale with white streaks. A patchy distribution of lesions is seen histologically, characterized by considerable fiber size variation with many round, atrophic fibers, phagocytosis, giant cells, and calcification. Histochemical distinction between type I and type II fibers is lost.

A stiff gait and dysphagia develop at 6 to 8 weeks of age. Affected animals are unable to jump or to support themselves on their pelvic limbs. The condition is progressive or may remain static, and animals have a low exercise tolerance. Skeletal muscles undergo atrophy and have increased tone, and there is initial resistance of passive joint movements.

Serum levels for creatine phosphokinase and aldolase are very high. Electromyography reveals continuous, bizarre, high frequency discharges (pseudomyotonia). Diagnosis is based on signalment, clinical, electrophysiological, serum muscle enzyme, and muscle biopsy data. Prognosis is poor. There is no treatment.

Identical clinical and pathological data occur in young, male golden retrievers. The condition is considered to be an autosomal recessive disease; however, breeding trials are lacking.

Acquired myotonic myopathy in mature dogs can be associated with endocrine disorders, such as hyperadrenocorticism and hypothyroidism. An adult form of myotonia and myopathy also occurs in Rhodesian ridgeback dogs (588). This myopathy is characterized by dysphagia, excessive muscle tone, percussion dimpling, and electrophysiological evidence of spontaneous myotonic potentials.

KEY DIAGNOSTIC AIDS: **Breed, Age, Clinical Signs, Electromyography**

Narcolepsy/Cataplexy

Episodic sleep, or narcolepsy, is an incurable central nervous system disorder characterized by excessive sleepiness in people. In dogs, however, the only clinical sign is cataplexy, which is characterized by sudden, paroxysmal attacks of flaccid paralysis that may last from a few seconds to several minutes (589–591). Respiratory and ocular muscles tend to be spared (592). The attacks may be induced by excitement, such as eating, playing, sexual activity, or the presence of the owner or of another dog. Attacks can be reversed by an external stimulus, such as petting or calling the animal's name. The frequency of attacks may vary from one every other day to several hundred per day. Signs generally appear in affected animals prior to 6 months of age (593). The pathogenesis of this disorder remains uncertain; however, an imbalance in neurotransmitters has been suggested resulting from depressed monoamine systems and hyperactive or hypersensitive acetylcholine systems (594).

Narcolepsy/cataplexy has been reported in many canine breeds, including Doberman pinscher, miniature poodle, Labrador retriever, dachshund, St. Bernard, and beagle. Isolated cases have been seen in the following breeds: afghan, Airedale, corgi, Irish setter, malamute, springer spaniel, standard poodle, wirehaired griffon, Australian shepherd mix, and Chihuahua terrier mix. The condition is considered to be an autosomal recessive trait in Doberman pinschers and is believed to be hereditary in poodles, dachshunds, and Labrador retrievers

(593). Diagnosis is typically based on clinical signs. Attacks can be induced in most affected animals by exercise or food eating. These signs can be alleviated for up to 45 minutes using an intravenous imipramine challenge test, at a dose of 0.5 mg/kg. The most common electrophysiological finding associated with narcolepsy/cataplexy in dogs is the REM (rapid eye movement) onset sleep and the shortened sleep cycle.

Prognosis is good. The disease is not in itself life threatening, and it will not get significantly worse with time. Animals can respond very favorably to imipramine. Recommended dosage ranges from 0.5 to 1.5 mg/kg orally two or three times a day. Side effects of this drug in dogs include nervousness and sleepiness, which appear to be dose related.

KEY DIAGNOSTIC AIDS: **Historical Data, Breed, Age, Clinical Signs**

Neoplasia

Neoplasia of the nervous system is no longer considered rare in animals (55, 60, 595–597). Indeed, nervous system tumors occur in dogs with a frequency and a variety similar to that in humans (595). Primary nervous system tumors originate from neuroectodermal, ectodermal, or mesodermal cells normally present in or associated with the brain, the spinal cord, or the peripheral nerves. Secondary tumors affecting the nervous system may originate from surrounding structures, such as bone and muscle, or from hematogenous metastasis of primary tumors in other organs. Tumor emboli can lodge and grow anywhere in the brain, the meninges, the choroid plexus, or the spinal cord. In animals, primary tumors rarely metastasize outside the cranial cavity or the vertebral canal (598–600).

Classification of nervous system tumors in animals has followed the criteria used for human tumors (595, 599, 601, 602). Classification is primarily based upon the characteristics of the constituent cell type, its pathological behavior, topographic pattern, and secondary changes seen within and surrounding the tumor. To a much lesser extent, classification is based on the biological behavior of the tumor. Although many animal neoplasms have characteristics analogous with corresponding tumors in humans, 15 to 20% of neuroectodermal tumors (especially gliomas) remain unclassified. Unlike the factors of age and breed, no gender predisposition for the various types of nervous system tumors has been detected (599, 603).

Pathogenesis

With intracranial tumors, accurate clinicopathological correlations are frequently impossible (604). The actual location of a tumor may be masked by secondary effects. Except in brain tissue actually infiltrated by a tumor, a mass lesion within the nonexpansible cranial cavity often leads to local necrosis, edema, subtentorial herniation of the cingulate gyrus, compression of the hypothalamus, and coning of the cerebellum as a result of herniation of the cerebellar vermis through the foramen magnum. Two other forms of brain herniation reported in dogs with brain tumors (605) are (*a*) herniation of portions of the temporal cortex ventral to the tentorium cerebelli ("caudal transtentorial" herniation), and (*b*) herniation of the rostral cerebellar vermis ventral to the tentorium cerebelli ("rostral transtentorial" herniation). Herniation combined with attenuation of the ventricular system, especially at the level of the mesencephalic aqueduct, can lead to hydrocephalus and elevated intracranial pressure; ischemic necrosis of herniated tissue can ensue (604, 606, 607). Immunoproliferative diseases such as macroglobulinemia-associated lymphocytic leukemia can also produce a spectrum of neurological abnormalities as a result of serum hyperviscosity (608). The transient signs and changing patterns have been attributed to increased intravascular erythrocyte aggregation and associated impaired blood flow in the vascular beds of affected areas.

Primary tumors usually have a slowly progressive growth pattern; bone tumors and secondary, highly malignant, metastatic tumors frequently demonstrate a more acute progression (609, 610).

Incidence

The incidence of neoplasia of the nervous system in domestic animals appears to vary according to the veterinary institution. Neoplasms of the nervous system occur more frequently in dogs than in any other domestic species (611). In one survey, 2.83% of 6175 dogs examined postmortem had intracranial neoplasms (612).

Brain Tumors

Primary tumors of the nervous system in animals occur more often in the brain than in the spinal cord or the peripheral nerves (55, 595, 599, 602, 613). The most frequent canine brain tumors are meningiomas, gliomas (astrocytomas, oligodendrogliomas) (Figs. 3.1–3.3), and undifferentiated sarcomas (614). Primary reticulosis (the focal form of granulomatous meningoencephalomyelitis), pituitary adenomas, and plexus papillomas (Figs. 3.4–3.5) are also commonly reported (602, 615–617). Metastatic brain tumors are relatively uncommon (Fig. 3.6). Dogs over 2 years old in the brachycephalic breeds with common ancestry— boxers, English bulldogs, and Boston terrier—have the highest incidence of brain tumors among domestic animals; of these tumors, the gliomas (including those that are unclassified) are the most numerous (599, 602, 603). The common locations of glial tumors (and other neoplasms of the nervous system) are outlined

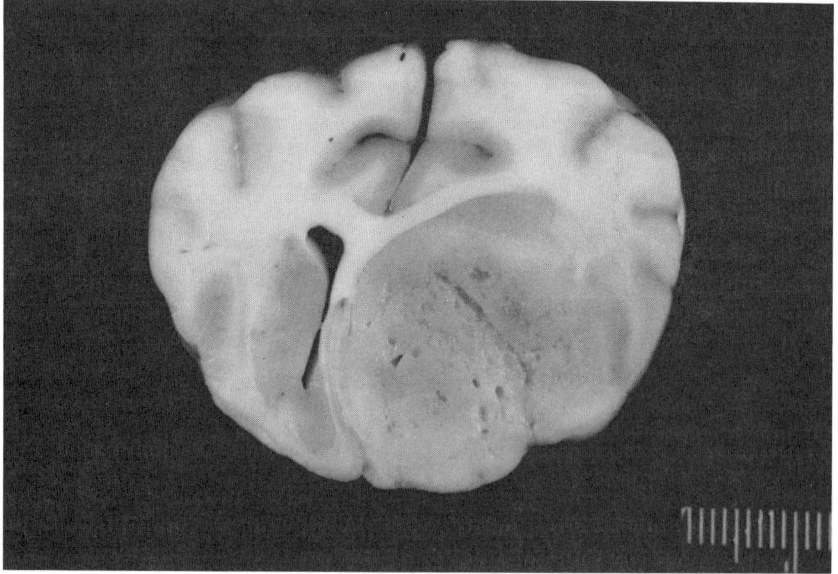

Figure 3.1. Astrocytoma located in the right cerebral hemisphere of a dog resulting in deviation of midline structures and compression of the left hemisphere. (Courtesy of Dr. Jorge Ribas.)

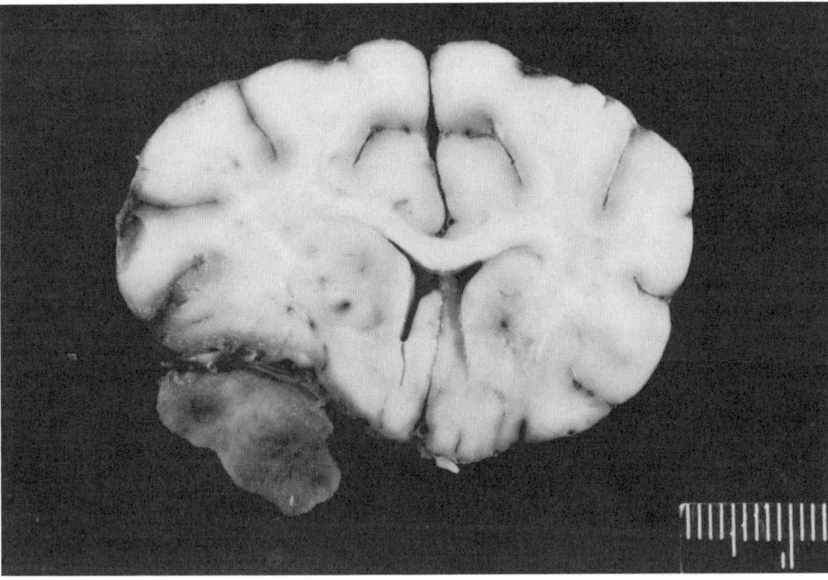

Figure 3.2. Basal meningioma from a dog with moderate shift of midline structures. (Courtesy of Dr. Jorge Ribas.)

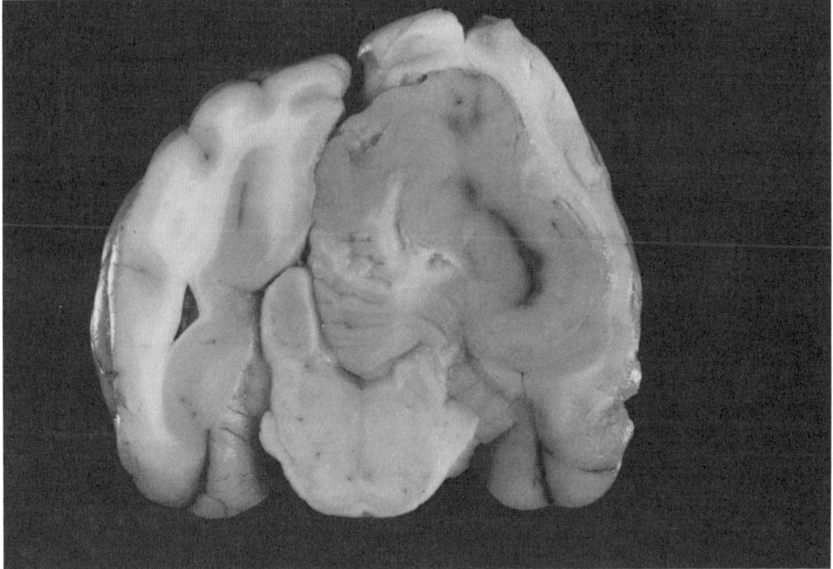

Figure 3.3. Malignant fibrous meningioma on the right side of the tentorium cerebelli of a dog. Much of the cerebellum and right occipital cortex have been replaced. (Courtesy of Dr. Jorge Ribas.)

in Table 3.2. Pituitary adenomas are also frequently reported in brachycephalic breeds, whereas meningiomas are observed more often in dolicocephalic breeds, such as German shepherds and collies. One study reported that 58% of meningiomas occurred on the ventral aspect of the brain (618).

Meningiomas are the most commonly reported feline primary brain tumors (619). Usual locations include the tela choroidea of the third ventricle and the supratentorial meninges (620–621). There is a high incidence of multiple meningiomas in cats.

Table 3.2. Classification of Tumors of the Nervous System

Tumor Type	Predilection Sites	Species/Breeds	Incidence
PRIMARY TUMORS			
1. Tumors of nerve cells			
Ganglioneuroma	Variable, e.g., cerebellum, cranial nerve roots, eye, cervical ganglion	Dogs	Rare
2. Tumors of neuroepithelium			
Ependymoma	Third and lateral ventricles	Dogs, cats	Rare
Neuroepithelioma	Meninges, thoracolumbar spinal cord	Dogs (German shepherd)	Uncommon
Choroid plexus papilloma	Fourth ventricle	Dogs	Common
3. Tumors of neuroglia			
Astrocytoma	Piriform area, convexity of cerebral hemispheres, thalamus, hypothalamus	Dogs (brachycephalic), cats	Common
Oligodendroglioma	Cerebral hemispheres	Dogs (brachycephalic)	Common
Glioblastoma	As for astrocytoma	Dogs (brachycephalic)	Uncommon
Spongioblastoma	Variable, e.g., ependymal surfaces, cerebellum, optic nerve/tracts	Dogs (brachycephalic)	Rare
Medulloblastoma	Cerebellum	Dogs, cats	Uncommon
Gliomas (unclassified)	Periventricular areas, especially in cerebral hemispheres	Dogs	Common
4. Tumors of peripheral nerves and nerve sheaths			
Nerve sheath tumors (schwannoma, neurofibroma, neurinoma)	Peripheral nerves	Dogs, cats	Common
5. Tumors of meninges, vessels, and other mesenchymal structures			
Meningiomas	Convexities of cerebral hemispheres and floor of the vault	Dogs (dilicocephalic), cats	Common
Angioblastoma	Variable	Dogs, cats	Rare
Sarcoma	Variable	Dogs, cats	Common
Focal granulomatous meningoencephalomyelitis (reticulosis)	Cerebral hemispheres and brainstem	Dogs, cats	Common (dogs)
6. Tumors of the pineal gland, pituitary gland and craniopharyngeal duct			
Pinealoma	Pineal body	Dogs	Rare
Pituitary edenoma	Pituitary gland	Dogs (brachycephalic), cats	Common
Craniopharyngioma	Hypophyseal-infundibular areas	Dogs	Rare
7. Tumors of heterotopic tissues (malformation tumors)			
Epidermoid, dermoid, teratoma	Variable (fourth ventricle and cerebellopontine angle for epidermoid)	Dogs	Rare

Table 3.2—*Continued*

Tumor Type	Predilection Sites	Species/Breeds	Incidence
SECONDARY TUMORS			
1. Metastatic tumors			
Mammary gland adenocarcinoma, pulmonary carcinoma, prostatic carcinoma, chemodectoma, malignant melanoma, lymphosarcoma, salivary gland adenocarcinoma, etc	Variable	Dogs, cats	Relatively common
2. Primary tumors from surrounding tissues			
Osteosarcoma, lipoma, chondrosarcoma, fibrosarcoma, nasal adenocarcinoma, hemangiosarcoma, multiple myeloma, calcifying aponeurotic fibromatosis, epidermoid cyst, etc	Variable	Dogs, cats	Relatively common

Brain tumors in dogs and cats tend to occur in mature adults, usually over 5 years of age.

Spinal Cord Tumors

In both dogs and cats, the incidence of primary nervous system tumors is much lower in the spinal cord than in the brain. The most frequently occurring types of canine spinal cord tumors are extradural, primary, malignant bone tumors (osteosarcoma, fibrosarcoma, hemangiosarcoma, myeloma) and tumors metastatic to bone and soft tissue (599, 609, 610, 622–624). The incidence of primary glial tumors is low, 15% in one study (610). In another canine study, approximately 30% of spinal tumors were primary with intramedullary sarcomas being prevalent (609). Neuroepithelioma are primary tumors with a predilection for the T10-L1 cord segments of young dogs, especially German shepherds. These tumors have an intradural-extramedullary position.

Primary vertebral tumors are rare in the cat with osteosarcoma being most commonly reported (625–627). Epidural lymphosarcomas are the most common feline spinal tumors (610, 628). Metastatic tumors affecting the spinal cord have been considered to be unusual in animals (599, 609, 610, 629), but an incidence of 16% has been reported in dogs (623).

The mean age of animals with spinal tumors is between 5 and 6 years, but age alone does not preclude a diagnosis of spinal tumor; 8 of 29 animals (30%) in one study of such tumors were 3 years of age or less (609). In that study, approximately 90% of the tumors occurred in large canine breeds.

Peripheral Nerve Tumors

Tumors of cranial and spinal nerves and nerve roots are not uncommon in dogs. In one study (611) peripheral nerve tumors represented 26.6% of canine nervous system tumors. The terminology given to these tumors has been confusing because of differing opinions regarding their cell of origin. Although "schwannoma," "neurilemoma," and "neurofibroma" are now accepted and used interchangeably, the designation "peripheral nerve sheath tumors" is probably more

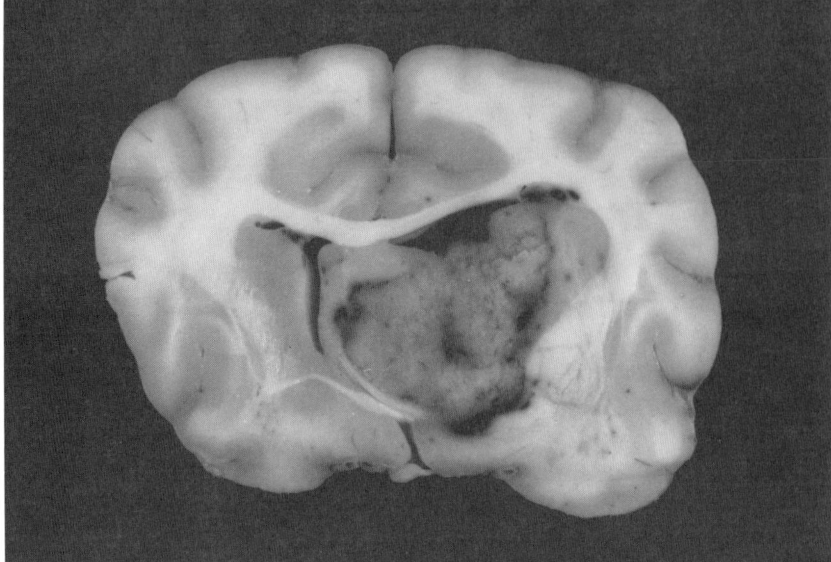

Figure 3.4. Malignant choroid plexus papilloma in the right lateral ventricle of a dog. This mass was associated with advanced hydrocephalus and midline shift. (Courtesy of Dr. Jorge Ribas.)

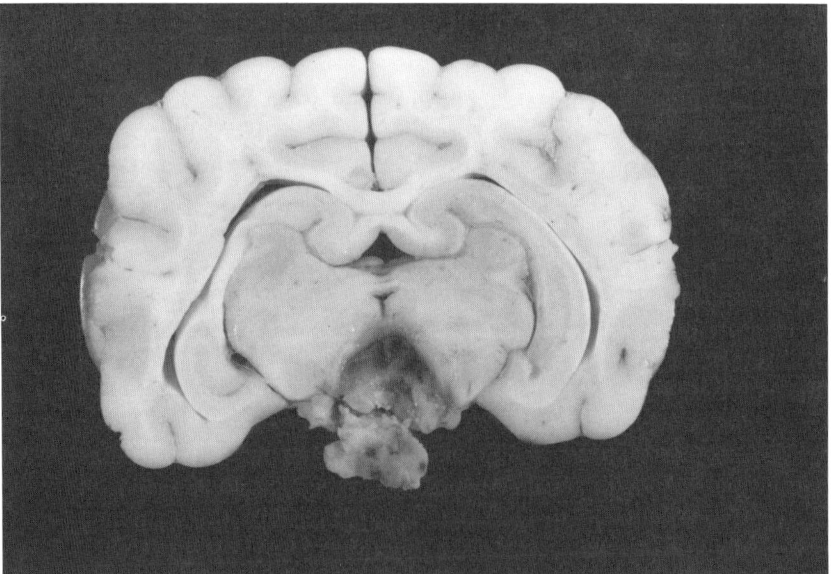

Figure 3.5. Pituitary carcinoma in a dog with destruction of most of the hypothalamus. (Courtesy of Dr. Jorge Ribas.)

appropriate until the neurohistological issue is settled. These tumors mainly involve the roots of the trigeminal nerve, the brachial plexus, cervical or thoracolumbar nerve roots. In one study, 72% of 18 nerve sheath tumors occurred in the cervical region (630). The neoplasms can extend along peripheral nerves, resulting in intradural-extramedullary spinal cord compression (609, 610, 615, 623, 630). Brainstem compression has also been reported (615, 631). Lymphosarcoma occasionally involves nerves and nerve roots (487, 632). Various tumors of the ear canal, such as squamous cell carcinoma, ceruminous adenocarcinoma,

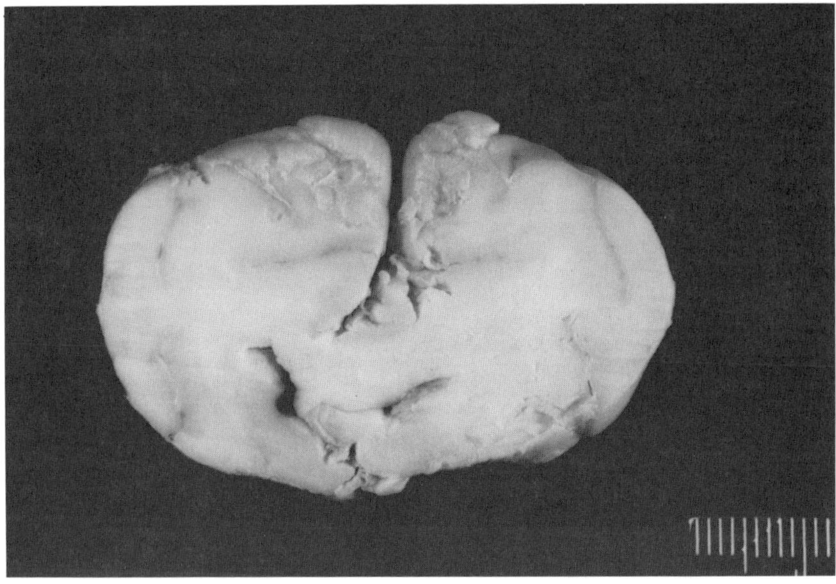

Figure 3.6. Metastatic nasal carcinoma involving the frontal lobes of a dog. The boundaries are ill defined, and most of the cortex is replaced by tumor cells. (Courtesy of Dr. Jorge Ribas.)

and fibrosarcoma, and osteosarcoma of the skull may involve the facial nerve or one of its branches (633).

Clinical Signs

Clinical signs of nervous system neoplasia vary according to the location of the tumor and any secondary effects (55, 605–607, 619, 634, 635). Onset of clinical signs can be acute or insidious, and the clinical course can progress rapidly or slowly.

In one recent study of spinal cord tumors in the dog and cat (609), intramedullary tumors had the shortest mean duration of clinical signs (1.7 weeks); the signs of extradural tumors had a mean duration of 3.4 weeks. Intradural-extramedullary tumors had the longest mean duration of signs (5.7 weeks). Accurate description of the temporal clinical course for the various brain tumors in animals, seemingly feasible from a retrospective study, is presently unknown. This situation probably results from the relatively low incidence of brain tumors in animals when compared with tumors of other organs or systems, from historical inaccuracies as to onset of clinical signs and subsequent clinical course, and finally to incomplete clinicopathological correlations.

Diagnosis

Diagnosis of a tumor of the nervous system is based on the animal's age and breed and on diagnostic aids which include plain-film radiography, contrast radiography (e.g., myelography), or specialized radiographic techniques, such as radionuclide imaging (scintigraphy) (636) and computerized axial tomography. Plain-film radiography detects evidence of bone neoplasia. Myelography can outline spinal tumors and may help to differentiate extradural, intradural-extramedullary, and intramedullary neoplasms (609, 610). Computerized axial tomography is the current method of choice for localizing brain tumors (637–641). This procedure is limited to institutions and some specialty practices.

Examination of cerebrospinal fluid can indicate an elevation in protein content, but this is a variable finding; tumor cells are rarely found in the cerebrospinal fluid (609, 642, 643). Peripheral nerve disorders can be diagnosed using electrophysiological techniques (electromyography, nerve conduction velocity determinations) in conjunction with surgical biopsy (removal of tumor and histopathological evaluation).

Prognosis and Treatment

Prognosis of animals with nervous system tumors is guarded to poor. Inability to localize a tumor mass in the brain accurately usually precludes surgical intervention; however, this situation should change with the advent of computerized axial tomography (CAT scan) (644). Although spinal cord tumors can be localized more definitively, intramedullary masses are not surgically resectable. Extradural tumors are either primary bone tumors (removal of which often results in decreased spinal stability, subluxation, or pathological fractures) or metastatic tumors, with possible sites elsewhere.

Although intradural-extramedullary tumors have been considered by some investigators to be benign, well encapsulated, and surgically correctable (610, 645), others have reported that only a small percentage is completely resectable and that the rate of recurrence is high (630).

Peripheral nerve and nerve root tumors can be resected, but it is sometimes necessary to remove the affected nerve and nerve root. Resection with anastomosis of the nerve is possible if the tumor is not too large. Complete amputation of the limb may be required if more than one root is involved, as is the usual finding, or if atrophy of all muscle groups is extreme (as may occur with a tumor of the brachial plexus). In veterinary medicine, the role of radiotherapy and chemotherapy in nervous system tumor management has been limited, primarily because of the expensive equipment required (e.g., cobalt 60 teletherapy and the use of clinical linear accelerators), although results of one study demonstrated that canine brain tumors may be treated effectively by use of megavoltage radiation (646). Another important factor is the emotionally charged issue of treating animals with profound neurological disease at the time of diagnosis. The success rate of chemotherapy on solid tumors in animals has been generally poor compared with that in humans. Corticosteroids may ameliorate clinical signs by reducing edema around the tumor and may produce temporary regression of lymphoid and reticulohistiocytic tumors.

KEY DIAGNOSTIC AIDS: **Breed, Age, Clinical Signs, CAT Scan, Myelography**

Neuroaxonal Dystrophy

Neuroaxonal dystrophy (NAD) is a degenerative neurological disease that has been reported in cats and dogs. NAD is transmitted as an autosomal recessive trait in cats and is suspected of being inherited in dogs. The disease is characterized by membrane-filled swellings ("spheroids") of distal axons within the central nervous system. The pathogenic mechanisms underlying the development of this type of axonal abnormality are not well understood. In general, clinical signs of cerebellar-like disease develop in young animals and typically are progressive. Ancillary laboratory tests, such as CSF analysis, skull-spinal radiography, and electrodiagnostics, are normal. There is no treatment. Prognosis is guarded due to the progressive nature of the disease.

Feline Hereditary Neuroaxonal Dystrophy

Domestic tricolor cats have been found to have an autosomal recessive condition that is characterized pathologically by gross atrophy of the cerebellar vermis and microscopically by marked ballooning of cell processes (spheroids) in nuclear groups extending from the medulla to the thalamus and cerebellar vermis (647). These changes are accompanied by loss of neurons, including Purkinje and granule cells of the cerebellar vermis. Inner ear lesions have been reported.

Clinical signs occur in kittens around 5 to 6 weeks of age, at which time head tremors and head shaking are observed. Signs progress to marked incoordination of gait and hypermetria. Affected kittens have a lilac color which darkens with age. Unaffected littermates are black.

Neuroaxonal Dystrophy in Rottweiler Dogs

A recessive mode of inheritance is suspected in rottweiler dogs with NAD (648, 649). The cerebellum is mildly atrophic and appearance may be small. Massive numbers of axonal spheroids are present in many regions of the neuraxis, especially in the dorsal horn of the spinal cord, nuclei gracilis and cuneatis, granular layer of the cerebellum, and vestibular nucleus. In some dogs, a marked loss of cerebellar Purkinje cells has been reported. Clinical signs are characterized by slowly progressive ataxia, hypermetria, and wide-based stance beginning in the first year of life. As the neurological deficit progresses, head intention tremors, postural and spontaneous nystagmus, and menace deficit may be noted. Some rottweilers have been observed up to 6 years of age.

Neuroaxonal Dystrophy in Collie Sheepdogs

A cerebellar neuroaxonal dystrophy in collie sheepdogs has been reported in New Zealand and Australia (650). The history of several affected pups in litters from successive mating of the same sire and dam is suggestive of an autosomal recessive mode of inheritance. Numerous spheroids, associated with mild wallerian degeneration, are present in the central cerebellar, adjacent peduncular and folia white matter, and associated cerebellar roof and lateral vestibular nuclei. Clinical signs develop from 2 to 4 months of age and include hypermetria, wide-based stance, difficulty in maintaining balance, intention tremor, and ataxia. Body growth, learning ability, and social behavior with other dogs appear to be normal.

Possible Neuroaxonal Dystrophy in Bull Mastiffs

It is possible that this disease in bull mastiffs may be another form of NAD. For a full description, see "**Cerebellar Degeneration.**"

KEY DIAGNOSTIC AIDS: **Breed/Species, Coat Color, Clinical Signs, Clinical Course**

Occipital Dysplasia

An abnormally large foramen magnum, which has been termed "occipital dysplasia," resulting from a defect in development of the occipital bone, has been described in small dogs (19, 651–654). The abnormality consists of a key-shaped dorsal midline extension of the foramen magnum into the occipital bone.

Clinical signs of cervical pain, personality changes, and seizures as described in the initial report (651) have not been substantiated by others (653). Varying degrees of enlargement of the foramen magnum occur normally in small and toy breed dogs (655). Frontal radiographs of the skull readily reveal the enlargement. Clinical evidence of neurological disease in such dogs (e.g., Yorkshire terrier, Pomeranian, Maltese, miniature and toy poodles, Chihuahuas, etc) most likely reflects some other intracranial disease, such as hydrocephalus (653). It is possible that dogs in which dorsal extension of the foramen magnum exists may have an increased potential for herniation of the brainstem through the foramen magnum.

KEY DIAGNOSTIC AIDS: **Breed, Skull Radiography**

Optic Nerve Hypoplasia

Bilateral hypoplasia of the optic nerve of unknown etiology has been reported in dogs (656–658) and cats (659). In several reports, optic nerve foramina have been reduced in diameter.

A malformation of parts of the eyeball occurs as a hereditary disease in collie dogs (660, 661). Abnormal development of optic nerve (and retina) may produce blindness. Pathologically, there is no stenosis of the optic canal, but there is a reduction in size of the optic nerve and atrophy and reduced number of optic nerve fibers. Vacuolation and paucity of neurons may be observed in ganglion cells of the retina.

Diagnosis is suggested by a history of visual impairment from birth. There is usually a menace deficit and reduced or absent pupillary reflexes in affected eyes. Prognosis is poor. There is no treatment.

KEY DIAGNOSTIC AIDS: **Age, Clinical Signs**

Optic Neuritis

Optic neuritis is an inflammatory condition of the optic nerve that results in loss of vision. It may be associated with primary ocular disease or can occur secondary to systemic inflammatory disease. The condition is not uncommon and affects dogs more frequently than cats.

In dogs, diagnostic considerations include canine distemper, ocular form of granulomatous meningoencephalomyelitis, systemic mycosis, toxoplasmosis, neoplasia, trauma, and acute toxicity (e.g., lead or chlorinated hydrocarbon toxicity).

Animals most frequently present with a history of unilateral or bilateral blindness of sudden onset in an apparently healthy animal. Pupils usually are unilaterally or bilaterally dilated and unresponsive to light stimulation. Ophthalmoscopically, the optic disk appears hyperemic and the vessels may be dilated. Focal hemorrhage may be present. The disk can be edematous and elevated. Active or inactive chorioretinitis may be detected. Atrophy of the optic nerve frequently follows episodes of acute optic neuritis. Optic neuritis is distinguished from papilledema in that vision is preserved in the latter condition.

Treatment is directed at the primary cause of the disease process that initiated the optic neuritis. The cause(s) is frequently undetermined, and the animal may be treated symptomatically with systemic corticosteroids (e.g., prednisolone at 2 mg/kg daily divided twice a day for 10 to 14 days, followed by half this dosage for 2 more weeks, and gradual reduction to maintenance therapy every other day for up to 1 year) and antibiotics. A diagnosis of idiopathic optic neuritis is made only after other causes have been ruled out. Prognosis is guarded, and clinical exacerbations may occur if treatment is stopped prematurely.

KEY DIAGNOSTIC AIDS: **History, Clinical Signs, Ophthalmoscopy**

Organophosphate/Carbamate Toxicity

Organophosphate and carbamate compounds are widely employed for control of external parasites in dogs and cats and for control of insects in the home and garden. Toxicosis may develop following ingestion of liquid concentrates or granules of these compounds or from excessive skin/hair coat dusting or painting (662, 663). Organophosphates and carbamates are acetylcholine esterase enzyme inhibitors (organophosphates are irreversible inhibitors of the enzyme, whereas carbamates are reversible inhibitors of acetylcholine esterase). This results in an accumulation of the neurotransmitter acetylcholine, causing overstimulation of the parasympathetic nervous system (salivation, lacrimation, pronounced gastrointestinal sounds, bradycardia, and pupillary constriction), skeletal muscle stimulation (muscle fasciculations, tremors, twitching, spasms, and hypertoxicity causing a stiff gait or rigid stance), and variable involvement of the central nervous system due to central cholinergic overstimulation (anxiety, restlessness, hyperactivity, and generalized seizures). Death from asphyxia may result from severe central respiratory depression, bronchial fluid accumulation, and bronchoconstriction. Clinical signs occur usually within minutes or hours. A delayed neurotoxicity may occur in cats days or weeks after minimal exposure. Lesions are associated with distal degeneration of motor nerves, beginning in the periphery and then following the motor nerves into the spinal cord (so-called dying-back axonopathy). Dogs appear to be more resistant to delayed neurotoxicity. Affected animals will manifest signs of a neuropathic syndrome.

Diagnosis is suggested by historical data, clinical signs, and response to therapy. Determination of blood cholinesterase may be useful. Atropine, at a dosage of 0.2 mg/kg of body weight, with about one-fourth of the dose given intravenously and the rest intramuscularly, usually results in a dramatic cessation of parasympathetic signs. Atropine blocks the effects of accumulated acetylcholine at muscarinic parasympathetic nerve endings. However, it does not affect the skeletal muscle (nicotinic) signs. Repeated doses of atropine can be given using one-half the initial dose. Overatropinization can cause behavioral excitation and signs of delirium.

These signs may be countered using a cholinesterase-reactivating oxime, such as 2-PAM (Protopam Chloride). This compound acts by forming a relatively nontoxic complex with the organophosphate and also reactivates acetylcholine esterase. 2-PAM works best in the presence of atropine, the dose of which may be reduced when 2-PAM is used. The dose of 2-PAM in small animals is 20 to 50 mg/kg given as a 10% solution intramuscularly or by slow intravenous injection. Oximes are of no benefit in treating carbamate toxicosis and may worsen the animal's condition. Orally administered activated charcoal in water can help to reduce absorption following ingestion of organophosphate/carbamate compounds.

KEY DIAGNOSTIC AIDS: **Historical Data, Clinical Signs, Response to Therapy**

Ossifying Myopathy

Ossifying myopathy (synonym is "myositis ossificans") is a rare myopathic disorder of animals that is characterized by heterotopic ossification of skeletal muscle and other soft tissues. Local and generalized forms of this disease have been reported in dogs and cats (664–666). The etiopathogenesis is uncertain. Trauma is often associated with localized ossifying myopathy, but it is not a prerequisite. The generalized form in people is suggested to be congenital or hereditary in nature. Fibrodysplasia ossificans of cats differs from localized ossifying myopathy in that it does not involve muscle and is multicentric, often symmetrical, and unrelated to trauma (667).

Histopathological lesions of ossifying myopathy in animals vary from mild interstitial fibrosis to complete replacement of muscle by fibrous tissue and heterotopic bone. Clinical signs are variable and include progressive weakness, stiffness, and palpable firm enlargements in affected muscles.

Radiographic studies reveal multiple radiopacities of irregular linear calcification. Prognosis is guarded. It has been reported that lesions may regress. Radical surgical excision has been performed successfully (667a). A high rate of recurrence can be expected in animals subjected to surgery.

KEY DIAGNOSTIC AIDS: **Clinical Signs, Radiography, Biopsy**

Paraneoplastic Neuromyopathy

Tumor-induced organ dysfunction not directly attributable to malignant invasion has been defined by such terms as "paraneoplastic," "carcinomatous," or "remote effects" syndrome. Polyneuropathies occurring in dogs with primary and metastatic neoplasia have been reported (629, 668, 669).

Paraneoplastic neuromyopathy may occur in animals with any form of systemic neoplasia. In people, the highest incidence occurs in patients with small cell anaplastic bronchogenic carcinoma (670). The veterinary literature probably does not reflect the incidence of paraneoplastic polyneuropathy in animals.

The pathogenesis of these disorders is not known, although several theories have beeen suggested (671): (*a*) elaboration of primary neuro- or myotoxic factors by the tumor; (*b*) an influence through alteration of homeostatic endocrine functions secondarily affecting muscle; (*c*) utilization or trapping of specific nutrients or factors required for normal neuromuscular function; and (*d*) stimulation of a host mechanism generating secondary neuro- or myoactive reactions.

Pathological changes in nerves include paranodal and segmental demyelination/remyelination, and occasional axonal degeneration. Skeletal muscle changes are observed and include focal myonecrosis, intrafascicular fatty infiltration, internal nuclei, and atrophy of fiber types (especially type 2 muscle fibers).

Clinical signs are variable, with the few cases reported being subclinical, as is also reported in people (672). A paraneoplastic effect should be considered in any older animal with neoplasia that manifests bizarre and/or vague neurological signs.

Electrodiagnostic testing may reveal slow nerve conduction velocities and spontaneous potentials including fibrillations, positive sharp waves, and high-frequency bizarre waves.

Diagnosis may be suggested by detection of a tumor, vague ill-defined neurological signs suggestive of a polyneuropathy, and electrodiagnostic and nerve/muscle biopsy data. Chest radiography can be useful for detection of tumor metastasis. Confirmation generally requires postmortem studies.

Prognosis is poor. There is no treatment.

KEY DIAGNOSTIC AIDS: **Age, Clinical Signs, Nerve/Muscle Biopsy, Chest Radiography**

Parasitic Migration

In contrast with large domestic animals, myiasis and helminthiasis involving the CNS in dogs and cats are rarely encountered clinically. Aberrant migration and growth of parasites can result in extensive damage to neural parenchyma,

Table 3.3. Parasitic Larval Migration in the Central Nervous System

Disease	Etiology	Species	Pathology	Clinical Signs	References
Cerebrospinal nematodiasis	1. *Dirofilaria immitis* (usually adults)	Dogs, cats	Focal, multifocal infarction and malacic tracts and granulomas in CNS; parenchymal compression if worms are in CSF pathways	Variable, e.g., seizures, visual impairment, depression, incoordination, paraparesis/ paraplegia	673–678
	2. *Toxocara canis* larvae	Dogs	As for dirofilariasis	Variable (refer to Dirofilariasis)	679, 680
	3. *Angiostrongylus cantonensis*	Dogs	As for dirofilariasis	Variable (refer to Dirofilariasis)	681
	4. *Ancylostoma caninum*	Dogs	As for dirofilariasis	Variable (refer to Dirofilariasis)	682
Cuterebriasis	*Cuterebra* sp. larvae	Dogs, cats	As for dirofilariasis	Variable (refer to Dirofilariasis)	683–686
Cerebral coenurosis	*Coenurus* sp.	Cats	Cysts within parenchyma	Variable (refer to Dirofilariasis)	687, 688
Cysticercosis	*Cysticercus cellulosae*	Dogs	Cysts within parenchyma	Variable (refer to Dirofilariasis)	689

including vascular rupture, necrosis, degeneration, atrophy, and proliferative (granulomatous) changes. In general, little is known of the route of migration of parasites that invade the brain, with the exception of hematogenous-borne *Dirofilaria immitis.* Apart from dirofilariasis, which occurs sporadically in mature dogs and cats, CNS parasitic invasion usually takes place in immature animals. Clinical signs are extremely variable depending on the location and nature of the lesion. The signs may reflect either a mass lesion or a multifocal disease process. Clinical diagnosis is difficult but may be suggested by the presence of an eosinophilic (together with neutrophilic and mononuclear cell) pleocytosis in cerebrospinal fluid; however, definitive diagnosis requires isolation and/or pathological demonstration of the parasite within the CNS.

The clinical course may be rapid or chronic, usually progressive, and follows an acute or insidious onset of signs. Prognosis is poor and treatment ineffective.

Clinical and pathological data for several parasitic larval diseases of the CNS of dogs and cats are outlined in Table 3.3.

KEY DIAGNOSTIC AIDS: **Age, Clinical Signs, CSF Analysis, Histopathology**

Parvovirus Encephalitis

There has been a recent report of a generalized form of canine parvovirus infection causing necrotizing vasculitis and leukomalacia, especially in the cerebrum in a 7.5-week-old dalmation puppy (690). Large basophilic inclusion bodies were observed in some cells of the vascular wall. In sections of the ileum, there was necrosis of crypt epithelum, with dilated, debris-laden crypts typical of the changes noted with canine parvovirus infection. Neurological signs were characterized by sudden onset of circling and blindness. The pathogenesis may be similar to that of feline panleukopenia virus in cats.

The clinician should be aware that infection with canine parvovirus may be manifested by a neurological syndrome as well as enteric and cardiac syndromes.

KEY DIAGNOSTIC AIDS: **Age, Clinical Signs, Virus Isolation, Serum Antibody Titer**

Polymyositis

Polymyositis is a relatively common myopathic disorder in dogs, the cause of which is unknown. It has been suggested that polymyositis, masticatory myositis, and other clinical variations, such as pharyngeal-esophageal and focal appendicular myositis, may represent different clinical and pathological expressions of a single primary muscle inflammatory disease (81).

The responsiveness of the disease to immunosuppressive therapy suggests that the pathogenesis is immune mediated. Histological findings in skeletal muscle (appendicular and masticatory) are focal/multifocal or diffuse myonecrosis, phagocytosis and lymphoplasmacytic cellular infiltrates, considerable fiber size variation, and areas of fiber regeneration. Deposition of immunoglobulin G on sarcolemmal membranes has been demonstrated (244).

Clinical signs are variable and are usually observed in larger breed, mature adults of either sex. Onset of signs may be acute or chronic. Signs include weakness of gait with rapid fatigue, abnormalities of deglutition with esophageal dilation and inhalation pneumonia, shifting lameness and/or stiffness of gait, muscle swelling and/or pain, pyrexia, muscle atrophy, voice change, and depression (244, 691). Neurological examination is normal. Early in the disease, serum levels of creatine phosphokinase and aldolase may be elevated.

Electrodiagnostic changes include polyphasic motor unit potentials, positive sharp waves, and fibrillation potentials. Some dogs have hypergammaglobulinemia, positive antinuclear antibodies, and circulating antimuscle antibodies. Polymyositis has been reported in dogs with autoimmune diseases—namely, systemic lupus erythematosus (245) and primary lymphocytic thyroiditis (81). Polymyositis is also a feature of a recently reported disease in collie dogs (135–137), familial canine dermatomyositis (see "**Dermatomyositis**"). This disease is believed to be autoimmune.

Prognosis is usually favorable for animals with polymyositis providing severe damage has not occurred in esophageal and laryngeal muscles. The disease is usually responsive to glucocorticoids, e.g., prednisone 0.5 to 1.0 mg/kg orally twice a day. The dose is reduced after remission and gradually withdrawn using alternate-day therapy. Repeated clinical episodes are not uncommon.

KEY DIAGNOSTIC AIDS: **Clinical Signs, Electromyography, Muscle Biopsy**

Porencephaly

This congenital disorder represents a circumscribed cerebral defect which communicates with the ventricular system. It is a rare disorder thought to be secondary to fetal vascular maldevelopment. Diagnosis is made at postmortem examination. Animals commonly are stillborn or die in the immediate neonatal period. There is no treatment.

KEY DIAGNOSTIC AIDS: **Age, Neuropathology**

Postvaccinal Distemper

Postvaccinal canine distemper encephalitis occurs in young animals, especially those less than 6 months of age. It has been recognized as a disease entity for a number of years and is believed to be associated with vaccination with live virus.

The pathogenesis of this disease is unclear. It may result from insufficient attenuation of the vaccine virus which causes subsequent infection of the central nervous system, from the triggering of a latent paramyxovirus infection by vaccination, or from an enhanced susceptibility of the animal. This disorder has been reported after combined distemper and infectious canine hepatitis vaccination in the dog (692–694).

Pathological changes in the brain are characterized by multifocal neuronal degeneration, neuronophagia, axonal degeneration, perivascular cuffing, and mild to moderate gliosis. The lesions are seen at all levels but tend to be most severe in the ventral pontine area where malacia may also be seen. Purkinje cells frequently remain unaffected. Intranuclear and intracytoplasmic inclusion bodies are present in many neuronal cells. Ultrastructural examination of the inclusion bodies reveals the presence of nucleocapsids with the features of the paramyxovirus group (692, 693).

Clinical signs are usually seen within 1 to 2 weeks after vaccination. They include anorexia, listlessness, and slight pyrexia. Neurological signs occur 1 to 3 days after the onset of these nonspecific signs. Sudden changes in temperament, viciousness (attacking owners, other dogs, and inanimate objects), aimless wandering, howling, incoordination, and terminal convulsions may be seen in acute cases of approximately 24 hours' duration. In subacute cases (a disease course of 2 to 3 days), pelvic limb incoordination, circling, depression, and visual impairment are frequently observed. CSF analysis may reveal elevated protein levels and a mononuclear pleocytosis.

This disorder differs from spontaneous distemper infection in young dogs. The clinical differences include an absence of systemic signs, and an alteration in personality to viciousness which is very similar in nature and clinical course to that seen in the furious form of rabies encephalitis. Pathologically, postvaccinal distemper encephalitis is distinguished from spontaneous distemper infection by the virtual absence of both visceral inclusions and demyelination in the area of the cerebellopontine angle, the presence of many neuronal inclusions, diffuse pontine tegmental malacia, and large numbers of degenerating axonal ovoids.

Prognosis is guarded, and treatment is symptomatic.

KEY DIAGNOSTIC AIDS: **Historical Data, Age, Clinical Signs, CSF Analysis**

Postvaccinal Rabies

A paralytic syndrome occasionally occurs in dogs and cats as a result of infection of the central nervous system by rabies modified live vaccine virus derived from chick embryos. Clinical signs appear within 7 to 21 days after vaccination (695, 696).

Pathological findings are incomplete. Acute nonsuppurative meningoencephalomyelitis has been reported (697). The lower motor neuron signs seen neurologically suggest that the tissue lesions are associated with polioencephalomyelitis. Negri bodies may not be found in the brain, and virus may not be detected in saliva; however, high levels of rabies virus antibody in serum and cerebrospinal fluid have been reported in dogs (696, 698). At present, there is no evidence to suggest that the vaccine virus reverts to its original virulence. Rabies virus has been isolated from brain, and rabies antigen has been demonstrated by fluorescent antibody techniques (696).

Clinicopathological correlations are not definitive, but ascending flaccid paralysis, beginning in the pelvic limbs following vaccination in the thigh, appears to be the most prominent neurological derangement. In this regard, the syndrome is similar to the dumb form of rabies. Paralysis of the cranial nerves as well as of attendant changes, such as the character of the bark and excessive salivary drooling, have been observed, and mental status may be depressed. Clinical recovery has been reported in dogs within 1 to 2 months (696, 698).

The clinical differentiation between postvaccinal syndrome and the naturally acquired form of rabies infection may be difficult and is therefore dependent on a history of possible natural exposure to rabies. Appropriate public health precautions need to be taken.

KEY DIAGNOSTIC AIDS: **Historical Data, Clinical Signs, Clinical Course**

Progressive Diffuse Myelomalacia

This destructive spinal cord lesion is one of the most undesirable sequela to spinal trauma. Synonyms include "hemorrhagic myelomalacia" and "hematomyelia." This condition may occur within a few hours to 1 day after the initiating injury, such as external spinal trauma or, more commonly, acute intervertebral disk extrusion. The thoracolumbar spinal cord is usually involved. The lesion is a combination of ischemic and hemorrhagic infarction of almost all parenchyma of the spinal cord. The underlying mechanism for the proposed occlusive vascular damage is uncertain; however, catecholamines are believed to play a role.

Clinical signs reflect the nature and level of the lesion. Initially, with a thoracolumbar cord lesion, an animal will show signs of acute onset, total paraplegia with exaggerated pelvic limb reflexes. As a result of edema and hemorrhage, the cord malacia can descend to involve the lumbosacral segments, and clinical signs of flaccid paraplegia with pelvic limb atonia and areflexia will develop within 2 to 3 days. The tail will be flaccid and the anus dilated and unresponsive to stimuli. Pain perception is absent in all these areas. As the disorder progresses rostrally, the thoracic limbs may become flaccid and analgesic, and bilateral Horner's syndrome may occur. If the spinal cord malacia ascends to lower or midcervical levels, respiratory paralysis will occur, followed by death.

Spinal cord damage is permanent. There is no treatment. It should be noted that this condition can develop even after immediate surgical decompression of acute disk extrusion.

KEY DIAGNOSTIC AIDS: **History, Clinical Signs, Clinical Course**

Protothecosis

Protothecosis is a rare disease caused by an acholoric genus of algae. Two species, *Prototheca wickerhamii* and *Prototheca zopfii*, have been shown to produce systemic disease in animals. Central nervous system involvement has been reported in dogs with both *Prototheca* species (699, 700).

The pathogenesis of protothecosis is uncertain. An alimentary route of exposure has been suggested. Failure of the host's immune competence may predispose to infection with this ubiquitous organism. Collie dogs seem to have a higher incidence of this disease compared with other breeds. It appears that *Prototheca* has a definite affinity for the eyes in dogs. Organisms and pyogranulomatous lesions have been described in eyes, brain, spinal cord, kidneys, muscle, heart, liver, spleen, and lungs. The cellular response in dogs is frequently minimal. Clinical neurological signs are variable, reflecting a multifocal disease process. They include visual impairment, paresis, tetraplegia, deafness, head tilt, facial hypalgesia, anosmia, and dementia. Acute blindness and deafness were the only signs observed in a recently reported case of protothecosis in a dog (701). An eosinophilic pleocytosis in CSF has been reported in one affected dog (700). Preretinal hemorrhage and chorioretinal scars have been noted ophthalmoscopically.

The organism has been cultured from CSF. The prognosis is poor, and treatment to date has been unrewarding.

KEY DIAGNOSTIC AIDS: **Clinical Signs, CSF Analysis and Culture**

Pseudorabies

This disease, also known as "Aujeszky's disease," "mad itch," and "infectious bulbar paralysis," affects most species of wild and domestic animals except horses (60). Swine are the natural host of this virus (Herpesvirus suis), and survivors may serve as inapparent carriers of infection. Aujeszky's disease in species other than swine, namely cattle, dogs, cats, and wildlife, is usually a fatal disease. The virus is believed to reach the central nervous system by traveling centripetally in the peripheral nerves, probably in the axoplasm (702, 703). The mode of transmission to dogs and cats is usually the consumption of virus-contaminated tissues of swine, cattle, rats, and mice (704). The virus may also gain entrance to the body via scratches or abrasions from contaminated objects.

The virus is highly neurotropic, and the most extensive brain changes in the dog and cat occur in the medulla, followed by the pons, thalamus, cerebellum, and cerebral cortex. Microscopically, a moderate meningoencephalitis is observed, with perivascular mononuclear infiltrations, proliferation of neuroglia and accompanying neutrophil leukocytes, as well as Cowdry type A intranuclear inclusions in glia, ganglia, and neurons (60, 705, 706).

The incubation period in the dog and cat ranges from 2 to 10 days. Death usually occurs within 24 to 48 hours after onset of clinical signs (707). Classically, the most characteristic clinical manifestations are intense localized pruritis of face or limbs, with scratching or chewing to the point of self-mutilation. However, pruritis may not always be a constant feature (702, 708–710). Early in the course of the disease, fever, restlessness, emesis, excessive salivation, and dyspnea may be noted, followed by incoordination, vocalization, anisocoria, ptosis, and facial tremors. Convulsions, coma, and death quickly ensue (704, 707). The course of the disease can be so rapid in cats that death may occur without any clinical signs. Treatment does not alter the course of the disease.

Clinical distinction from rabies can be made by the presence of intense pruritis and/or observing that affected animals are not aggressive to animate and inanimate objects. Diagnosis may be suggested by clinical and histological data, substantiated by neuropathological findings and confirmed by fluorescent antibody test of brain tissue, by laboratory animal (usually rabbit) inoculation with tissue extracts, or by virus isolation in cell culture.

KEY DIAGNOSTIC AIDS: **Historical Data, Clinical Signs, Laboratory Animal Inoculation**

Pug Dog Encephalitis

This is a chronic progressive neurological disease recognized in pug dogs, male and female, 9 months to 4 years of age (81). The course of the disease varies from 1 to 6 months. The etiology is unknown. Pathologically, a granulomatous encephalitis is observed affecting white and gray matter, primarily in the cerebrum often with associated lymphocytic meningitis. Perivascular cuffs consist of lymphocytes and histiocytes.

The most common clinical signs are seizures (generalized and partial). Circling, visual deficits, and intermittent screaming have also been observed in some affected dogs. Death is often preceded by coma or status epilepticus. The clinical course may span a few days to several months.

Cerebrospinal fluid has moderate pleocytosis (mononuclear), and protein levels may be slightly increased. Prognosis is poor. Seizures are often refractory to anticonvulsant drugs, and glucocorticoids are ineffectual.

KEY DIAGNOSTIC AIDS: **Breed, Clinical Signs, CSF Analysis**

Pyogranulomatous Meningoencephalomyelitis

Pyogranulomatous meningoencephalomyelitis is an acute, rapidly progressive disease of 2 to 3 weeks' duration that, to date, has been recognized only in mature pointers (M Vandevelde, unpublished information; 193).

The cause of the meningoencephalomyelitis is unknown. Special histological stains for microorganisms, cultures of blood and cerebrospinal fluid, and studies of animal inoculations have all been negative. Clinical and pathological data suggest a bacterial etiology.

Pathological changes are found throughout the brain and spinal cord but are most severe in the upper segments of the cervical spinal cord and in the lower brainstem. These changes are characterized by extensive mononuclear (plasma, lymphocytic cells) and polymorphonuclear inflammatory infiltrations in the leptomeninges and parenchyma. Large perivascular cuffs are seen. In some cases, central necrosis of gray matter and edema are found in segments of the cervical cord along with infiltration of macrophages, monocytes, neutrophils, and plasma cells. These changes are probably secondary to impaired spinal circulation from the meningeal reaction. An increased population of reticuloendothelial cells is occasionally observed among the perivascular cells. Focal ependymitis may be present along ventricular pathways.

Clinical signs include cervical rigidity, kyphosis, nose held close to the ground, reluctance to move, incoordination, head tilt, falling/rolling, spontaneous and positional nystagmus, and seizures. Occasionally, bradycardia, vomiting, and atrophy of the cervical muscles are seen. Signs of parenchymal involvement include paralysis of the trigeminal and facial nerves, and Horner's syndrome.

Marked, predominantly neutrophilic pleocytosis (500 to 1000 white blood cells/ mm^3) and an increased concentration of protein (sometimes over 700 mg/dl) are found on examination of the cerebrospinal fluid of affected animals.

In this small series of cases so far observed, prognosis has been poor. Temporary remission of signs has resulted following antibiotic therapy.

KEY DIAGNOSTIC AIDS: **Breed, Clinical Signs, CSF Analysis**

Rabies

All warm-blooded mammals are susceptible to rabies encephalitis; however, there is considerable interspecies susceptibility. Wildlife are the chief natural reservoir of rabies. In most northern countries, such as Canada, Greenland, and the USSR, foxes are the main vectors. In other parts of the world, wolves (Iran), mongooses (the Caribbean), skunks and raccoons (USA), and bats (Latin America) play important roles in transmitting rabies (711). In the US, dogs play a relatively small part in current epizootics. Dog vaccination helped to bring down cases of canine rabies in the US from 5000 in 1946 to 180 in 1973, thus eliminating the major route of rabies transmission to humans.

Rabies is caused by a rhabdovirus which is destroyed by lipid solvents and low pH (712). Transmission most often occurs through bite wounds from infected animals that are secreting virus in their saliva. Infection may also occur by wound/abrasion contamination from infected saliva or other infected material. Airborne transmission and infection through mucous membranes may also occur.

The incubation period is variable, depending on the amount of virus transmitted, site of inoculation, and nature of the wound (713).

Rabies virus is highly neurotropic and reaches the central nervous system (CNS) via passive centripetal movement in the axoplasmic compartment of peripheral nerves (714, 715). Following the entry of the virus into CNS, usually spinal cord, its ascending course to the brain is rapid (716, 717). In man and animals, rabies infection is usually extremely widespread in the brain. The virus has a significantly higher tropism for neurons than for glia (718). Negri bodies (viral antigen aggregates) are often largest in the largest neurons, such as in the pyramidal cells of the hippocampus, ganglionic neurons of pontine nuclei, and Purkinje cells of the cerebellum (717). Centrifugal spread of virus to sites involved in bite transmission is via peripheral nerves and involves target cells exposed to body surfaces. Salivary gland mucous epithelium is the major source of virus shed into secretions in species which maintain rabies in nature. These include the dog, fox, skunk, raccoon, and bat (717). Results of recent experimental studies indicate that dogs can excrete rabies virus in the saliva up to 13 days before clinical signs are exhibited (719), thus necessitating a longer observation period in prospectively rabid dogs than the 10 days currently recommended.

Pathologically, rabies is characterized by a multifocal, mild polioencephalomyelitis with mononuclear perivascular infiltrates, diffuse glial proliferation, regressive changes in neuronal cells, and glial nodules (60). There is a predilection for localization in the brainstem, especially the substantia nigra, red nucleus, and periaqueductal gray matter of the midbrain; the pontine nuclei; the reticular formation; the floor of the fourth ventricle; and the hypothalamus. Other areas commonly affected include the gray matter of the spinal cord, hippocampus, globus pallidus, and thalamic nuclei. Intracytoplasmic Negri bodies are usually most numerous in hippocampal neurons and Purkinje cells.

Initial clinical signs tend to be nonspecific and include apprehension, restlessness, anorexia, and vomiting. A change in temperament may be noted at this stage, and excessive salivation may occur. These signs, which may be present for 2 to 5 days, are followed either by the dumb or the furious form of the disease (55, 60). Approximately 25 to 30% of affected animals exhibit the furious form (713) which is characterized by increased restlessness, wandering, viciousness (attack of animals, man, or inanimate objects), howling, polypnea, drooling of saliva, and sometimes convulsions. Death usually occurs between 4 and 8 days after the onset of clinical signs. It is usually the furious form of rabies that occurs in cats.

The dumb or paralytic form of rabies encephalomyelitis is more common and is characterized by progressive ascending spinal paresis or paralysis, paralysis of the lower jaw, pharyngeal and hypoglossal paralysis (resulting in difficulty in eating and drinking, and drooling of saliva), and facial paralysis. In dogs, a noticeable change in the character of the bark occurs as a result of the pharyngeal paralysis. Death as a result of respiratory failure occurs between 3 and 6 days after the onset of clinical signs.

Recently, dogs infected with rabies experimentally have developed clinical signs and recovered. Previously, rabies was considered invariably fatal in the dog. These findings place an increased responsibility on the veterinarian in managing animals with encephalitis.

It should be noted that clinical signs associated with rabies in dogs are often so variable that a distinction between the furious and dumb forms may be unjustified (720). As a result, the diagnosis of rabies must be based on laboratory confirmation; histopathological examinations of brain sections/smears for presence of an acute meningoencephalitis and identification of Negri bodies; fluorescent antibody test on tactile facial hair follicles obtained from skin biopsy or on brain samples, and mouse inoculation. Mouse inoculation has the disadvantage of a 3-week observation period to establish a negative diagnosis. The rabies fluorescent antibody test is widely used for it is an extremely accurate and rapid technique. Also, a focus-forming inhibition assay to detect rabies antibodies in serum is available. A moderate mononuclear pleocytosis (40 to 60 white blood cells/mm^3) and slight protein elevation (50 to 70 mg/dl) may be found on CSF analysis. Electroencephalographic tracings may be abnormal and suggestive of an encephalitis.

There is no treatment. Animals exposed to rabies that have not been immunized should be euthanatized. If the animal is current on rabies vaccination and exposed (and the owners do not want euthanasia), the animal should be revaccinated and closely confined under observation for at least 30 days.

KEY DIAGNOSTIC AIDS: **Historical Data, Clinical Signs, Fluorescent Antibody Test**

Rickettsial Meningoencephalitis

Rickettsial diseases—such as Rocky Mountain spotted fever (RMSF) caused by *Rickettsia rickettsii*, and ehrlichiosis caused by *Ehrlichia canis*—sporadically involve the central nervous system of dogs, where they produce a meningoencephalitis (721, 722). Lesions are characterized by vasculitis and perivascular inflammatory cell infiltrates. Both diseases are characterized by fever, depression, lymphadenopathy, and neurological signs that include depression, paraparesis or tetraparesis, vestibular dysfunction, and generalized or localized hyperesthesia (722). Seizures, cranial nerve deficits, and coma have been reported in dogs with RMSF. Fundic lesions, including retinal hemorrhage, chorioretinal exudate, and/or retinal detachment, can occur with either disease. Analysis of CSF from dogs with either disease may reveal slight to moderate elevations in protein content (38 to 159 mg/dl) and variable, predominantly mononuclear pleocytosis (10 to 130 white blood cells/mm^3). Thrombocytopenia occurs with both diseases. Rising serum titers or positive direct fluorescence for *R. rickettsii* in skin biopsy specimens will confirm a diagnosis of RMSF, whereas a single serum titer for *E. canis* can suffice for a diagnosis of ehrlichiosis (722).

The treatment of choice for both diseases is tetracycline, using a dosage of 22 mg/kg orally three times a day.

While dogs without neurological disease can show a dramatic response to treatment, the prognosis is guarded for those animals with neurological signs. Recovery may be prolonged with residual neurological deficits from irreversible brain damage.

KEY DIAGNOSTIC AIDS: **Clinical Signs, CSF Analysis, Serology**

Sacrococcygeal Dysgenesis

Congenital malformations of the sacrocaudal spinal cord and vertebrae have been well described in tailless Manx cats, in which the disease is transmitted as an autosomal dominant trait (723–725). A synonym for this disease is "caudal dysgenesis."

Pathologically, subcutaneous cyst formation, meningocele, myelomeningocele, syringomyelia, dystematomyelia, shortening of the spinal cord and absence of cauda equina, and anomalies of the dorsal horn have been described in affected animals (723, 726–729). Affected animals may steadily deteriorate after birth and become paraplegic, or a partial disability may remain stationary (727). Neurological signs including plantigrade posture, hopping gait, pelvic limb paresis/paraplegia, fecal and urinary incontinence, and perianal sensory loss are associated with agenesis or dysgenesis of caudal vertebrae, and in some cats, severe sacral dysgenesis and spina bifida.

Prognosis is guarded. There is no treatment. Mildly affected animals may attain longevity if fecal and urinary incontinence are managed.

A similar disorder has been reported in a Maltese kitten (730).

KEY DIAGNOSTIC AIDS: **Breed, Age, Clinical Signs, Radiography**

Scotty Cramp

Scotty cramp (synonym is "hyperkinesis") is an inherited paroxysmal neurological disorder with a recessive mode of transmission in Scottish terrier dogs (731–733). The condition is also variously described as muscular hypertonicity, muscular cramping, and hyperkinesis. Although there are no structural changes observed in the central or peripheral nervous systems or in muscle, physiological studies have demonstrated that the defect appears to be in those neuronal systems that control or moderate muscle contraction. Pharmacological studies suggest that the disorder may be associated with serotonic transmitters, since antiserotonin agents markedly increase the severity of clinical signs.

Clinical signs may be elicited by exercise, excitement, stress, and poor health. The condition may occur in animals at any age; however, signs tend to be more prevalent in young dogs. Affected dogs appear normal when at rest or on initial exercise. As the excercise continues, clinical signs are usually observed which progressively increase in severity. Initial signs may be abduction of the thoracic limbs or arching of the lumbar spine, followed by pelvic limb stiffness, occasional catapulting of the pelvic limbs into the air, falling and curling into a ball, with the tail and pelvic limbs tightly flexed against the body. Respiration may momentarily cease, and facial muscles may be contracted. Animals do not lose consciousness. Signs usually remit within 10 minutes. Multiple episodes may occur over a 24-hour period. The disorder is usually nonprogressive.

Diagnosis is based on the clinical signs, since all laboratory tests are within normal limits. Historical information may reveal a family history of hyperkinesis. Signs can be induced using methysergide, a serotonin antagonist. The drug is administered orally at a dosage of 0.3 mg/kg, and the animal is exercised 2 hours later.

Treatment consists of daily oral dosing of acepromazine maleate (0.1 to 0.75 mg/kg every 12 hours) or diazepam (0.5 mg/kg every 8 hours). Vitamin E (125 IU/kg/day) may also be effective. Sometimes, behavioral modification or environmental change may be sufficient.

A similar condition has been reported in young dalmation dogs (734) and in Norwich terriers (735).

KEY DIAGNOSTIC AIDS: **Breed, Age, Clinical Signs, Normal Laboratory Tests, Response to Medication**

Seizures

Seizures (synonyms are "convulsion," "epilepsy," "fit") are paroxysmal disorders of the nervous system that have a tendency to recur. The actual attack is called the "ictus." Sometimes, a preictal aura may occur seconds to minutes before the seizure, during which time the animal can appear apprehensive and restless and may seek out the owner or hide and act fearful. The postictal period is the time interval during which recovery occurs. It can be manifested as depression, visual impairment, protracted sleep, or other disturbances of behavior and may last from several minutes to 1 hour, up to 1 day, or more.

The pathogenesis of seizures is believed to be associated with neuronal hyperexcitability resulting from imbalance in neurotransmitter activity and/or altered cell metabolism or membrane properties (736). Seizural disorders are more common in dogs than cats.

Seizures have been broadly classified as partial or generalized (737, 738). Partial seizures are characterized clinically by various combinations of the following signs: somnolence, apparent blindness, tonus or clonus of one or more limbs, head turning, viciousness, senseless screaming or barking, attacking inanimate objects, generalized trembling, fear, chewing or licking movements, tail or flank biting, and snapping at imaginary objects ("fly catching"). Partial seizures can become generalized.

Generalized seizures (synonym "grand mal seizures"), which are much more common than partial seizures, typically are characterized by loss of consciousness, opisthotonus, limb rigidity, and clonic activity, followed by paddling or running limb movements. Urination, defecation, and salivation may occur. The attacks usually last from a few seconds to 3 to 5 minutes. In some animals, repeated seizures occur without intervening periods of consciousness. This state, called "status epilepticus," is life threatening and requires prompt treatment in order to avoid permanent laminar necrosis of the cerebral cortex (190) and death from hyperthermia, circulatory and respiratory collapse, acidosis, and hypoxia.

Seizures can occur in association with one of the following categories:

1. Intracranial disease, such as malformations (e.g., hydrocephalus), inflammatory disorders (e.g., distemper encephalitis), nutritional deficiency (e.g., thiamine), neoplasia, cranial trauma, and cerebral infarction. Affected animals typically present with progressive neurological disease.

2. Metabolic diseases, such as hypoglycemia, hepatic encephalopathy, renal disease, and hyperlipoproteinemia. Affected animals may show clinical signs of the primary organ dysfunction but usually are normal neurologically between seizure episodes.

3. Intoxications. Following exposure to toxins or poisons (e.g., lead, organophosphates, or excessive chocolate consumption), healthy animals manifest acute onset of seizure activity. It is not uncommon for mildly intoxicated animals to have a single attack.

4. Idiopathic epilepsy. In several breeds of dogs, and also in cats, paroxysmal seizural attacks occur which are considered to have a hereditary or familial basis. Such breeds include German shepherds, keeshonds and Belgian Tervurens, colony-bred beagles, Irish setters, St. Bernards, standard and miniature poodles, wirehaired fox terriers, cocker spaniels, Labrador retrievers, and golden retrievers. These animals are clinically and neurologically normal between seizures. Onset of the first seizure occurs usually between 1 and 3 years of age. The male:female ratio in both purebred and mixed breeds of dogs with idiopathic epilepsy has been estimated to be 60:40 (GC Farnbach, unpublished information). Several of the larger breed dogs have a tendency toward clusters of generalized seizures. In smaller breeds, seizures can be generalized but milder, sometimes without loss of consciousness, and are characterized by spasticity and generalized trembling and collapse with crawling attempts toward the owner.

Animals with idiopathic epilepsy tend to have recurring attacks, often at regular intervals (weeks or months). It is not uncommon for the frequency of attacks to increase with age. Some of these animals have abnormal electroencephalograms (EEGs) in the interictal period. Diagnosis of idiopathic epilepsy is based on historical and signalment data and on rule-out of intracranial and metabolic causes. Results of CSF analysis, hematology, and skull radiographs are within normal limits, and EEG traces can be normal in many animals. Animals with idiopathic epilepsy should not be used for breeding purposes.

Evidence of acquired seizures (brain disease, metabolic disorder, intoxication) can be assessed using historical data, physical and neurological examinations, CSF analysis (pressure, cell count, and protein concentration), EEG examination, fasting blood glucose content, complete blood count, blood urea nitrogen, serum alanine aminotransferase, serum alkaline phosphatase, sulfobromophthalein, and bilirubin.

Treatment must be directed at the primary cause. The treatment of choice for animals with idiopathic epilepsy is anticonvulsant drug medication. The three most commonly used anticonvulsant drugs are phenobarbital, primidone, and phenytoin.

Phenobarbital. This drug is a very effective anticonvulsant in dogs and cats. Barbiturates reduce neuronal excitability. The dose is 2 to 4 mg/kg in dogs, given orally two or three times a day. In cats, the dose is 1 to 2 mg/kg, at the same frequency. Effective control of seizures in dogs has been documented only when between 15 and 45 μg/ml of serum concentrations of phenobarbital are given (739). Side effects include ataxia, sedation/depression, polyphagia, polydipsia and polyuria, restlessness, and sometimes behavior change (excitability or aggression). Sedation and ataxia tend to disappear when the dose is reduced. Long-term usage results in elevated alkaline phosphatase levels secondary to hepatic microsomal induction. Barbiturate dependence occurs, so abrupt withdrawal of phenobarbital should be avoided. Gradual dose reduction over several weeks is recommended if the drug is to be discontinued.

Primidone (Mylepsin, Mysoline). This drug also is a very effective anticonvulsant in dogs. It is reportedly contraindicated in cats; however, recent studies have indicated that this drug can be used safely in cats using a total daily dose of up to 40 mg/kg, divided three times daily (AJ Parker, unpublished information). Primidone in dogs is largely metabolized to phenobarbital and phenylethylmalonamide, also an anticonvulsant (740). The dosage is 30 to 60 mg/kg orally daily, given in three divided doses. Seizure control in dogs given primidone is closely correlated with serum phenobarbital concentrations, which should be maintained between 15 to 45 μg/ml to achieve clinical efficacy in from 50 to 70% of epileptic dogs (739). Side effects include ataxia, sedation/depression, polyphagia, polydipsia, polyuria, and behavior change. All these effects appear to be dose related (741). Long-term usage results in elevated alkaline phosphatase levels, similar to phenobarbital, and can produce biochemical and histological evidence of hepatic dysfunction (742–744). Test results that are abnormal most often are alanine transaminase activity and sulfobromophthalein (BSP) excretion. Hepatic cirrhosis associated with long-term (7 years) primidone therapy in a dog has recently been reported (745). Primidone medication should never be abruptly terminated because of the potential for withdrawal seizures. According to one report, there is no advantage to the use of primidone over the use of phenobarbital for the control of seizures in most dogs (746).

Phenytoin (Diphenylhydantoin, Dilantin). Clinical trials are needed to assess the efficacy of this drug and to define the optimal blood level needed in seizure control (747). Due to the variable rapid rate of metabolism of phenytoin in dogs, dosage ranges from 35 to 80 mg/kg three times a day. Side effects include mild ataxia in dogs and sedation, anorexia, and ataxia in cats. This drug has not been approved by the Food and Drug Administration for use in cats. Intention tremors, ataxia, and hypermetria can occur in dogs when chloramphenicol and phenytoin are administered concurrently (748). These signs of phenytoin toxicity result from prolongation of phenytoin half-life by chloramphenicol. Clinical liver dysfunction has been reported in dogs receiving phenytoin and primidone in combination (743). Hepatitis, jaundice and death due to phenytoin toxicity have been reported in a 3-year-old collie dog (749).

The time-honored drug for the treatment of **status epilepticus** is diazepam (Valium) at a dose of 5 to 10 mg intravenously every 15 minutes until seizures cease. Supportive care includes insertion of an endotrachial tube, oxygen if needed, intravenous fluids and electrolytes, and maintenance of normal body temperature by cooling or warming as needed. Intravenous pentobarbital or phenobarbital, 3 to 15 mg/kg to effect, can be used if three to four doses of diazepam do not control the seizures.

It should be noted that status epilepticus not infrequently occurs following abrupt withdrawal of anticonvulsant medication. It also can occur with inappropriate anticonvulsant medication, toxicities or metabolic abnormalities, and progressive brain disease. Status epilepticus is a constant threat in animals that have clusters of seizures.

The prognosis of animals with idiopathic epilepsy is guarded for seizure control. Anticonvulsant medication can be a lifelong ordeal, and dosage adjustment may be frequent, depending on side effects and seizure frequency. Total control or elimination of seizures is unlikely in most patients. Thus, the goal of anticonvulsant therapy is to reduce the frequency and severity of attacks to a level acceptable to the owner and patient, without excessive drug-related side effects. Relapses are to be expected even in well-controlled patients. It may be necessary to use one or more drugs in trial periods to achieve successful control of seizures. When changing drugs, it is important to allow sufficient time for the new drug to become effective before discontinuing the former drug (e.g., a 50% decrement every week). Lapses in medication, either by forgetfulness of the owner or regurgitation by the animal, usually will precipitate seizures.

In some animals, especially larger breed dogs, such as German shepherds, St. Bernards, and Irish setters, seizures can be severe, often occur in clusters, and may be totally refractory to any medication. These animals are frequently euthanatized.

There probably is little justification for preventive therapy for a single seizure. Also, animals that have a mild seizure every few months may not require preventive therapy, if the owner can tolerate the attacks. Medication should begin if the frequency of attacks increases.

There is no well-defined correlation between severity and duration of seizures and underlying disease. In fact, seizures can be more severe and longer in dogs with idiopathic epilepsy compared to dogs with brain tumors or encephalitis.

It should be noted that anticonvulsant medication may be of little benefit in dogs with either progressive brain disease or metabolic dysfunction. In such animals, it is imperative that treatment be aimed at the underlying disorder.

KEY DIAGNOSTIC AIDS: **History, Breed, Age, Interictal Signs, Blood Biochemistry, Urinalysis, CSF**

Sensory Neuronopathy

A new sensory disorder has recently been reported in adult dogs of different breeds, including a 1.5-year-old Doberman pinscher, a 2-year-old Siberian husky, a 5-year-old whippet, a 6-year-old Scottish terrier, and a 4-year-old golden retriever (750; JE Steiss, unpublished information). The term "neuronopathy" refers to a type of peripheral nerve disease in which the primary changes appear in the nerve cell body. The cause has not been determined. Pathologically, the disease is characterized by pronounced degeneration and loss of dorsal root ganglion cells (and probably cells of sensory ganglia of cranial nerves), sometimes accompanied by mononuclear cell infiltration. As a result of the ganglion cell loss, dorsal nerve roots show a marked loss of larger diameter myelinated fibers, and there is a selective loss of myelinated fibers in the dorsal columns of the spinal cord. Similar degenerative changes may occur in sensory pathways of cranial nerves, such as the descending tracts of the trigeminal nerves.

The clinical course is usually insidiously progressive over several months or years. Clinical signs are variable and include proprioceptive deficits, generalized ataxia with preservation of muscle strength, and depression or absence of tendon reflexes, such the patellar reflex. Muscle atrophy is not a feature. Occasionally, an animal may develop an abnormal extension of a pelvic limb, have difficulty prehending and swallowing food, have paresthesia or abnormal sensation about the face or trunk, and demonstrate reduced deep and superficial pain sensation.

Hematological values, cerebrospinal fluid analysis, and radiographic studies are within normal limits.

Electromyographic findings are normal; however, motor nerve conduction velocity of appendicular nerves may be slower than normal. Prognosis is poor. There is no treatment.

Another example of a neuropathy affecting primary sensory neurons is that which occurs in English pointer dogs in which the salient deficit is nociceptive (pain) loss (see "**Mutilating Neuropathy**").

KEY DIAGNOSTIC AIDS: **Clinical Signs, Clinical Course, Sensory Nerve Biopsy**

Sensory Trigeminal Neuropathy

Sensory trigeminal neuropathy has been reported in a 2-year-old rough collie dog (751). The cause was not determined. Pathological abnormalities were limited to the three major branches of both trigeminal nerves and the gasserian ganglia. There was partial loss of myelinated nerve fibers in each branch and also in the spinal tract of the fifth nerve in the brainstem. It was considered that the primary abnormality was in the gasserian ganglion. Clinical signs of acute onset of excessive salivation, coughing, and dysphagia were believed to be associated with bilateral loss or absence of tactile sensation and deep pain from the face, tongue, and oral mucosa. The condition in this dog remained relatively unchanged over an 18-month period.

KEY DIAGNOSTIC AIDS: **Clinical Signs**

Sphingomyelinosis

Sphingomyelinosis (synonym is "Niemann-Pick disease") is a rare and presumably heritable lysosomal storage disease that has been reported in a 5-month-old miniature poodle dog (752) and in 3- to 4-month-old Siamese cats (753–755). The disease results from a profound deficiency of lysosomal sphingomyelinase activity, with resultant accumulations of sphingomyelin, cholesterol, and gangliosides in neurons and visceral cells of the mononuclear phagocyte system. Pathological lesions are characterized by widespread cytoplasmic swelling and vacuolation of neurons in central and peripheral nervous systems, and foamy macrophages in the lung, spleen, lymph nodes, liver, adrenal glands, and intestine. Changes are most marked in Purkinje cells of the cerebellum and neurons of the cerebellar roof nuclei and hippocampus, and in dorsal root and peripheral ganglion cells. Most lymphocytes and monocytes in blood smears contain cytoplasmic vacuoles.

Clinical signs include ataxia, hypermetria, continuous head tremors, and loss of equilibrium. Signs can progress to visual impairment, total paresis, and death. A neurogenic syndrome, without central nervous system signs, has recently been observed (JE Steiss, PA Cuddon, unpublished information). Signs in affected animals include absent conscious proprioception, severely depressed to absent spinal reflexes, hypotonia, and a palmigrade/plantigrade stance with only an ability to crawl rather than to walk or run. Pain perception and cranial nerve function are normal. Motor nerve conduction velocities are markedly depressed, and positive sharp waves and fibrillation potentials can be recorded in many appendicular muscles. While little changes are present in skeletal muscles, peripheral nerves show widespread myelin degeneration associated with many vacuolated macrophages interspersed within the nerve fibers. Necropsy examination indicated widespread infiltration of virtually every body system with sphingomyelin-laden macrophages.

Premortem diagnosis can be established by assays for leukocyte sphingomyelinase levels. Postmortem diagnosis is made most reliably by enzyme assay of brain or liver.

Prognosis is poor. There is no treatment.

KEY DIAGNOSTIC AIDS: **Breed, Age, Clinical Signs, Enzyme Assays**

Spina Bifida

This anomaly results from failure of fusion of the halves of the dorsal spinous processes with or without protrusion of the spinal cord or its membranes, or both. Spina bifida manifesta, cystica, and operta are synonymous subclassifications indicating presence of meningocele, myelocele, or meningomyelocele (756). Spina bifida occulta is characterized by a bony defect without visible protrusion of enclosed vertebral canal structures (55). Myelodysplasia, consisting of gliosis, hydromyelia (dilation of the central canal), syringomyelia (cavitations within the spinal cord) or abnormal position of the central gray matter, and anomalies of dorsal and ventral horns can also occur with spina bifida (55, 756).

The embryonic pathogenesis of this anomaly is controversial. One theory is that there is overgrowth of cells of the dorsal neural tube which interferes with fusion of the neural tube and vertebral arches (757). Another theory suggests that vertebral arches fail to fuse as a result of a neuroschistic bleb (758).

Spina bifida has been commonly reported in dogs and cats (55, 60, 361, 652, 759–764). There is a high incidence of spina bifida in young English bulldogs (652, 756). The condition may occur anywhere along the spinal column but is most common in the lumbar region. Clinical signs are often noticed when affected animals begin to ambulate and may include pelvic limb ataxia and paresis, fecal and urinary incontinence, perineal analgesia, and flaccid anal sphincter. The site of the bony defect may be marked by dimpling of the overlying skin, streaming of hair coat, and palpable cavitation in the dorsal spinous process (55, 756). Plain radiographs will demonstrate abnormalities ranging from nonfusion of dorsal laminae to a cleft spinous process. However, myelography may demonstrate protrusion of spinal cord, meninges, or both.

Prognosis is guarded to poor. Treatment is usually not attempted.

KEY DIAGNOSTIC AIDS: **Breed, Age, Clinical Signs, Radiography/Myelography**

Spinal Dysplasia

This congenital myelodysplasia most commonly occurs in weimaraner dogs and is considered to be an inherited condition transmitted by a co-dominant gene with reduced penetrance and variable expression (765). The disorder has also been reported in other breeds of dogs (81, 765–768). Prenatal studies have shown that dysraphic changes, resulting from abnormal migration of mantle cells, are evident in embryos (24 to 28 days of gestation) obtained by mating severely dysraphic weimaraner dogs (769, 770).

Pathologically, the malformation includes hydromyelia, duplication of central canal or an absent central canal, syringomyelia, usually in dorsal columns, chromatolysis and loss of nerve cell bodies in gray matter, aberrations in the dorsal median septum and ventral median tissue, and gray matter ectopias (767, 771). These morphological changes tend to present in varying degrees in various cord segments in an affected animal.

Clinical signs usually appear by 4 to 6 weeks of age; however, abnormal spinal reflexes reportedly are observed in newborn dysraphic pups (772). Affected animals have a symmetrical "bunny hopping" pelvic limb gait, wide-based stance, and overextension of pelvic limbs with depressed proprioception. Less constant signs include scoliosis, abnormal hair streams in the dorsal neck region, and koilosternia (gutter-like depression of the chest) (767). Clinical signs neither progress nor retrogress. Routine hematology, radiology, and CSF tests are usually within normal limits. Animals can lead a normal life. There is no treatment.

KEY DIAGNOSTIC AIDS: **Breed, Age, Clinical Signs**

Spinal Muscular Atrophy

Spinal muscular atrophy refers to premature degeneration and death of various neuronal cell populations in the spinal cord and/or brainstem. This form of neuronal abiotrophy has been reported in dogs and cats. Clinical signs usually are progressive. Prognosis is guarded to poor, and there is no treatment.

Spinal Muscular Atrophy of Swedish Lapland Dogs

An autosomal recessive disease has been reported in Swedish Lapland dogs (773, 774). Degeneration of Purkinje cells and spinal ganglion cells occurs together with diffuse axonal degeneration in the medullary rays of the cerebellum and projections of the dorsal roots and cranial nerves 2, 5 and 7 and in the dorsal funiculus of the spinal cord and spinocerebellar tracts. Neuronal degeneration and loss are observed in the ventral gray matter in cervical and lumbar intumescences.

Only the spinal cord lesions are detected clinically. Signs appear in affected puppies at 5 to 7 weeks of age. The onset is marked by thoracic or pelvic limb weakness that progresses rapidly to tetraparesis. Subsequent muscle wasting and deformity are most pronounced in distal portions of the limbs. Spinal reflexes are reduced or absent, and electromyographic examination reveals denervation potentials.

Spinal Muscular Atrophy of Brittany Spaniels

Hereditary spinal muscular atrophy is a dominantly inherited lower motor neuron disease in Brittany spaniels. The motor neurons of selected brainstem nuclei and ventral horn of the spinal cord are characterized by chromatolysis, neuronal depletion, and neurofibrillary abnormalities in perikarya, dendrites, and proximal axons (775–777). Three phenotypic variants have been recognized: (*a*) Early onset. Pups become weak by 1 month of age and are tetraparetic by 3 to 4 months. (*b*) Intermediate onset. Clinical signs develop between 4 and 6 months of age. Pups are tetraparetic by 2 to 3 years. (*c*) Late onset. This is characterized by slowly progressive disease with dogs surviving well into adult life.

In all three phenotypes muscle weakness first appears in proximal muscles of limb girdles and trunk. Animals walk in a waddling fashion. Progressive atrophy ensues in proximal muscles of pelvic limbs and lumbar paraspinal muscles. In some dogs, cranial nerve abnormalities are observed and include weakness and atrophy of facial muscles (causing wrinkling of facial skin and wide palpebral fissures), depressed gag reflex, and decreased muscle tone in the tongue. Severely affected animals remain in lateral recumbency and are unable to raise their heads (778).

Electromyography reveals sporadic fibrillations, fasciculations, and occasional polyphasic potentials. Nerve conduction studies are normal. Degenerative changes in peripheral nerves result in neurogenic atrophy in more proximal skeletal muscles.

Spinal Muscular Atrophy of Pointer Dogs

A hereditary disorder has been described in young pointer dogs in Japan (779). The mode of inheritance remains to be determined. Axonal degeneration is found in peripheral nerves (780). Chronic degenerative atrophy occurs in skeletal muscle. Numerous accumulated lipid-like granules are present in ventral horn cells of the spinal cord and in hypoglossal and spinal accessory nuclei of the brainstem.

Clinical signs of weakness, dysphonia, and diminished tendon reflexes are observed in affected dogs at about 5 months of age. Progressive muscular atrophy occurs in all limbs and trunk, particularly in the shoulder region. Muscle fasciculations are present. Animals eventually become tetraplegic. On electromyographic examination, fibrillation potentials and positive sharp waves are noted in epaxial and proximal and distal appendicular muscles. The clinical course of this progressive disease is 3 to 4 months. Routine hematology and radiography tests are within normal limits.

Spinal Muscular Atrophy of Giant-Breed Crosses

This rare degenerative condition (synonym is "Stockard's paralysis") was produced in 1936 by cross-breeding Great Danes with bloodhounds and St. Bernards. Pathological changes include degeneration and depletion of motor and preganglionic sympathetic neurons in ventral and intermediolateral horns of lumbar spinal cord (781). The disease is transmitted through an inheritable multiple factor involving at least three dominant genes.

Clinical signs occur at 3 months of age and are characterized by sudden onset of paresis and posterior paralysis and atrophy of pelvic limb appendicular muscles.

Similar disorders have been reported sporadically in young collie sheepdogs (782), a 10-week-old domestic shorthair kitten (783), a 12-week-old collie puppy (784), and Siamese kittens (58).

KEY DIAGNOSTIC AIDS: **Breed, Age, Clinical Signs, Electrodiagnostics**

Spinal Trauma

Spinal trauma of sufficient magnitude to cause vertebral fractures, luxation/subluxations, or traumatic disk extrusion usually results in serious spinal cord concussion and/or laceration. Spinal injury of this type is one of the more frequent neurological disorders seen in clinical practice. Common causes include automobile accidents, falls, gunshot wounds, and fight injuries. Fractures and luxations of the spine generally occur at the junction of movable and stable spinal segments, such as atlanto-occipital, cervicothoracic, thoracolumbar, and lumbosacral areas. The thoracic vertebrae reportedly comprise the most immobile portion of the spinal column (109, 785), and the most frequent site of spinal fracture and/or luxation in the dog is the thoracolumbar junction. Cervical spinal subluxation at the C5-C6 level has been reported in several dogs as a result of fight injuries, suggesting a possible anatomical predisposition for this type of injury (786, 787). Traumatic injuries of the spinal column have been arbitrarily divided into (*a*) ventral compartment injuries involving the vertebral body, intervertebral disk, dorsal/ventral longitudinal ligaments, and intertransverse ligaments; and (*b*) dorsal compartment injuries involving the lamina, pedicles, dorsal spinous processes, articular processes, and supraspinous/interspinous/interarcuate ligaments (788). Combined compartment injuries are often seen in animals following spinal trauma.

Spinal cord trauma usually is immediate. Aside from the obvious mechanical injury to the cord at the time of spinal trauma, a sequence of events may be initiated (possibly by prostaglandins and biogenic amines such as 5-hydroxytryptamine and norepinephrine) that results in a progressive autodestructive process within the cord. In severe spinal cord injury this inherent process will be irreversible with resultant permanent paralysis. Impact injuries of less magnitude can induce transient spinal cord dysfunction, probably associated with such reversible changes as tissue ischemia, hypoxia, edema, and varying degrees of demyelination.

Spinal cord injuries are characterized pathologically by variable degrees of ischemia, edema, hemorrhagic necrosis of central gray matter with adjacent neuronal degeneration, demyelination, and focal malacia. Localized edema may result in pronounced cord swelling and collapse of the subarachnoid space. After several days, lipid macrophages are observed in necrotic areas. More chronic cases are characterized by cystic spaces and increased density of astrocytic and microglial cells, and gray matter can appear fenestrated due to loss of neurons and fibers.

Clinical signs typically are acute in onset, usually nonprogressive, and either stable or improve with time. In rare cases in which clinical signs are progressive, continued bleeding and/or excessive bony movement at the site of injury should be suspected. Clinical syndromes seen with spinal fractures and luxations are cervical, cervicothoracic, thoracolumbar, or lumbosacral. Localization of the lesion in such cases usually can be determined with the animal in lateral recumbency. The animal should be handled carefully with minimal manipulation so as to avoid further cord injury from the unstable vertebrae.

Radiography usually will demonstrate obvious fractures and luxations of the vertebral column. The degree of luxation has no prognostic value. In some animals, the degree of luxation that is seen radiographically may have been much worse at the time of the injury, e.g., a severe luxation resulting in spinal cord transection may return to normal immediately after the accident. Traumatic disk extrusion sometimes occurs with spinal injury and may be suggested radiographically by the presence of a narrowed disk space. Rarely, severe spinal cord contusion can occur in the absence of verterbal or disk damage. In such cases, myelographic studies may help to delineate an area of spinal cord swelling which may be present up to 36 hours after the injury. The entire vertebral column should be evaluated radiographically to rule out more than one site of vertebral fracture, luxation, or traumatic disk extrusion.

Prompt medical and surgical treatment is mandatory. Dexamethasone at a dose of 2 to 4 mg/kg intravenously, repeated at 6- to 8-hour intervals, should be administered for up to 36 hours. Thereafter, the dose can be gradually reduced on a twice-daily basis over 3 to 5 days. Mannitol should also be given at a dose of 1 to 2 gm/kg intravenously, slowly over 10 minutes and repeated once or twice at 3- to 4-hour intervals. Medical management is usually combined with prompt surgical decompression of the spinal cord (e.g., dorsolateral hemilaminectomy), vertebral reduction, and internal stabilization (e.g., using a vertebral body plate) in patients with fractures and luxations. Animals with luxations and mild paresis may require only stabilization without decompression. Paretic animals without evidence of vertebral column injury can be managed with medical treatment and strict cage rest for 1 to 2 weeks.

Prognosis of animals with acute spinal cord injury is always guarded. In general (following medical and surgical treatment), animals that are paretic or paralyzed but have normal pain sensation may have a favorable prognosis. Clinical signs can be expected to improve within 2 to 3 weeks. Animals that are paralyzed with reduced pain sensation have a guarded or poor prognosis. Any clinical improvement should be seen within 3 to 6 weeks. Paralyzed animals with loss of pain sensation have a grave prognosis. Early decompressive surgery (e.g., within 4 hours of the accident) in conjunction with medical treatment will have a positive effect on the return of clinical function and on the rate of recovery of animals with severe paresis/paralysis but with normal pain sensation. Animals with cervicothoracic or lumbosacral syndromes can have a more guarded prognosis than animals with cervical or thoracolumbar syndromes due to potential involvement of irreversible gray matter lesions and, hence, of permanent damage to nerves that innervate the limb muscles and/or vital structures, such as the bladder.

KEY DIAGNOSTIC AIDS: Historical Data, Clinical Signs, Radiography

Spondylosis Deformans

This is a degenerative disorder of the vertebral column characterized by the presence of vertebral osteophytes at intervertebral spaces, resulting in the formation of spurs or complete bony bridges (154, 789–791). While the condition is believed to be associated with degenerative changes in the annus fibrosus of the intervertebral disks, it is rarely observed in chondrodystrophoid breeds that are frequently affected with disk diseases.

Spondylosis deformans has been reported in dogs and cats, usually middle-aged but some as early as 2 years of age. In one comprehensive canine study, five large breeds of dogs (flat-coated retriever, Irish setter, boxer, bloodhound, and Rhodesian ridgeback) were identified as having a high risk of spondylosis deformans, and females had a significantly higher incidence than males (792). The incidence increases with age. In dogs, vertebral sites most often affected are T9-T10 and L7-S1. The distribution at these areas of maximal spinal mobility in dogs (154, 793) suggests that mechanical factors may play a role in the pathogenesis.

Osteophytes tend to develop on ventral, lateral, or dorsolateral aspects of vertebral margins. Osteophytic projections into the spinal canal with compression of the spinal cord are rare.

Spondylosis deformans in dogs and cats tends to be a subclinical disorder. Localized pain or lameness may occur in association with fracture of bony spurs or bridges. Diagnosis is based on radiographic findings. Osteophytes have a smooth ventral border and a curved beak-like appearance. Treatment is symptomatic. Prognosis is good.

KEY DIAGNOSTIC AIDS: **Age, Clinical Signs, Radiography**

Spongiform Degeneration

Rare, variable spongiform degenerative conditions, possibly hereditary in nature, have been recognized in young dogs and cats.

A suspected genetic disorder occurs in the Egyptian Mau breed of cat (a small breed derived from the Siamese cat) (794). There is widespread vacuolation of white and gray matter of brain and spinal cord. There is no evidence of myelin breakdown. Clinical signs are first noticed in kittens at 7 weeks of age and are characterized by pelvic limb ataxia and hypermetria. Subsequent signs include intermittent periods of severe depression and reduced activity, with frequent flicking movements of distal pelvic limbs when at full flexion. The condition may improve with age.

Spongiform degeneration has also been described in the dog. In a Samoyed puppy, a generalized vacuolation of white matter throughout brain and spinal cord has been reported, with most severe changes being found in the cerebellum (795). Pelvic limb tremors were observed at 12 days of age, progressing to generalized tremors over the next 5 days. A similar spongiform change is described in the cerebral and cerebellar white matter, but not in spinal cord, of silky terrier puppies (796). A large number of Alzheimer type II protoplasmic astrocytes are found in severely affected areas. Clinical signs are noted at birth and consist of uncontrolled intermittent contractures of the vertebral column, especially muscles of the thoracolumbar region at intervals of approximately 2/second. Occasionally the pelvic limbs are lifted off the ground during these contractures. The episodes are intensified with excitement. Low-intensity contractions continue during sleep. Signs do not appear to be progressive.

Spongiform degeneration of the white matter of the CNS and peripheral nervous system, with most prominent lesions in cerebellar peduncle, deep cerebellar white matter to cerebral white matter, has been observed in two young female Labrador retriever littermates, between 4 and 6 months of age (797). Clinical signs are characterized by progressive ataxia and dysmetria of head, trunk, and limbs, hyporeflexia with clonus, and extensor rigidity with episodes of exaggerated rigidity and episthotonus and muscle atrophy. Clinical signs were noted between 4 and 6 months of age. Routine hematology, blood chemistries, urinalysis, and CSF tests are all within normal limits. Prognosis of dogs with this disorder appears to be guarded to poor. Treatment with acepromazine (0.25 mg/kg intramuscularly) may reduce the episodes of extensor rigidity. Phenobarbital, 5 mg/kg/day orally may produce temporary improvement of signs.

KEY DIAGNOSTIC AIDS: **Breed, Age, Clinical Signs**

Steroid Myopathy

This myopathy is associated with exogenous administration of glucocorticoids resulting in iatrogenic hyperadrenocorticism (417, 418). Clinical, electrophysiological, and pathological data are identical to those described for spontaneous hyperadrenocorticism.

KEY DIAGNOSTIC AIDS: **History, Clinical Signs, Plasma Cortisol Levels, Muscle Biopsy**

Strychnine Poisoning

Strychnine is a poison used for control of squirrels, gophers, rabbits, and other wild carnivora. Dogs, and infrequently cats, become poisoned when they eat strychnine baits intended for mammalian pests (798, 799). Dogs also are commonly poisoned maliciously. Strychnine acts at the brainstem and spinal cord level by blocking the motor inhibitory neurotransmitter, glycine. Clinical signs of poisoning are manifested by uncontrolled impulses reaching skeletal muscles and are characterized by retraction of the corners of the mouth, drawing together of the ears, stiffness of muscles of the neck, chest, and abdomen, stiffness of gait, and assumption of a "sawhorse" stance followed by tonic extension of the limbs, opisthotonus, vocalization, and difficult respiration. Affected animals are hypersensitive to auditory and tactile stimui. Consciousness is not lost during initial "seizural" attacks. After several minutes, the attack(s) may subside, only to be followed by further episodes. Eventually, the respiratory muscles may be unable to function. Apnea can lead to cerebral anoxia, loss of consciousness, and death. The entire course may last from 30 minutes to 1 to 2 hours, if the animal is untreated.

A presumptive diagnosis is based on a history of ingestion and characteristic clinical signs. Chemical confirmation can be made from stomach contents and/or vomitus. Prognosis is guarded, depending on the amount of poison ingested and/or the promptness of treatment. The main objectives of treatment are to keep the muscles relaxed and to prevent asphyxia. Muscle relaxants recommended include glyceryl guaiacolate ether given in an intravenous dose of 110 mg/kg in either a 5 or $33\frac{1}{3}\%$ solution (800). This drug controls "seizures" for up to 60 minutes. It can be safely repeated as needed. Methocarbamol (Robaxin) also can be used, at a dose of 150 mg/kg intravenously, repeated as needed. Supportive treatment includes prompt gastric or enterogastric lavage using 1 to 2% tannic acid or 1:2000 potassium permanganate and enemas. Forced diuresis with 5% mannitol in isotonic saline and acidification of urine with 150 mg/kg of body weight of ammonium chloride orally will enhance urinary elimination of strychnine. If the animal survives 24 hours, prognosis for complete recovery is very good.

KEY DIAGNOSTIC AIDS: **History, Clinical Signs, Analysis of Vomitus/Stomach Contents**

Syncope

Syncope (synonym "fainting") refers to a sudden loss of consciousness resulting from paroxysmal episodes of cerebral deprivation of oxygen and/or glucose. The incidence of syncope in animals is believed to be low. Syncope most commonly occurs secondary to decreased cerebral perfusion, e.g., arrhythmias (cardiac conduction defects, tachyarrhythmias, bradyarrhythmias), cardiac malformation (tetralogy of Fallot, patent ductus arteriosus, septal defects, aortic stenosis, and chronic valvular fibrosus), and rarely to increased intracranial pressure due to edema, tumors, hemorrhage, or inflammation (801, 802). Sick sinus syndrome, associated with abnormally long (e.g., 2- to 6-second) intervals of sinus arrest, occurs frequently in middle-aged miniature schnauzers and boxers. Chlorpromazine can be given slowly intravenously in doses of up to 1 mg/kg in order to enhance the ECG abnormality.

Syncope also can be associated with heartworm disease, coughing, hypoglycemia, acid-base imbalance, severe anemia, polycythemia, and such iatrogenic factors as digitalis intoxication.

Clinical signs typically have an abrupt onset and are characterized by ataxia, collapse, and loss of consciousness. Attacks sometimes are accompanied by uncoordinated involuntary muscle activity, defecation, and/or urination as a result of cerebral ischemia. The entire episode may last no more than 15 to 20 seconds, after which the animal quickly recovers to a normal state. Attacks may or may not be preceded by periods of excitement. Syncope due to cardiac malformations usually is associated with exercise.

Clinical examination frequenty reveals signs of disease sufficient to explain the syncopal episodes. Diagnosis can be substantiated by electrocardiographic, hematological, and chest radiographic studies.

Prognosis is guarded depending upon the underlying cause. Arrhythmias can respond favorably to medication, and certain cardiac malformations are readily amenable to surgical correction. Metabolic abnormalities usually are reversible.

KEY DIAGNOSTIC AIDS: **Historical Data, Clinical Signs, ECG**

Tetanus

Tetanus is a bacterial disease caused by *Clostridium tetani* that can affect all domestic animals and man (55). Disease occurs as a result of localization of tetanus spores in an anaerobic environment such as a necrotic wound, with conversion to a vegetative, toxin-producing form. The organisms produce an exotoxin within 4 to 8 hours, which travels via peripheral nerves to the central nervous system (803). A transsynaptic migration of tetanus toxin occurs in spinal cord motor neurones (804). Toxin binds the release of inhibitory neurotransmitter from interneurons, resulting in release of motor neurons (especially alpha) from inhibition and subsequent hyperexcitability.

Considerable species differences exist in susceptibility to tetanus. The dog is much less susceptible than the horse. Tetanus in the cat is very rare. Clinical signs usually are observed within 5 to 10 days of infection (55, 805–807a) and include stiffness of gait with extensor rigidity in all limbs, dyspnea, and spasms of the masticatory and pharyngeal muscles resulting in trismus and dysphagia. The tail may be elevated, facial muscles may be contracted to give a sneering expression ("risus sardonicus") with wrinkling of the forehead, and the third eyelid may be protruded. Ear flaps are usually held in an erect fashion. In severe disease, the animal may be recumbent and opisthotonic. Death results from respiratory failure. Affected animals are hypersensitive to external stimuli.

Diagnosis of the severe form of tetanus is largely based on characteristic clinical data. Mild forms of the disease may be difficult to diagnose since there are no specific ancillary aids available. There is a lack of the usually observed electrical silence following needle insertion in electromyograhic studies. Nerve conduction studies are normal.

Prognosis is usually favorable with treatment, which consists of aqueous penicillin G (20,000 to 50,000 IU/kg four times a day in dogs) and immediate administration of tetanus antitoxin (TAT) at 100 to 500 IU/kg intravenously (808). A test dose (e.g., 0.1 ml) of antitoxin can be given subcutaneously 20 minutes prior to the intravenous dosage and the animal observed for any allergic reaction. In cats, penicillin is used at a dosage of about 80,000 units/kg intramuscularly once a day for a minimum of 5 days. If a wound is present, radical debridement and excision of all infected or necrotic-appearing tissue should be performed, along with peroxide irrigation to reverse the anaerobic state, and local instillation of 10,000 units of TAT and 1,000,000 units of aqueous penicillin G.

Complete remission of clinical signs in dogs and cats may take 30 days or longer; however, there are no permanent aftereffects.

KEY DIAGNOSTIC AIDS: **Historical Data, Clinical Signs**

Thiamine Deficiency

Thiamine or vitamin B_1 deficiency (synonym is "Chastek paralysis") occurs sporadically in dogs and cats if their rations are naturally low in thiamine or if their food is cooked before feeding. In cats especially, thiamine deficiency may occur with an all-fish diet that contains thiaminase (809, 810). Many freshwater and saltwater fish contain thiaminase, the activity of which is highest in viscera.

The critical enzymatic effect in thiamine deficiency is in the oxidative decarboxylation of pyruvic acid. This reaction is essential for complete oxidation of glucose through the citric acid cycle. Tissues dependent on glucose or lactate-pyruvate for energy, such as the brain and heart, are particularly compromised in thiamine deficiency.

Pathological findings in dogs and cats are similar and are characterized by bilaterally symmetrical spongy changes, necrosis, and hemorrhage of upper brainstem nuclei, primarily in periventricular gray matter. The inferior colliculi are consistently involved. Foci of myofiber necrosis can be found on the heart.

Clinical signs in dogs include anorexia, depression, progressive spastic paraparesis, torticollis, circling, exophthalmos, generalized seizures, recumbency, and death (811, 812). In cats, vestibular signs, ataxia, seizures, ventroflexion of the head, and dilated, poorly responsive pupils can be observed (809). In advanced cases, semicoma, persistent crying, opisthotonus, and limb spasticity and death may occur (810, 813).

In the early stages of the disease prompt administration of thiamine hydrochloride can result in complete remission of clinical signs. Parenteral (subcutaneously, intramuscularly, or intravenously) thiamine therapy for dogs is 5 to 50 mg, and for cats is 1 to 20 mg.

KEY DIAGNOSTIC AIDS: **Dietary History, Clinical Signs**

Tick Paralysis

This is a flaccid, afebrile ascending motor paralysis in domestic and wild animals and man, produced by a neurotoxin generated by some but not all strains of certain species of ticks. Not all infested animals become paralyzed. The common wood tick, *Dermacentor variabilis*, and *Dermacentor andersoni* are incriminated most often. In Australia, *Ixodes holocyclus* is the most important species. Adult ticks, especially female, produce a salivary neurotoxin that circulates in the host animal and interferes with acetylcholine liberation at the neuromuscular junction.

Onset of clinical signs is gradual, paralysis first becoming evident as an incoordination in the pelvic limbs resulting in an unsteady gait. Altered voice, cough, and dysphagia can be early signs. Dogs become recumbent in 24 to 72 hours. Reflexes are lost but sensation is preserved. Jaw muscle weakness and facial paresis may be present. Death may occur in several days from respiratory paralysis.

Electromyographic studies reveal absence of spontaneous potentials and lack of motor unit action potentials. No muscle response follows direct nerve stimulation. Nerve conduction velocity may be slower than normal.

Prognosis is usually good with recovery occurring in 1 to 3 days following tick removal or dipping the animal in an insecticide solution. In Australia, a hyperimmune serum is used to treat humans and dogs affected with paralysis caused by *I. holocyclus.* The prognosis for this form of tick paralysis is guarded even with tick removal, insecticide treatment, and administration of hyperimmune serum (814).

KEY DIAGNOSTIC AIDS: **History, Clinical Signs, Response to Tick Removal/Dipping**

Toxoplasmosis

Toxoplasmosis is an infectious condition caused by the protozoal parasite *Toxoplasma gondii* and occurs in acquired and congenital forms in man and animals (815, 816). Cats are the definitive host for this parasite. The three known infective stages of *Toxoplasma* are bradyzoites, tachyzoites, and sporozoites. The three modes of transmission are carnivorism, fecal contamination, and transplacental or congenital infection. These modes of transmission involve the different infective stages as follows: carnivorous ingestion of bradyzoites, tachyzoites, or both; contamination with feline feces containing sporozoites of sporulated oocysts; transplacental infection of the fetus with tachyzoites after ingestion of encysted bradyzoites or sporulated oocysts by the mother (817). *Toxoplasma* oocysts are shed in feline feces unsporulated and are not infective until sporulated (1 to 5 days). Sporulated oocysts can survive in soil for several months. Land snails, earthworms, flies, and cockroaches may serve as transport hosts for oocysts. Most mammals become intermediate hosts through ingestion of oocysts.

T. gondii is highly adapted to transmission by encysted bradyzoites via carnivorism. This applies particularly to cats. Man, sheep, pigs, dogs, and (rarely) cats are known to transmit *T. gondii* transplacentally. In man, congenital infection occurs only when a woman becomes infected during pregnancy (818). Congenitally infected children may have signs of retinochoroiditis, hydrocephalus, seizures, and cerebral calcification.

The incidence of clinical toxoplasmosis is low in dogs and cats. Toxoplasmosis is a systemic infection affecting most organs and the CNS in particular (819–821). Pathologically, perivascular cuffing, diffuse and focal infiltration of meninges by lymphocytes, plasma cells, and histiocytes, hemorrhage, edema, necrosis, and neuronal degeneration have been described throughout the CNS. In some instances, a granulomatous reaction may be observed. *Toxoplasma* organisms may be found extracellularly and/or in cysts. It has been hypothesized that immaturity and concurrent distemper infection contribute to an increased susceptibility of dogs to toxoplasmosis (822, 823).

Clinical neurological signs associated with toxoplasmosis are variable and may reflect a focal or multifocal disease process. In dogs signs include hyperexcitability, depression, intention tremor, paresis, paralysis, and seizures (821–824). Clinically apparent encephalomyelitis is uncommon in cats. Pneumonia is the most important clinical manifestation of feline toxoplasmosis (825–827). Ocular toxoplasmosis also has been reported (827).

Cerebrospinal fluid is usually abnormal with elevated protein content and a mixed monocytic-polymorphonuclear pleocytosis. Xanthochromia will be present if hemorrhage has occurred.

Several serological procedures are available for detection of antibodies of *T. gondii*. The most specific, and most expensive, is the cytoplasm modifying or "dye" test of Sabin and Feldman. Other tests include the indirect fluorescent antibody, indirect hemagglutination, agglutination, and complement fixation.

Prognosis is guarded once animals manifest neurological signs. Sulfonamides and pyrimethamine are two drugs widely used for therapy of systemic toxoplasmosis.

KEY DIAGNOSTIC AIDS: **Age, Clinical Signs, Serology**

Toxoplasma Myositis

This is probably the most commonly reported infectious myositis in small animals, even through the incidence is low (822, 824, 828–830). The disease tends to be more severe in young dogs, especially those less than 6 months of age. The exact pathogenesis of toxoplasmosis is speculative. While the predilection for the neuromuscular system is accepted, its myotropism in congenital and chronic infections remain enigmatic. Exacerbations of disease may reflect depression of immune mechanisms. Histological changes include variation in fiber size as a result of pronounced fiber atrophy, severe multifocal or diffuse myonecrosis, and mononuclear granulomatous inflammation. Free *Toxoplasma* organisms are frequently seen within muscle fibers. Interstitial fibrosis is pronounced in chronic cases.

Toxoplasma myositis results in progressive pelvic limb paresis, synchronous hopping gait, and bilateral rigidity of the pelvic limbs. Rigid pelvic limb muscles are nonpainful on palpation and slowly become atrophic. A fulminating disease resulting in tetraplegia over 1 week has been observed in two mature dogs (between 4 and 5 years of age) with toxoplasmosis (KG Braund, unpublished information). Extremely severe myonecrosis and mononuclear cell infiltrations were found in all skeletal muscles. *Toxoplasma* organisms were identified in muscle and CNS.

Diagnosis is based on clinical data, positive serological evidence, and histological demonstration of the organism in lesions from muscle biopsy samples (831). Prognosis is poor when signs of pelvic limb spasticity are observed. Furthermore, many affected animals have concomitant lesions in the central nervous system.

KEY DIAGNOSTIC AIDS: **Age, Clinical Signs, Serology, Muscle Biopsy**

Traumatic Neuropathy

Trauma to peripheral nerves (usually spinal rather than cranial) is the most common cause of neuropathies in animals. Nerve injuries may result from mechanical blows, gunshot, fractures, pressure, and stretching (see "Brachial Plexus Avulsion") (832–834). Iatrogenic causes include crushing, cutting, spearing the nerve with an intramedullary pin, compression by casts or splints, and injecting agents into or adjacent to the nerve.

Nerve damage may be defined in terms of structural damage. "Neurotmesis" is complete severance of all structures of the nerve with wallerian degeneration (axonal necrosis and myelin fragmentation) of the distal stump. "Axonotmesis" consists of damage to the nerve fibers resulting in degeneration; however, the endoneurial and Schwann cell sheaths remain intact and provide a framework for axonal regeneration. "Neuropraxia" is an interruption in the function and conduction of a nerve, without structural damage.

The regenerative ability of a nerve is directly proportional to the amount of continuity of connective tissue structures of the nerve. In neuropraxic and axonotmesic lesions where the endoneurial connective tissue and Schwann cells remain intact, the potential for axonal regeneration is good. In neurotmesis, axonal regeneration is usually frustrated by lack of connective tissue scaffold or growth tubes. Also, scar tissue tends to interfere with sprouting axons, resulting in neuroma formation (835). Once an axon has grown past the point of injury and penetrates a Schwann tube in the distal nerve stump, remyelination occurs. Axonal regeneration is considered to occur at a rate of 1 to 4 mm/day.

Clinical signs of cranial and spinal nerve dysfunction are outlined in Table 3.4.

Diagnosis of traumatic neuropathy is usually based on history and clinical signs. Electrodiagnostic data may be helpful in evaluating nerve integrity and severity of damage and in monitoring progress/regeneration. Approximately 5 to 7 days postinjury are required before increased insertional activity and spontaneous potentials (positive sharp waves and fibrillation potentials) are detected. Nerve integrity may be easily assessed by nerve stimulation proximal and distal to the site of the lesion. Exploratory surgery has been advocated as another method for direct evaluation of peripheral nerve damage.

Prognosis is guarded with peripheral nerve injury. Lesions characterized by neuropraxia and axonotmesis have a better prognosis than those of neurotmesis.

The closer the nerve injury is to the muscle it must reinnervate the better the prognosis. Self-mutilation can be a major complication that results from abnormal sensation in an affected area produced by regeneration of sensory nerves.

Treatment may involve surgical anastomosis or neurolysis. In those instances where nerve damage is chronic, high, or severe, procedures for muscle relocation and muscle tendon transfers have been described (836, 837). Physical therapy, such as whirlpool bath, may help to overcome circulation problems and delay muscle atrophy.

KEY DIAGNOSTIC AIDS: **History, Clinical Signs**

Trigeminal Neuritis

Bilateral paralysis of muscles of mastication occurs in dogs and cats and is characterized by acute onset of inability to close the jaw (838). Pathologically, a bilateral nonsuppurative neuritis is found in all motor branches of the trigeminal nerve and ganglion, associated with demyelination and occasional fiber degeneration. Sensory perception of the head is normal. The disease appears to be self-limiting, and recovery usually occurs in 2 to 3 weeks.

KEY DIAGNOSTIC AIDS: **Clinical Signs, Clinical Course**

Vitamin E/Selenium-Responsive Myopathy

Vitamin E/selenium-responsive myopathies (synonyms are "white muscle disease," "nutritional myopathy," and "selenium-responsive myopathy") have been reported in sheep, cattle, pigs, horses, and poultry but only rarely in dogs (839–

Table 3.4.   Spinal Nerve Dysfunction

Nerve	Spinal Cord Origin	Muscles Innervated	Clinical Signs of Dysfunction
		THORACIC LIMB	
1. Suprascapular	C6–C7	Supraspinatus Infraspinatus	Loss of shoulder extension; muscle atrophy with prominent spine of scapula
2. Axillary	C7–C8	Deltoideus Teres major Teres minor	Reduced shoulder flexion; deltoid atrophy; reduced sensation over lateral surface of shoulder
3. Musculocutaneous	C6–C8	Biceps brachii Brachialis Coracobrachialis	Reduced elbow flexion; loss of bicipital reflex; reduced sensation over medial surface of forearm
4. Radial	C7–T2	Triceps brachii Extensor carpi radialis Ulnaris lateralis Lateral digital extensor Common digital extensor	Reduced extension of elbow, carpus, and digits; loss of extensor postural thrust and limb support (with high radial damage, i.e., above the elbow); loss of triceps reflex; reduced sensation over dorsal surface of paw and craniolateral surface of forearm
5. Median	C8–T2	Flexor carpi radialis Superficial digital flexor	Reduced flexion of carpus and digits; reduced sensation over palmar surface of paw
6. Ulnar	C8–T2	Flexor carpi ulnaris Deep digital flexor	Reduced flexion of carpus and digits; reduced senation over caudal surface of forearm
		PELVIC LIMB	
1. Femoral	L4–L6	Iliopsoas Quadriceps Sartorius	Inability to extend stifle or bear weight on affected limb; loss of patellar reflex; reduced sensation over medial surface of paw, hock, stifle, and thigh (via sensory saphenous nerve)
2. Obturator	L5–L6	External obturator Pectineus Gracilis	Inability to adduct hip or thigh (animal "does the splits" on a smooth surface)
3. Sciatic	L6–S1	Biceps femoris Semimembranosus Semitendinosus	Inability to flex stifle; loss of flexor reflex (for other dysfunction see branches of sciatic nerve—tibial and common peroneal nerves)
(a) Tibial	L7–S1	Gastrocnemius Popliteus Deep digital flexor Superficial digital flexor	Inability to extend hock or flex digits; reduced sensation over plantar surface of paw; loss of gastrocnemius reflex

Table 3.4—*Continued*

Nerve	Spinal Cord Origin	Muscles Innervated	Clinical Signs of Dysfunction
(b) Common peroneal	L6–L7	Peroneus longus Lateral digital extensor Long digital extensor Cranial tibial	Inability to flex hock or extend digits; knuckling of dorsal paw; reduced sensation over craniodorsal surface of paw, hock, and stifle
4. Pudenal	S1–S3	External anal sphincter Striated urethral muscle	Loss of anal reflex and bulbocavernosus reflex (males only); reduced sensation of perineum
5. Pelvic (parasympathetic)	S1–S3	Smooth muscle of bladder and rectum	Urinary incontinence

841). This myopathy is associated with low dietary levels of selenium and/or vitamin E. The pathogenesis of the disorder is unknown. Skeletal muscle lesions tend to be bilaterally symmetrical and may affect individual or several muscle groups. Grossly the affected muscle is paler than normal and may show distinct chalky longitudinal striations. Histological findings are characterized by necrosis, phagocytosis, proliferation of sarcolemmal nuclei, loss of striations, and fiber regeneration.

Clinical signs include weakness, dysphagia, sialosis, dysphonia, stiff-stilted gait, and difficulty in rising from a recumbent position. Sudden death is reported in newborn puppies. Signs may be exacerbated with exercise. Muscle enzymes are often elevated.

Diagnosis is based on historical, clinical, and pathological data. Animals usually recover after selenium and/or vitamin E replacement therapy.

A confirmed case of a myopathy due to a deficiency of vitamin E has been reported in a cat that was fed a diet consisting almost entirely of boiled Norwegian coley (842). Muscles in the pelvic limbs were swollen, hot, and very painful on palpation. Muscle changes were similar to those reported in dogs. Complete clinical recovery occurred within 14 days following correct dietary management.

KEY DIAGNOSTIC AIDS: **Dietary History, Clinical Signs, Muscle Biopsy**

References

1. Bestetti G, Buhlmann V, Nicolet J, Fankhauser R: Paraplegia due to *Actinomyces viscosus* infection in a cat. *Acta Neuropathol* 39:231–235, 1977.
2. Heavner JE, Pierce M: Brain abscess in a dog. *Vet Med Small Anim Clin* 76:785–793, 1976.
3. Mccandlish IAP, Ormerod EJ: Brain abscess associated with a penetrating foreign body. *Vet Rec* 102:380–381, 1978.
4. Rhoades HE, Reynolds HA, Rahn DP, Small E: Nocardiosis in a dog with multiple lesions of the central nervous system. *J Am Vet Med Assoc* 142:278–281, 1963.
5. Stowater JL, Codner EC, McCoy JC: Actinomycosis in the spinal canal of a cat *Feline Pract* 8:26–27, 1978.
6. Allen PBR, Speakman TJ: Brain abscess: an evaluation of current treatment. *Can Med Assoc J* 86:852–854, 1962.
7. Jarvis CA, Burkhart RL, Koprowski H: Demyelinating encephalomyelitis in the dog associated with antirabies vaccination. *Am J Hyg* 50:14–26, 1949.
8. Gage ED, Hoerlein BF, Bartels JE: Spinal cord compression resulting from a leptomeningeal cyst in the dog. *J Am Vet Med Assoc* 152:1664–1670, 1968.
9. Parker AJ, Adams WM, Zachary JF: Spinal arachnoid cysts in the dog. *J Am Anim Hosp Assoc* 19:1001–1008, 1983.

10. Gage ED: Atlanto-axial subluxation. In Bojrab MJ (ed): *Current Techniques in Small Animal Surgery.* Philadelphia, Lea and Febiger, 1975, p 376.

11. Geary JC: Canine spinal lesions not involving disks. *J Am Vet Med Assoc* 155:2038–2044, 1969.

12. Geary JC, Oliver JE, Hoerlein BF: Atlanto-axial subluxation in the canine. *J Small Anim Pract* 8:577–582, 1967.

13. Ladds P, Guffy M, Blauch B, Splitter G: Congenital odontoid process separation in two dogs. *J Small Anim Pract* 12:463–471, 1970.

14. Parker AJ, Park RD: Atlanto-axial subluxation in small breeds of dogs. Diagnosis and pathogenesis. *Vet Med Small Anim Clin* 68:1133–1137, 1973.

15. Cook JR, Oliver JE: Atlantoaxial luxation in the dog. *Comp Cont Educ* 3:242–252, 1981.

16. Richter K, Lorenzana R, Ettinger SJ: Traumatic displacement of the dens in a cat: case report *J Am Anim Hosp Assoc* 19:751–753, 1983.

17. Watson AG: Congenital occipitoatlantoaxial malformation (OAM) in a dog. *Anat Histol Embryol* 8:187, 1979.

18. Watson AG, Hall MA, de Lahunta A: Congenital occipitoatlantoaxial malformation in a cat. *Comp Cont Educ* 7:245–254, 1985.

19. Morgan JP: *Radiology in Veterinary Orthopedics.* Philadelphia, Lea and Febiger, 1972.

20. Oliver JE, Lewis PE; Lesions of the atlas and axis in dogs. *J Am Anim Hosp Assoc* 9:304–313, 1973.

21. Gage ED, Hoerlein BF: Surgical repair of cervical subluxation and spondylolisthesis in the dog. *J Am Anim Hosp Assoc* 9:385–390, 1973.

22. Gage ED, Smallwood JE; Surgical repair of atlanto-axial subluxation in a dog. *Vet Med Small Anim Clin* 65:583–592, 1970.

23. Kishigami M: Application of an atlantoaxial retractor for atlantoaxial subluxation in the cat and dog. *J Am Anim Hosp Assoc* 20:413–419, 1984.

24. Gilmore DR: Nonsurgical management of four cases of atlantoaxial subluxation in the dog. *J Am Anim Hosp Assoc* 20:93–96, 1984.

25. Whitney JC: Atrophic myositis in a dog: the differentiation of this disease from eosinophilic myositis. *Vet Rec* 69:130–131, 1957.

26. Whitney JC; A case of cranial myodegeneration (atrophic myositis) in a dog. *J Small Anim Pract* 11:735–742, 1970.

27. Farnbach GC: Myositis in the dog. *Comp Cont Educ* 1:183–188, 1979.

28. Purchase HS; Cerebral babesiosis in dogs. *Vet Rec* 59:269–270, 1947.

29. Okoh AEJ: A case of cerebral babesiosis in the dog. *Bull Anim Health Prod Afr* 26:118–119, 1978.

30. Blakemore WF, Rees-Evans ET, Wheeler PEG: Botulism in foxhounds. *Vet Rec* 100:57, 1977.

31. Darke PGG, Roberts TA, Smart JL, Bradshaw PR: Suspected botulism in foxhounds. *Vet Rec* 99:98–99, 1976.

32. Pilet C, Cazabat H, Ardonceau R: Une nouvelle enzootic de botulisme chez le chien de meute *Bull Acad Vet Fr* 32:297–303, 1959.

33. Barsanti JA, Walser M, Hatheway CL, Bowen JM, Crowell W: Type C botulism in American foxhounds. *J Am Vet Med Assoc* 172:809–813, 1978.

34. Cornelissen JM, Haagsma J, van Nes JJ: Type C botulism in five dogs. *J Am Anim Hosp Assoc* 21:401–404, 1985.

35. Kao I, Drachman DB, Price DL; Botulinum toxin: mechanism of presynaptic blockade. *Science* 193:1256–1258, 1976.

36. van Nes JJ, van der Most, van Spijk D: Electrophysiologic evidence of peripheral nerve dysfunction in six dogs with botulism type C. *Res Vet Sci* in press.

37. Griffiths IR, Duncan ID, Barker J: A progressive axonopathy of boxer dogs affecting the central and peripheral nervous systems. *J Small Anim Pract* 21:29–43, 1980.

38. Wright JA, Brownlie S: Progressive ataxia in a Pyrenean Mountain dog. *Vet Rec* 116:410–411, 1985.

39. Griffiths IR; Avulsion of the brachial plexus. 1. Neuropathology of the spinal cord and peripheral nerves. *J Small Anim Pract* 15:165–176, 1974.

40. Griffiths IR, Duncan ID, Lawson DD: Avulsion of the brachial plexus. 2. Clinical aspects. *J Small Anim Pract* 15:177–182, 1974.

41. Steinberg HS; The use of electrodiagnostic techniques in evaluating traumatic brachial plexus root injuries. *J Am Anim Hosp Assoc* 15:621–626, 1979.
42. Alexander JW, de Lahunta A, Scott DW: A case of brachial plexus neuropathy in a dog. *J Am Anim Hosp Assoc* 10:515–516, 1974.
43. Cummings JF, Lorenz MD, de Lahunta A, Washington LD: Canine brachial plexus neuritis: a syndrome resembling serum neuritis in man. *Cornell Vet* 63:589–617, 1973.
44. Bright RM, Crabtree BJ, Knecht CD: Brachial plexus neuropathy in the cat: a case report *J Am Anim Hosp Assoc* 14:612–615, 1978.
45. de Lahunta A, Averill DR: Hereditary cerebellar cortical and extrapyramidal nuclear abiotrophy in Kerry Blue terriers. *J Am Vet Med Assoc* 168:1119–1124, 1976.
46. Cork LC, Troncoso JC, Price DL: Canine inherited ataxia. *Ann Neurol* 9:492–499, 1981.
47. de Lahunta A: Comparative cerebellar disease in domestic animals. *Comp Cont Educ* 2:8–19, 1980.
48. de Lahunta A: Diseases of the cerebellum. *Vet Clin North Am* 10:91–102, 1980.
49. de Lahunta A: Comparative cerebellar disease in domestic animals. In *American College of Veterinary Internal Medicine, Scientific Proceedings,* July 23, 1979, p 10.
50. de Lahunta A, Fenner WR, Indrieri RJ, Mellick PW, Gardner S, Bell JS: Hereditary cerebellar cortical abiotrophy in the Gordon setter. *J Am Vet Med Assoc* 177:538–541, 1980.
51. Troncoso JC, Cork LC, Price DL: Canine inherited ataxia: ultrastructural observations. *J Neuropathol Exp Neurol* 44:165–175, 1985.
52. Hartley WJ, Barker JSF, Wanner RA, Farrow BRH: Inherited cerebellar degeneration in the rough coated collie. *Aust Vet Pract* 8:79–85, 1978.
53. Gill JM, Hewland ML: Cerebellar degeneration in the border collie. *NZ Vet J* 8:170, 1980.
54. Carmichael S, Griffiths IR, Harvey MJA: Familial cerebellar ataxia with hydrocephalus in bull mastiffs. *Vet Rec* 112:354–358, 1983.
55. McGrath JT: *Neurologic Examination of the Dog,* ed 2. Philadelphia, Lea and Febiger, 1960.
56. Cordy DR, Snelbaker HA; Cerebellar hypoplasia and degeneration in a family of Airedale dogs. *J Neuropathol Exp Neurol* 11:324–328, 1952.
57. Dow RW: Partial agenesis of the cerebellum in dogs. *J Comp Neurol* 72:569–586, 1940.
58. Frauchiger E, Fankhauser R: *Vergleichende Neuropathologie des Menschen und der Tiere.* Berlin, Springer Verlag, 1957.
59. Kay WJ, Budzelovich GN: Cerebellar hypoplasia and agenesis in the dog. *J Neuropathol Exp Neurol* 29:156, 1970.
60. Innes JRM, Saunders LZ: *Comparative Neuropathology.* New York, Academic Press, 1962.
61. Kronevi T, Ostensson K, Lesser J: A case of partial cerebellar hypoplasia in a cat. *Nord Vet Med* 30:221–222, 1978.
62. Bradfield T: A dalmation with partial aplasia of cerebral hemispheres. *Southwest Vet* 22:323–324, 1969.
63. Kilham L, Margolis G, Colby ED: Congenital infections of cats and ferrets by feline panleukopenia virus manifested by cerebellar hypoplasia. *Lab Invest* 17:465–480, 1967.
64. Johnson RH, Margolis G, Kilham L: Identity of feline ataxia virus on the feline panleukopenia virus. *Nature* 214:175, 1967.
65. Patel V, Koppang N, Patel B, Zeman W: Phenylene diamine-mediated peroxidase deficiency in English setters with neuronal ceroid-lipofuscinosis. *Lab Invest* 30:366–368, 1974.
66. Koppang N: Neuronal ceroid-lipofuscinosis in English setters. *J Small Anim Pract* 10:639–644, 1970.
67. Koppang N; Canine ceroid-lipofuscinosis. A model for human neuronal ceroid-lipofuscinosis and aging. *Mech Ageing Devel* 2:421–445, 1973/1974.
68. Koppang N: Juvenile amaurotic idiocy by English setter in Norway. *Acta Pathol Microbiol Scand* 64:158–159, 1965.
69. Rac R, Giesecke PR: Lysosomal storage disease in Chihuahuas. *Aust Vet J* 51:403–404, 1975.

70. Jolly RD, Hartley WJ: Storage diseases of domestic animals. *Aust Vet J* 53:1–8, 1977.
71. Cummings JF, de Lahunta A: An adult case of canine neuronal ceroid-lipofuscinosis. *Acta Neuropathol (Berl)* 39:43–51, 1977.
72. Vandevelde M, Fatzer R: Neuronal ceroid-lipofuscinosis in older dachshunds. *Vet Pathol* 17:686–692, 1980.
73. Hoover DM, Little PB, Cole WD: Neuronal ceroid-lipofuscinosis in a mature dog. *Vet Pathol* 21:359–361, 1984.
74. Appleby EC, Longstaffe JA, Bell FR: Ceroid lipofuscinosis in two saluki dogs. *J Comp Pathol* 92:375–380, 1982.
75. Hartley WJ, Canfield PJ, Donnelly TM: A suspected new canine storage disease. *Acta Neuropathol (Berl)* 56:225–232, 1982.
76. Fankhauser R: Degenerative lipidiotische Erkrankung des Zentralnervensystems bei zwei Hunden. *Schweiz Arch Tierheilkd* 107:73–87, 1965.
77. Hanichen T, Puschner H: Generalized lipofuscinosis with neural complications in a dog. *Vet Med Rev* 1:27–39, 1971.
78. Nimmo Wilkie JS, Hudson EB: Neuronal and generalized ceroid-lipofuscinosis in a cocker spaniel. *Vet Pathol* 19:623–628, 1982.
79. Greene PD, Little PB: Neuronal ceroid-lipofuscin storage in Siamese cats. *Can J Comp Med* 38:207–210, 1974.
80. Schmidt U: Generalisierte Lipofuscinose bei einer Katze. *Berl Munch Tierarztl Wochenschr* 4:70–73, 1974.
81. de Lahunta A: *Veterinary Neuroanatomy and Clinical Neurology*, ed 2. Philadelphia, WB Saunders, 1983.
82. Dueland R, Furneaux RW, Kaye MM: Spinal fusion and dorsal laminectomy for midcervical spondylolisthesis in a dog. *J Am Vet Med Assoc* 162:366–369, 1973.
83. Parker AJ, Park RD, Cusick PK, Jeffers CB: Cervical vertebral instability in the dog. *J Am Vet Med Assoc* 163:71–74, 1973.
84. Selcer RR, Oliver JE; Cervical spondylopathy-wobbler syndrome in dogs. *J Am Anim Hosp Assoc* 11:175–179, 1975.
85. Wright F, Rest JR, Palmer AC: Ataxia of the Great Dane caused by stenosis of the cervical vertebral canal: comparison with similar conditions in the bassett hound, Doberman pinscher, Ridgeback, and the thoroughbred horse. *Vet Rec* 92:1–6, 1973.
86. Hedhammer A, Wu F-M, Krook L, Schryver HF, de Lahunta A, Whalen JP, Kallfelz FA, Nunez EA, Hintz HF, Sheffy BE, Ryan GB: Overnutrition and skeletal disease: an experimental study in growing Great Dane dogs. *Cornell Vet* 64 (Suppl 5):1–160, 1974.
87. Mason TA: Cervical vertebral instability (wobbler syndrome) in the Doberman. *Aust Vet J* 53:440–445, 1977.
88. Seim HB, Withrow SJ: Pathophysiology and diagnosis of caudal cervical spondylomyelopathy with emphasis on the Doberman pinscher. *J Am Anim Hosp Assoc* 18:241–251, 1982.
89. Denny HR, Gibbs C, Gaskell CJ: Cervical spondylopathy in the dog—a review of thirty-five cases. *J Small Anim Pract* 18:117–132, 1977.
90. Olsson S-E, Starenborn M, Hoppe F: Dynamic compression of the cervical spinal cord: a myelographic and pathologic investigation in Great Dane dogs. *Acta Vet Scand* 23:65–78, 1982.
91. Wright JA: A study of the radiographic anatomy of the cervical spine in the dog. *J Small Anim Pract* 18:341–357, 1977.
92. Palmer AC, Wallace ME: Derformation of cervical vertebrae in bassett hounds. *Vet Rec* 80:430, 1967.
93. Palmer AC: *Introduction to Animal Neurology*, ed 2. Oxford, Blackwell Scientific, 1976.
94. Hatch RC: Poisons causing nervous stimulation or depression. In Booth NH, McDonald LE (eds): *Veterinary Pharmacology and Therapeutics*, ed 5. Ames, Iowa State University Press, 1982, p 999.
95. Cummings JF, de Lahunta A: Chronic relapsing polyradiculoneuritis in a dog. A clinical light- and electron-microscopic study. *Acta Neuropathol (Berl)* 28:191–204, 1974.
96. Flecknell PA, Lucke VM: Chronic relapsing polyradiculoneuritis in a cat. *Acta Neuropathol (Berl)* 41:81–84, 1978.
97. Cummings JF, Haas DC: Coonhound paralysis: an acute idiopathic polyradiculoneu-

ritis in dogs resembling the Landry-Guillain-Barré syndrome. *J Neurol Sci* 4:51–81, 1967.

98. Northington JW, Brown MJ: Acute canine idiopathic polyneuropathy. A Guillain-Barré-like syndrome in dogs. *J Neurol Sci* 56:259–273, 1982.

99. Northington JW, Brown MJ, Farnbach GC, Steinberg SA: Acute idiopathic polyneuropathy in the dog. *J Am Vet Med Assoc* 179:375–379, 1981.

99a. Holmes DF, Schultz RD, Cummings JF, de Lahunta A: Experimental coonhound paralysis: animal model of Guillain-Barré syndrome. *Neurology* 29:1186–1187, 1979.

100. Cummings JF, de Lahunta A, Holmes DF, Schultz RD: Coonhound paralysis: further clinical studies and electron microscopic observations. *Acta Neuropathol (Berl)* 56:167–178, 1982.

101. Holmes DF, de Lahunta A: Experimental allergic neuritis in the dog and its comparison with the naturally occurring disease; coonhound paralysis. *Acta Neuropathol (Berl)* 30:329–337, 1974.

102. Trayser CV, Marshall AE: A mild form of polyradiculoneuritis in a dog. *J Am Vet Med Assoc* 164:150–151, 1974.

103. Blackmore JA, Schaer M: Idiopathic polyradiculoneuritis and impaired ventilation in a dog: a case report. *J Am Anim Hosp Assoc* 20:487–490, 1984.

104. Klatzo I: Neuropathological aspects of brain edema. *J Neuropathol Exp Neurol* 26:1–14, 1967.

105. Fishman RA: Brain edema. *N Engl J Med* 293:706–711, 1975.

106. Palmer AC: Concussion: the result of impact injury to the brain. *Vet Rec* 111:575–578, 1982.

107. Smith DR, Ducker TB, Kempe LG: Experimental in vivo microcirculatory dynamics in brain trauma. *J Neurosurg* 30:664–672, 1969.

108. Palmer AC: The accident case. IV. The significance and estimation of damage to the central nervous system. *J Small Anim Pract* 5:25–33, 1964.

109. Hoerlein BF: *Canine Neurology—Diagnosis and Treatment*, ed 3. Philadelphia, WB Saunders, 1978.

110. Duncan ID, Griffiths IR, Munz M: The pathology of a sensory neuropathy affecting long haired dachshund dogs. *Acta Neuropathol (Berl)* 58:141–151, 1982.

111. Bjerkas I: Hereditary "cavitating" leukodystrophy in dalmation dogs. *Acta Neuropathol (Berl)* 40:163–169, 1977.

112. Chrisman CL: Distal polyneuropathy of Doberman pinschers. In *Proceedings of the 3rd Annual Medical Forum, American College of Veterinary Internal Medicine*, San Diego, June 1, 1985, p 164.

113. Adams EW: Hereditary deafness in a family of foxhounds. *J Am Vet Med Assoc* 128:302–303, 1956.

114. Igarashi M, Alford BR, Cohn AM, Saito R, Watanabe T: Inner ear anomalies in dogs. *Ann Otol Rhinol Laryngol* 81:249–255, 1972.

115. Lurie MH; The membranous labyrinth in the congenitally deaf collie and dalmation dog. *Laryngoscope* 58:279–287, 1948.

116. Hayes HM, Wilson GP, Fenner WR, Wyman M: Canine congenital deafness: epidemioligic study of 272 cases. *J Am Anim Hosp Assoc* 17:473–476, 1981.

117. Bergsma DR, Brown KS: White fur, blue eyes and deafness in the domestic cat. *J Hered* 62:171–185, 1971.

118. Johnston DE, Cox B: The incidence in purebred dogs in Australia of abnormalities that may be inherited. *Aust Vet J* 46:465–474, 1970.

119. Sims MH, Shull-Selcer E: Electrodiagnostic evaluation of deafness in two English setter littermates. *J Am Vet Med Assoc* 187:398–404, 1985.

120. Bosher SK, Hallpike CS: Observations on the histologic features, development and pathogenesis of the inner ear degeneration of the deaf white cat *Proc R Soc (Biol) Ser B* 162:147–170, 1965.

121. Rebillard G, Rebillard M, Carlier E, Pujol R: Histo-physiological relationships in the deaf white cat auditory system. *Acta Otolaryngol* 82:48–56, 1976.

122. Wolff D: Three generation of deaf white cats. *J Hered* 33:39–43, 1942.

123. Hudson WR, Ruben RJ; Hereditary deafness in the dalmation dog. *Arch Otolaryngol* 75:213–219, 1962.

124. Griffiths IR, Duncan ID: Chronic degenerative radiculomyelopathy in the dog. *J Small Anim Pract* 16:461–471, 1975.

125. Bichsel P, Vandevelde M: Degenerative myelopathy in a family of Siberian husky

dogs. *J Am Vet Med Assoc* 183:998–1000, 1983.
126. Matthews NS, de Lahunta A: Degenerative myelopathy in an adult miniature poodle. *J Am Vet Med Assoc* 186:1213–1215, 1985.
127. Averill DR: Degenerative myelopathy in the aging German shepherd dog: clinical and pathologic findings. *J Am Vet Med Assoc* 162:1045–1051, 1973.
128. Braund KG, Vandevelde M: German shepherd dog myelopathy. A morphologic and morphometric study. *Am J Vet Res* 39:1309–1315, 1978.
129. Waxman FJ, Clemmons RM, Hinrichs DJ: Progressive myelopathy in older German shepherd dogs. II. Presence of circulating suppressor cells. *J Immunol* 124:1216–1222, 1980.
130. Waxman FJ, Clemmons RM, Johnson G, Evermann JF, Johnson MI, Roberts C, Hinrichs DJ: Progressive myelopathy in older German shepherd dogs. I. Depressed response to thymus-dependent mitogens. *J Immunol* 124:1209–1215, 1980.
131. Williams DA, Sharp NJH, Batt RM: Enteropathy associated with degenerative myelopathy in German shepherd dogs. In *Scientific Proceedings, American College of Veterinary Internal Medicine*, New York, July 18, 1983, p 40.
132. Mesfin GM, Kusewitt D, Parker A: Degenerative myelopathy in a cat. *J Am Vet Med Assoc* 176:62–64, 1980.
133. Douglas SW, Palmer AC: Idiopathic demyelination of brain-stem and cord in a miniature poodle puppy. *J Pathol Bacteriol* 82:67–71, 1961.
134. Steinberg SA, Rhodes WH, Marshak RR, McGrath JT: Clinico-pathologic conference. *J Am Vet Med Assoc* 143:404–410, 1963.
135. Hargis AM, Haupt KH, Hegreberg GA, Prieur DJ, Moore MP: Familial canine dermatomyositis: initial characterization of the cutaneous and muscular lesions. *Am J Pathol* 116:234–244, 1984.
136. Kunkle GA, Chrisman CL, Gross TL, Fadok V, Werner LL: Dermatomyositis in collie dogs. *Comp Cont Educ* 7:185–192, 1985.
137. Hargis AM, Haupt KH, Prieur DJ, Moore MP: A skin disorder in three shetland sheepdogs: comparison with familial canine dermatomyositis of collies. *Comp Cont Educ* 7:306–315, 1985.
138. Selcer EA, Helman RG, Selcer RR: Dermoid sinus in a Shih Tzu and a boxer, *J Am Anim Hosp Assoc* 20:634–636, 1984.
139. Burns M, Fraser MN: *Genetics of the Dog*. Philadelphia, Lippincott, 1966, p 84.
140. Antin IP: Dermoid sinus in a Rhodesian ridgeback dog. *J Am Vet Med Assoc* 157:961–962, 1970.
141. Hofmeyr CFB: Dermoid sinus in the ridgeback dog. *J Small Anim Pract* 4 (Suppl):5–8, 1963.
142. Leyh R, Carithers RW: Dermoid sinus in a Rhodesian ridgeback. *Iowa St Univ Vet* 41:36–39, 1979.
143. Braund KG, Dillon AR, Pidgeon GL, August JR: Neuromuscular changes in dogs with spontaneous diabetes mellitus. In *Scientific Proceedings, American College of Veterinary Internal Medicine*, St. Louis, July 20, 1981, p 53.
144. Braund KG, Steiss JE; Distal neuropathy in spontaneous diabetes mellitus in the dog. *Acta Neuropathol (Berl)* 57:263–269, 1982.
145. Katherman AE, Braund KG: Polyneuropathy associated with diabetes mellitus in a dog. *J Am Vet Med Assoc* 182:522–524, 1982.
146. Steiss JE, Orsher AN, Bowen JM: Electrodiagnostic analysis of peripheral neuropathy in dogs with diabetes mellitus. *Am J Vet Res* 42:2061–2064, 1981.
147. Kramek BA, Moise NS, Cooper B, Raffe MR: Neuropathy associated with diabetes mellitus in the cat. *J Am Vet Med Assoc* 184:42–45, 1984.
148. Johnson CA, Kittleson MD, Indrieri RJ: Peripheral neuropathy and hypotension in a diabetic dog. *J Am Vet Med Assoc* 183:1007–1009, 1983.
149. Thomas PK, Eliasson SG: Diabetic neuropathy. In Dyck PJ, Thomas PK, Lambert EH (eds): *Peripheral Neuropathy*. Philadelphia, WB Saunders, 1975, pp 956–981.
150. Thomas PK: Metabolic neuropathies. In Aguayo AJ, Karpati G (eds): *Current Topics in Nerve and Muscle Research*. Amsterdam, Excerpta Medica, 1979, pp 255–261.
151. Clements RS: Diabetic neuropathy—new concepts of its etiology. *Diabetes* 28:604–611, 1979.
152. Spencer PS, Schaumburg HH: Ultrastructural studies of the dying-back process. IV. Differential vulnerability of PNS and CNS fibers in experimental central-peripheral distal axonopathies. *J Neuropathol Exp Neurol* 36:300–320, 1977.

153. Spencer PS, Sabri MI, Schaumburg HH, Moore CL: Does a defect of energy metabolism in the nerve fiber underlie axonal degeneration of polyneuropathies? *Ann Neurol* 5:501–507, 1979.

154. Hansen H-J: A pathologic-anatomical study on disk degeneration in the dog. *Acta Orthop Scand* (Supply 11), 1952.

155. Braund KG: Canine intervertebral disk disease. In Bojrab MJ (ed): *Pathophysiology in Small Animal Surgery*. Philadelphia, Lea and Febiger, 1981, p 739.

156. Braund KG, Ghosh P, Taylor TKF, Larsen LH: Morphological studies on the canine intervertebral disk. The assignment of the beagle to the achondroplastic classification. *Res Vet Sci* 19:167–172, 1975.

157. Ghosh P, Taylor TKF, Yarroll JM, Braund KG, Larsen LH: Genetic factors in the maturation of the canine intervertebral disk. *Res Vet Sci* 19:304–311, 1975.

158. Priester WA: Canine intervertebral disk disease—occurrence by age, breed, and sex among 8117 cases. *Theriogenol* 6:293–303, 1976.

159. Goggin JE, Li AS, Franti CE: Canine intervertebral disk diseases; characterization by age, sex, breed, and anatomical site of involvement. *Am J Vet Res* 31:1687–1692, 1970.

160. King AS, Smith RN: Disc protrusion in the cat: distribution of dorsal protrusions along the vertebral column. *Vet Rec* 72:335–337, 1960.

161. King AS, Smith RN: Disc protrusion in the cat: incidence of dorsal protrusions. *Vet Rec* 72:381–383, 1960.

162. Griffiths IR: Some aspects of the pathology and pathogenesis of the myelopathy caused by disc protrusions in the dog. *J Neurol Neurosurg Psychiatry* 35:403–413, 1972.

163. Wright F, Palmer AC: Morphological changes caused by pressure on the spinal cord. *Pathol Vet* 6:355–368, 1969.

164. Prata RG: Neurosurgical treatment of thoracolumbar disks: the rationale and value of laminectomy with concomitant disk removal. *J Am Anim Hosp Assoc* 17:17–26, 1981.

165. Hoerlein BF, Spano JS: Non-neurological complications following decompressive spinal cord surgery. *Arch Am Coll Vet Surg* 4:11–16, 1975.

166. Moore RW, Withrow SJ: Gastrointestinal hemorrhage and pancreatitis associated with intervertebral disk disease in the dog. *J Am Vet Med Assoc* 180:1443–1447, 1982.

167. Toombs JP, Caywood DD, Lipowitz AJ, Stevens JB: Colonic perforation following neurosurgical procedures and corticosteroid therapy in four dogs. *J Am Vet Med Assoc* 177:68–72, 1980.

168. Bellah JR; Colonic perforation after corticosteroid and surgical treatment of intervertebral disk disease in a dog. *J Am Vet Med Assoc* 183:1002–1003, 1983.

169. Norsworthy GD: Discospondylitis as a cause of posterior paresis. *Feline Pract* 9:39–40, 1979.

170. Henderson RA, Hoerlein BF, Kramer TT, Meyer ME: Discospondylitis in three dogs infected with *Brucella canis*. *J Am Vet Med Assoc* 165:451–455, 1974.

171. Johnson DE, Summers BA: Osteomyelitis of the lumbar vertebrae in dogs caused by grass-seed foreign bodies *Aust Vet J* 47:289–294, 1971.

172. Kornegay JN, Barber DL: Diskospondylitis in dogs. *J Am Vet Med Assoc* 177:337–341, 1980.

173. Kornegay JN, Barber DL, Earley TD: Cranial thoracic diskospondylitis in two dogs. *J Am Vet Med Assoc* 174:192–194, 1979.

174. LaCroix JA: Vertebral body osteomyelitis: a case report. *Am Vet Radiol J* 14:17–21, 1973.

175. Bennett D, Carmichael S, Griffiths IR: Discospondylitis in the dog. *J Small Anim Pract* 22:539–547, 1981.

176. Patnaik AK, Liu S-K, Wilkins RJ, Johnson GF, Seitz PE: Paecilomycosis in a dog. *J Am Vet Med Assoc* 161:806–813, 1972.

177. Wood GL, Hirsh DC, Selcer RR, Rinaldi MG, Boorman GA: Disseminated aspergillosis in a dog. *J Am Vet Med Assoc* 172:704–707, 1978.

178. Johnson RG, Prata RG: Intradiskal osteomyelitis: a conservative approach. *J Am Anim Hosp Assoc* 19:743–750, 1983.

179. Hurov L, Troy G, Turnwald G: Diskospondylitis in the dog: 27 cases. *J Am Vet Med Assoc* 173:275–281, 1978.

180. Van Bree H, de Rick A, Verschooten F, Mattheeuws D: Successful conservative

treatment of cervical discospondylitis in a dog. *J Small Anim Pract* 22:59–65, 1981.

181. Gage ED: Treatment of diskospondylitis in the dog. *J Am Vet Med Assoc* 166:1164–1169, 1975.

182. Griffiths IR, Duncan ID: Distal denervating disease: a degenerative neuropathy of the distal motor axon in dogs. *J Small Anim Pract* 20:579–592, 1979.

183. Braund KG, Luttgen PJ, Redding RW, Rumph PF: Distal symmetrical polyneuropathy in a dog. *Vet Pathol* 17:422–435, 1980.

184. Dillon AR, Braund KG: Distal polyneuropathy after canine heartworm disease therapy complicated by disseminated intravascular coagulation. *J Am Vet Med Assoc* 181:239–242, 1982.

185. Imagawa DT, Goret P, Adams JM: Immunological relationships of measles distemper and rinderpest viruses. *Proc Natl Acad Sci* 46:1119–1123, 1959.

186. Appel MJ, Glickman LT, Raine CS, Tourtellotte WW: Canine viruses and multiple sclerosis. *Neurology* 31:944–949, 1981.

187. Appel MJG: Pathogenesis of canine distemper. *Am J Vet Res* 30:1167–1182, 1969.

188. Appel MJG, Gillespie JH; Canine distemper virus. *Virol Monogr* 11:1–96, 1972.

189. Summers BA, Greisen HA, Appel MJG: Possible initiation of viral encephalomyelitis in dogs by migrating lymphocytes infected with distemper virus *Lancet* 2:187–190, 1978.

189a. Hartley WJ: Polioencephalomalacia in dogs. *Acta Neuropathol (Berl)* 2:271–281, 1963.

190. Braund KG, Vandevelde M: Polioencephalomalacia in the dog. *Vet Pathol* 16:661–672, 1979.

191. Lisiak JA, Vandevelde M: Polioencephalomalacia associated with canine distemper virus infection. *Vet Pathol* 16:650–660, 1979.

192. Finnie JW, Hooper PT: Polioencephalomalacia in dogs with distemper encephalitis. *Aust Vet J* 61:407–408, 1984.

193. Braund KG: Encephalitis and meningitis. *Vet Clin North Am* 10:31–56, 1980.

194. Vandevelde M, Kristensen B, Braund KG, Greene CE, Swango LJ, Hoerlein BF: Chronic distemper virus encephalitis in mature dogs. *Vet Pathol* 17:17–29, 1980.

195. Braund KG, Crawley RR, Speakman C: Hippocampal necrosis associated with canine distemper virus infection. *Vet Rec* 109:122–123, 1981.

196. McGovern VJ, Steel JD, Wyke BD, Dodson ME: Canine encephalitis causing a syndrome characterized by tremor. *Aust J Exp Biol Med Sci* 28:433–447, 1950.

197. Cordy DR: Canine encephalomyelitis. *Cornell Vet* 32:11–28, 1942.

198. Adams JM, Brown WJ, Snow HD, Lincoln SD, Sears AW, Barenfus M, Holliday TA, Cremer NE, Lennette EH: Old dog encephalitis and demyelinating diseases in man *Vet Pathol* 12:220–226, 1975.

199. Lincoln SD, Gorham JR, Davis WC, Ott RL: Studies of old dog encephalitis. II. Electron microscopic and immunohistologic findings. *Vet Pathol* 10:124–129, 1973.

200. Lincoln SD, Gorham JR, Ott RL, Hegreberg GA: Etiologic studies of old dog encephalitis. I. Demonstration of canine distemper viral antigen in the brain in two cases. *Vet Pathol* 8:1–8, 1971.

201. Koestner A: Animal model of human disease: subacute sclerosing panencephalitis multiple sclerosis. Animal model: distemper-associated demyelinating encephalomyelitis. *Am J Pathol* 78:361–364, 1975.

202. Hall WW, Imagawa DT, Choppin PW: Immunological evidence for the synthesis of all canine distemper virus polypeptides in chronic neurological diseases in dogs. Chronic distemper and old dog encephalitis differ from SSPE in man. *Virology* 98:283–287, 1979.

203. Cutler RWP, Averill DR: Cerebrospinal fluid gamma globulins in canine distemper encephalitis. *Neurology* 19:1111–1114, 1969.

204. Long JF, Jacoby RO, Olson M, Koestner A: Beta-glucuronidase activity and levels of protein and protein fractions in serum and cerebrospinal fluid of dogs with distemper associated demyelinating encephalopathy *Acta Neuropathol (Berl)* 25:179–187, 1973.

205. Hagen WA, Bruner DW, Gillespie JH: *Hagen's Infectious Diseases of Domestic Animals*, ed 6. Ithaca, NY, Cornell University Press, 1973.

206. Fischer CA: Retinal and retinochoroidal lesions in early neuropathic canine distemper. *J Am Vet Med Assoc* 158:740–752, 1971.

207. Jubb KV, Saunders LZ, Coates HV: The intraocular lesions in canine distemper. *J*

Comp Pathol 67:21–29, 1957.
208. Kristensen B, Vandevelde M: Immunofluorescence studies of canine distemper encephalitis on paraffin-embedded tissue. *Am J Vet Res* 39:1017–1021, 1978.
209. Vandevelde M, Kristensen B: Observations on the distribution of canine distemper virus in the central nervous system of dogs with demyelinating encephalitis. *Acta Neuropathol (Berl)* 40:233–236, 1977.
210. Koestner A, McCullough B, Krakowka GS, Long JF, Olsen RG: Canine distemper, a virus-induced demyelinating encephalomyelitis. In Zeman W, Lenette E (eds): *Slow Virus Diseases*. Baltimore, Williams & Wilkins, 1974, pp 86–101.
211. Imagawa DT, Howard EB, van Pelt LF, Ryan CP, Bui HD, Shapshak P: Isolation of canine distemper virus from dogs with chronic neurological diseases. *Proc Soc Exp Biol Med* 164:355–362, 1980.
212. Cook SD, Dowling PC: A possible association between house pets and multiple sclerosis. *Lancet* 1:980–982, 1977.
213. Cook SD, Natelson BH, Levin BE, Chavis PS, Dowling PC: Further evidence of a possible association between house dogs and multiple sclerosis. *Ann Neurol* 3:141–143, 1978.
214. Bauer HF, Wikstrom J: Multiple sclerosis and house pets. Lancet 2:1029, 1977.
215. Krakowka S, Koestner A: Canine distemper virus and multiple sclerosis. Lancet 1:1127, 1978.
216. Kurtzke JF, Priester WA: Dogs distemper and multiple sclerosis in the United States. *Acta Neurol Scand* 60:312–319, 1979.
217. Winston J: Clinical problems pertaining to neurotoxicity of streptomycin group of drugs. *Arch Otolaryngol* 58:55–61, 1953.
218. Hawkins JE, Lurie MH: The ototoxicity of dihydrostreptomycin and neomycin in the cat. *Ann Otol Rhinol Laryngol* 62:1128–1148, 1953.
219. McGee TM, Olszewski J: Streptomycin sulfate and dihydrostreptomycin toxicity. *Arch Otolaryngol* 75:295–311, 1962.
220. Morgan JP, Coulter DB, Marshall AE, Goetsch DD: Effects of neomycin on the waveform of auditory-evoked brain stem potentials in dogs. *Am J Vet Res* 41:1077–1081, 1980.
221. Morgan JP; Spinal dural ossification in the dog: incidence and distribution based on a radiographic study. *J Am Vet Radiol Soc* 10:43–48, 1969.
222. Sandersleben J, el Sergany MA: Ein Beitrag zur sogenannten Pachymeningitis spinalis ossificans des Hundes unter Berucksichtigung pathogenetischer und atiologischer Gesichtspunkte. *Zentralbl Veterinaermed* A13:526, 1966.
223. Wilson JW, Greene HJ, Leipold HW: Osseous metaplasia of the spinal dura mata in a Great Dane. *J Am Vet Med Assoc* 167:75–77, 1975.
224. Basson PA, McCully RM, Warnes WEJ: Nosematosis: report of a canine case in the Republic of South Africa. *J S Afr Vet Med Assoc* 37:3–9, 1966.
225. Botha WS, van Dellen AF, Stewart CG: Canine encephalitozoonosis in South Africa. *J S Afr Vet Med Assoc* 50:135–144, 1979.
226. Plowright W: An encephalitis-nephritis syndrome in the dog probably due to congenital encephalitozoon infection. *J Comp Pathol* 62:83–92, 1952.
227. Plowright W, Yeoman G: Probable encephalitozoon infection of the dog. *Vet Rec* 64:381–383, 1952.
228. Shadduck JA, Bendele R, Robinson GT: Isolation of the causative organism of canine encephalitozoonosis. *Vet Pathol* 15:449–460, 1978.
229. Shadduck JA, Pakes SP: Encephalitozoonosis (nosematosis) and toxoplasmosis. *Am J Pathol* 64:657–671, 1971.
230. Stewart CG, van Dellen AF, Botha WS: Canine encephalitozoonosis in kennels and the isolation of *Encephalitozoon* in tissue culture. *J S Afr Vet Med Assoc* 50:165–168, 1979.
231. van Dellen AF, Botha WS, Boomker J, Warnes WEJ: Light and electron microscopic studies on canine encephalitozoonosis: cerebral vasculitis. *Onderstepoort J Vet Res* 45:165–186, 1978.
232. van Rensburg IBJ, du Plessis JL: Nosematosis in a cat: a case report. *J S Afr Vet Med Assoc* 42:327–331, 1971.
233. Rogers WA, Fenner WR, Sherding RG: Electromyographic and esophagomanometric findings in clinically normal dogs and in dogs with idiopathic megaesophagus. *J Am Vet Med Assoc* 174:181–183, 1979.

234. Harvey CE, O'Brien JA, Durie VR, Miller DJ, Veenema R: Megaesophagus in the dog: a clinical survey of 79 cases. *J Am Vet Med Assoc* 165:443–446, 1974.

235. Clifford DH, Lee MO, Lee DC, Ross JN: Classification of congenital neuromuscular dysfunction of the canine esophagus. *J Am Vet Radiol Soc* 17:98–100, 1976.

236. Schwartz A, Ravin CE, Greenspan RH, Schoemann RS, Burt JK: Congenital neuromuscular esophageal disease in a litter of Newfoundland puppies. *J Am Vet Radiol Soc* 17:101–104, 1976.

237. Cox VS, Wallace LJ, Anderson VE, Rushmer RA: Hereditary esophageal dysfunction in the miniature schnauzer dog. *Am J Vet Res* 41:326–330, 1980.

238. Clifford DH, Waddell ED, Patterson DR, Wilson CF, Thompson HL: Management of esophageal achalasia in miniature schnauzers. *J Am Vet Med Assoc* 161:1012–1021, 1972.

239. Osborne CA, Clifford DH, Jessen C: Hereditary esophageal achalasia in dogs. *J Am Vet Med Assoc* 151:572–581, 1967.

240. Clifford DH, Soifer FK, Wilson MD, Guillord GL: Congenital achalasia of the esophagus in 4 cats of common ancestry. *J Am Vet Med Assoc* 158:1554–1560, 1971.

241. Duncan ID, Griffiths IR, Nash AS: Myotonia in canine Cushing's disease. *Vet Rec* 100:30–31, 1977.

242. Feldman EC, Tyrrell JB: Hypoadrenocorticism. *Vet Clin North Am* 7:555–581, 1977.

243. Griffiths IR, Duncan ID: Myotonia in the dog: a report of four cases. *Vet Rec* 93:184–188, 1973.

244. Kornegay JN, Gorgacz EJ, Dawe DL, Bowen JM, White NA, DeBuysscher EV: Polymyositis in dogs. *J Am Vet Med Assoc* 176:431–438, 1980.

245. Krum SH, Cardinet GH, Anderson BC, Holliday TA: Polymyositis and polyarthritis associated with systemic lupus erythematosus in a dog. *J Am Vet Med Assoc* 170:61–64, 1977.

246. Lorenz MD, de Lahunta A, Alstrom DH: Neostigmine-responsive weakness in the dog similar to myasthenia gravis. *J Am Vet Med Assoc* 161:795–800, 1972.

247. Palmer AC: Myasthenia gravis. *Vet Clin North Am* 10:213–221, 1980.

248. Higgs B, Kerr FWL, Ellis FH; The experimental production of esophageal achalasia by electrolytic lesions in the medulla. *J Thorac Cardiovasc Surg* 50:613–625, 1965.

249. Diamant N, Szczepanski M, Mui H: Idiopathic megaesophagus in the dog: reasons for spontaneous improvement and a possible method of medical therapy. *Can Vet J* 15:66–71, 1974.

250. Boudrieau RJ, Rogers WA: Megaesophagus in the dog: a review of 50 cases. *J Am Anim Hosp Assoc* 21:33–40, 1985.

251. Bartsch RC, McConnell EE, Imes GD, Schmidt JM: A review of exertional rhabdomyolysis in wild and domestic animals and man. *Vet Pathol* 14:314–324, 1977.

252. Spangler WL, Muggli FM: Seizure-induced rhabdomyolysis accompanied by acute renal failure in a dog. *J Am Vet Med Assoc* 172:1190–1194, 1978.

253. Davis PE, Paris R: Azoturia in a greyhound: clinical pathology aids to diagnosis. *J Small Anim Pract* 15:43–54, 1974.

254. Gannon JR: Exertional rhabdomyolysis (myoglobinuria) in the racing greyhound. In Kirk RW (ed): *Current Veterinary Therapy. VIII. Small Animal Practice.* Philadelphia, WB Saunders, 1983.

255. Bjotvedt G, Hendricks GM, Weems CW: Exertional rhabdomyolysis in a racing greyhound: a case report *Vet Med Small Anim Clin* 78:1215–1220, 1983.

256. Fox JG, Averill DR, Hallett M, Schunk K: Familial reflex myoclonus in Labrador retrievers. *Am J Vet Res* 45:2367–2370, 1984.

257. Key TJA, Gaskell CJ: Puzzling syndrome in cats associated with pupillary dilation. *Vet Rec* 110:160, 1982.

258. Sharp NJH, Nash AS, Griffiths IR: Feline dysautonomia (the Key-Gaskell syndrome): a clinical and pathological study of forty cases. *J Small Anim Pract* 25:599–615, 1984.

259. Nash AS, Griffiths IR, Sharp NJH: The Key-Gaskell syndrome—an autonomic polyganglionopathy. *Vet Rec* 111:307–308, 1982.

260. Griffiths IR, Nash AS, Sharp NJH: The Key-Gaskell syndrome: the current situation. *Vet Rec* 111:532–533, 1982.

261. Griffiths IR, Sharp NJH, McCulloch MC: Feline dysautonomia (the Key-Gaskell

syndrome): an ultra structural study of autonomic ganglia and nerves. *Neuropathol Appl Neurobiol* 11:17–29, 1985.

262. Rochlitz L, Bennett AM: Key-Gaskell syndrome in a bitch. *Vet Rec* 112:614–615, 1983.

263. O'Reilly KJ, Fishman B, Hitchcock LM: Feline infectious peritonitis: isolation of a coronavirus. *Vet Rec* 104:348, 1979.

264. Wolf LG, Griesemer RA: Feline infectious peritonitis. *Pathol Vet* 3:255–270, 1966.

265. Wolf LG, Griesemer RA: Feline infectious peritonitis: review of gross and histopathologic lesions. *J Am Vet Med Assoc* 158:987–993, 1971.

266. Slausen DO, Finn JP: Meningoencephalitis and panophthalmitis in feline infectious peritonitis. *J Am Vet Med Assoc* 160:729–734, 1972.

267. Pedersen NC: Feline infectious peritonitis: something old, something new. *Feline Pract* 6:42–51, 1976.

268. Pedersen NC: Serologic studies of naturally occurring feline infectious peritonitis. *Am J Vet Res* 37:1449–1453, 1976.

269. Barlough JE, Summers BA: Encephalitis due to feline infectious peritonitis virus in a twelve-week-old kitten. *Feline Pract* 14:43–46, 1984.

270. Krum S, Johnson K, Wilson J: Hydrocephalus associated with the noneffusive form of feline infectious peritonitis. *J Am Vet Med Assoc* 167:746–748, 1975.

271. Kornegay JN: Feline infectious peritonitis: the central nervous system form. *J Am Anim Hosp Assoc* 14:580–584, 1978.

272. Fatzer R: Meningitis und Chorio-Ependymitis granulomatosa bei Katzen. *Schweiz Arch Tierheilkd* 117:633–640, 1975.

273. Legendre AM, Whitenack DL: Feline infectious peritonitis with spinal cord involvement in two cats *J Am Vet Med Assoc* 167:931–932, 1975.

274. McGrath JT, Batt R: A leukodystrophy in the dog. *J Neuropathol Exp Neurol* 34:78, 1975.

275. McGrath JT: Fibrinoid lekodystrophy (Alexander's disease). In Andrews EJ, Ward BC, Altman NH (eds): *Spontaneous Animal Models of Human Disease.* vol. II. New York, Academic Press, 1979. p 147.

276. Moore RW, Rouse GP, Piermattei DL, Ferguson HR: Fibrotic myopathy of the semitendinosus muscle in four dogs *Vet Surg* 10:169–174, 1981.

277. Vaughan LC: Muscle and tendon injuries in dogs. *J Small Anim Pract* 20:711–736, 1979.

278. Darling PR: Lysosomal storage diseases in animals. In Dingle JT, Dean RT, Sly W (eds): *Lysosomes in Biology and Pathology.* Amsterdam, Elsevier, 1984, pp 347–379.

279. Kelly WR, Clague AE, Barnes RJ, Bate MJ, MacKay BM: Canine L-fucosidosis: a storage disease of springer spaniels. *Acta Neuropathol (Berl)* 60:9–13, 1983.

280. Littlewood JD, Herrtage ME, Palmer AC: Neuronal storage disease in English springer spaniels. *Vet Rec* 112:86, 1983.

281. Blakemore WF, Palmer AC: Cerebral lipidoses and leucodystrophies in animals. *Vet Ann* 12:129–135, 1971.

282. Jolly RD: Lysosomal storage diseases. *Neuropathol Appl Neurobiol* 4:419–427, 1978.

283. Jolly RD, Blakemore WF: Inherited lysosomal storage diseases: an essay in comparative medicine. *Vet Rec* 92:391–400, 1973.

284. Read DH, Harrington DD, Keenan TW, Hinsman EJ: Neuronal-visceral GM1 gangliosidosis in a dog with β-galactosidase deficiency. *Science* 194:442–445, 1976.

285. Blakemore WF: GM1 Gangliosidosis in a cat. *J Comp Pathol* 82:179–185, 1972.

286. Baker HJ: Inherited metabolic disorders of the nervous system in dogs and cats. In Kirk RW (ed): *Current Veterinary Therapy V.* Philadelphia, WB Saunders, 1974, p 700.

287. Baker HJ, Lindsey JR: Animal model of human disease: human GM1 gangliosidosis. Animal model: feline GM1 gangliosidosis. *Am J Pathol* 74:649–652, 1974.

288. Baker HJ, Lindsey JR, McKann GM, Farrell DF: Neuronal GM1 gangliosidosis in a Siamese cat with β-galactosidase deficiency. *Science* 174:838–839, 1971.

289. Baker HJ, Mole JA, Lindsey JR, Creel RM: Animal models of human ganglioside storage diseases. *Fed Proc* 35:1193–1201, 1976.

290. Baker HJ, Reynolds GD, Walkley SU, Cox NR, Baker GH: The gangliosidoses: comparative features and research applications. *Vet Pathol* 16:635–649, 1979.

291. Karbe E, Schiefer B: Familial amaurotic idiocy in male German shorthair pointers. *Pathol Vet* 4:223–232, 1967.

292. Karbe E: Animal model of human disease: GM2-gangliosidosis (amaurotic idiocies) types I, II, and III. Animal model: canine GM2-gangliosidosis. *Am J Pathol* 71:151–154, 1973.

293. McGrath JT, Kelly AM, Steinberg SA: Cerebral lipidosis in the dog. *J Neuropathol Exp Neurol* 27:141, 1968.

294. Cummings JF, Wood PA, Walkley SU, de Lahunta A, De Forest ME: GM2 gangliosidosis in a Japanese spaniel. *Acta Neuropathol* 67:247–253, 1985.

295. Cork LC, Munnell JF, Lorenz MD, Murphy JF, Baker HJ, Rattazzi MC: GM2 ganglioside lysosomal storage disease in cats with β-hexosaminidase deficiency. *Science* 196:1014–1017, 1977.

296. Cork LC, Munnell JF, Lorenz MD: The pathology of feline GM2 gangliosidosis. *Am J Pathol* 90:723–734, 1978.

297. Van den Berg PB, Baker MK, Lange AL: A suspected lysosomal storage disease in Abyssinian cats. Part I: genetic, clinical and clinical pathological aspects. *J S Afr Vet Assoc* 48:195–199, 1977.

298. Lange AL, Van den Berg PB, Baker MK: A suspected lysosomal storage disease in Abyssinian cats. Part II: histopathological and ultrastructural aspects. *J S Afr Vet Assoc* 48:201–209, 1977.

299. Duncan ID, Griffiths IR: Canine giant axonal neuropathy. *Vet Rec* 101:438–441, 1977.

300. Duncan ID, Griffiths IR: Peripheral nervous system in a case of canine giant axonal neuropathy. *Neuropathol Appl Neurobiol* 5:25–39, 1979.

301. Duncan ID, Griffiths IR: Canine giant axonal neuropathy; some aspects of its clinical pathological and comparative features. *J Small Anim Pract* 22:491–501, 1981.

302. Duncan ID, Griffiths IR, Carmichael S, Henderson S: Inherited canine giant axonal neuropathy. *Muscle Nerve* 4:223–227, 1981.

303. Griffiths IR, Duncan ID: The central nervous system in canine giant axonal neuropathy. *Acta Neuropathol (Berl)* 46:169–172, 1979.

304. Griffiths IR, Duncan ID, McCulloch M, Carmichael S: Further studies of the central nervous system in canine giant axonal neuropathy. *Neuropathol Appl Neurobiol* 6:421–432, 1980.

305. Howell JMcC, Palmer AC: Globoid leukodystrophy in two dogs. *J Small Anim Pract* 12:633–642, 1971.

306. Fankhauser R, Luginbuhl H, Hartley WJ: Leukodystrophie von Typus Krabbe beim Hund. *Schweiz Arch Tierheilkd* 105:198–207, 1965.

306a. McGrath JT, Schutta H, Yaseen A, Steinberg S: A morphologic and biochemical study of canine globoid cell leukodystrophy. *J Neuropathol Exp Neurol* 28:171, 1969.

307. Fletcher TF, Kurtz HJ, Low DG: Globoid cell leukodystrophy (Krabbe type) in the dog. *J Am Vet Med Assoc* 149:165–172, 1966.

308. Fletcher TF, Kurtz HJ, Stadlan EM: Experimental wallerian degeneration in peripheral nerves of dogs with globoid cell leukodystrophy. *J Neuropathol Exp Neurol* 30:593–602, 1971.

309. Fletcher TF, Lee DG, Hammer RF: Ultrastructural features of globoid-cell leukodystrophy in the dog. *Am J Vet Res* 32:177–181, 1971.

310. Fletcher TF, Kurtz HJ: Animal model for human disease: globoid cell leukodystrophy, Krabbe's disease. *Am J Pathol* 66:375–378, 1972.

311. Suzuki Y, Austin J, Armstrong D, Suzuki K, Schlenker J, Fletcher T: Studies in globoid leukodystrophy: enzymatic and lipid findings in the canine form. *Exp Neurol* 29:65–75, 1970.

312. Suzuki Y, Miyatake T, Fletcher TF, Suzuki K: Glycosphingolipid β-galactosidases. 1. Canine form of globoid cell leukodystrophy; comparison with the human disease. *J Biol Chem* 249:2109–2112, 1974.

313. Hirth RS, Nielsen SW: A familial canine globoid cell leukodystrophy ("Krabbe type"). *J Small Anim Pract* 8:569–575, 1967.

314. Johnson GR, Oliver JE, Selcer R: Globoid cell leukodystrophy in a beagle. *J Am Vet Med Assoc* 167:380–384, 1975.

315. Zaki F, Kay WJ: Globoid cell leukodystrophy in a miniature poodle. *J Am Vet Med Assoc* 163:248–250, 1973.

316. Luttgen PJ, Braund KG, Storts RW: Globoid cell leukodystrophy. *J Small Anim Pract* 24:153–160, 1983.

317. Boysen BG, Tryphonas L, Harries NW: Globoid cell leukodystrophy in the bluetick hound dog. 1. Clinical manifestations. *Can Vet J* 15:303–308, 1974.
318. Selcer EA, Selcer RR: Globoid cell leukodystrophy in two West Highland white terriers and one Pomeranian. *Comp Cont Educ* 6:621–624, 1984.
319. Johnson KH: Globoid leukodystrophy in the cat. *J Am Vet Med Assoc* 157:2057–2064, 1970.
320. Roszel JF: Membrane filtration of canine and feline cerebrosinal fluid for cytologic evaluation. *J Am Vet Med Assoc* 160:720–725, 1972.
321. Hartley WJ, Blakemore WF: Neurovisceral glucocerebroside storage (Gaucher's disease) in a dog. *Vet Pathol* 10:191–201, 1973.
322. Van De Water NS, Jolly RD, Farrow BRH: Canine Gaucher disease—the enzymatic defect. *Aust J Exp Biol Med Sci* 57:551–554, 1979.
323. Walvoort HC, van Nes JJ, Stokhof AA, Wolvekamp WTC: Canine glycogen storage disease type II: a clinical study of four affected Lapland dogs. *J Am Anim Hosp Assoc* 20:279–286, 1984.
324. Walvoort HC, Kowter JF, Reuser AJJ: Heterozygote detection in a family of Lapland dogs with a recessively inherited metabolic disease: canine glycogen storage disease type II. *Res Vet Sci* 38:174–178, 1985.
325. Rafiquzzaman M, Svenkerud R, Strande A, Hauge JG: Glycogenosis in the dog. *Acta Vet Scand* 17:196–209, 1976.
326. Ceh L, Hauge JG, Svenkerud R, Strande A: Glycogenesis type III in the dog. *Acta Vet Scand* 17:210–222, 1976.
327. Hegreberg GA, Norby DE: An inherited storage disease of cats. *Fed Proc* 32:821, 1973.
328. Mackenzie CD, Johnson RP; Lafora's disease in a dog. *Aust Vet J* 52:144, 1976.
329. Hegreberg GA, Padgett GA: Inherited progressive epilepsy of the dog with comparisons to Lafora's disease of man. *Fed Proc* 35:1202–1205, 1976.
330. Tomchick TL: Familial Lafora's disease in the beagle dog. *Fed Proc* 32:8–21, 1973.
331. Edmonds HL, Hegreberg GA, van Gelder NM, Sylvester DM, Clemmons RM, Chatburn CG: Spontaneous convulsions in beagle dogs. *Fed Proc* 38:2424–2428, 1979.
332. Holland JM, Davis WC, Prieur DJ, Collins GH: Lafora's disease in the dog. *Am J Pathol* 58:509–529, 1970.
333. Cusick PK, Cameron AM, Parker AJ: Canine neuronal glycoproteinosis—Lafora's disease in the dog. *J Am Anim Hosp Assoc* 12:518–521, 1976.
334. Montgomery DL, Lee AC: Brain damage in the epileptic beagle dog. *Vet Pathol* 20:160–169, 1983.
335. Braund KG: Granulomatous meningoencephalomyelitis. *J Am Vet Med Assoc* 186:138–141, 1985.
336. Braund KG, Vandevelde M, Walker TL, Redding RW: Granulomatous meningoencephalomyelitis in six dogs. *J Am Vet Med Assoc* 172:1195–1200, 1978.
337. Cordy DR: Canine granulomatous meningoencephalomyelitis. *Vet Pathol* 16:325–333, 1979.
338. Palmer AC: Pathogenesis and pathology of the cerebello-vestibular syndrome. *J Small Anim Pract* 11:167–176, 1970.
339. Koestner A: Primary lymphoreticuloses of the nervous system in animals. *Acta Neuropathol* (Suppl VI):85–89, 1975.
340. Koestner A, Zeman W: Primary reticuloses of the central nervous system in dogs. *Am J Vet Res* 23:381–392, 1962.
341. Cuddon PA, Smith-Maxie L: Reticulosis of the central nervous system in the dog. *Comp Cont Educ* 6:23–33 1984
342. Glastonbury JRW, Frauenfelder AR: Granulomatous meningoencephalomyelitis in a dog. *Aust Vet J* 57:186–189, 1981.
343. Alley MR, Jones BR, Johnstone AC: Granulomatous meningoencephalomyelitis of dogs in New Zealand. *NZ Vet J* 31:117–119, 1983.
344. Russo ME; Primary reticulosis of the central nervous system in dogs. *J Am Vet Med Assoc* 174:492–500, 1979.
345. Fankhauser R, Fatzer R, Luginbuhl H, McGrath JT: Reticulosis of the central nervous system (CNS) in dogs. *Adv Vet Sci Comp Med* 16:35–71, 1972.
346. Vandevelde M: Primary reticulosis of the central nervous system. *Vet Clin North Am* 10:57–63, 1980.
347. Vandevelde M, Fatzer R, Fankhauser R: Immunohistologic studies in primary reticulosis of the canine brain. *Vet Pathol* 18:577–588, 1981.

348. Cameron AM, Conroy JD; Rabies-like neuronal inclusions associated with a neoplastic reticulosis in a dog. *Vet Pathol* 11:29–37, 1974.
349. Vandevelde M, Kristensen B, Greene CE: Primary reticulosis of the central nervous system in the dog. *Vet Pathol* 15:673–675, 1978.
350. Fischer CA, Jones GT: Optic neuritis in dogs. *J Am Vet Med Assoc* 160:68–79, 1972.
351. Fischer CA, Liu S-K: Neuro-ophthalmic manifestations of primary reticulosis of the central nervous system in a dog. *J Am Vet Med Assoc* 158:1240–1248, 1971.
352. Garmer NL, Naeser P, Bergman AJ: Reticulosis of the eyes and the central nervous system in a dog. *J Small Anim Pract* 22:39–45, 1981.
353. Smith JS, de Lahunta A, Riis RC; Reticulosis of the visual system in a dog. *J Small Anim Pract* 18:643–652, 1977.
354. Morgan JP: Congenital anomalies of the vertebral column of the dog: a study of the incidence and significance based on a radiographic and morphometric study. *J Am Vet Radiol Soc* 9:21–29, 1968.
355. Bailey CS: An embryological approach to the clinical significance of congenital vertebral and spinal cord abnormalities. *J Am Anim Hosp Assoc* 11:426–434, 1975.
356. Schmorl G, Junghanns H: *The Human Spine in Health and Disease*, ed 2. New York. Grune and Stratton, 1971.
357. Done SH, Drew RA, Robins GM, Lane JG: Hemivertebra in the dog: clinical and pathological observations. *Vet Rec* 96:313–317, 1975.
358. Drew RA: Possible association between abnormal vertebral development and neonatal mortality in bulldogs. *Vet Rec* 94:480–481, 1974.
359. Dahme E, Schroder B: Kongophile Angiopathie cerebrovascular Mikroaneurysmen und cerebrale Blutungen beim alten Hund. *Zentralbl Veterinarmed* A26:601–613, 1979.
360. Cordy DR: Vascular malformations and hemangiomas of the canine spinal cord. *Vet Pathol* 16:275–282, 1979.
361. Fankhauser R, Luginbuhl H: *Pathologische Anatomie des Zentralen und Peripheren Nervensystems der Haustiere.* Berlin, Paul Parey, 1968.
362. Fankhauser R, Luginbuhl H, McGrath JT: Cerebrovascular disease in various animal species. *Ann NY Acad Sci* 127:817–860, 1965.
363. Zaki FA: Vascular malformation (cavernous angioma) of the spinal cord in a dog. *J Small Anim Pract* 20:417–422, 1979.
364. Strombeck DR, Meyer DJ, Freedland RA: Hyperammonemia due to a urea cycle enzyme deficiency in two dogs. *J Am Vet Med Assoc* 166:1109–1111, 1975.
365. Strombeck DR, Weiser MG, Kaneko JA: Hyperammonemia and hepatic encephalopathy in the dog. *J Am Vet Med Assoc* 166:1105–1108, 1975.
366. Strombeck DR, Krum S, Rogers Q: Coagulopathy and encephalopathy in a dog with acute hepatic necrosis. *J Am Vet Med Assoc* 169:813–816, 1976.
367. Strombeck DR, Breznock EM, McNeel S: Surgical treatment for portosystemic shunts in two dogs. *J Am Vet Med Assoc* 170:1317–1319, 1977.
368. Vulgamott JC: Hepatic encephalopathy associated with acquired portocaval shunt in a dog. *J Am Vet Med Assoc* 175:724–726, 1979.
369. Twedt DC: Jaundice hepatic trauma and hepatic encephalopathy. *Vet Clin North Am* 11:121–145, 1981.
370. Griffiths GL, Lumsden JH, Valli VEO: Hematologic and biochemical changes in dogs with portosystemic shunts. *J Am Anim Hosp Assoc* 17:705–710, 1981.
371. Vulgamot JC, Turnwald GH, King GK, Herring DS, Hansen JF, Boothe HW: Congenital portocaval anomalies in the cat: two case reports. *J Am Anim Hosp Assoc* 16:915–919, 1980.
372. Levesque DC, Oliver JE, Cornelius LM, Mahaffey MB, Rawlings CA, Kolata RJ: Congenital portocaval shunts in two cats: diagnosis and surgical correction. *J Am Vet Med Assoc* 181:143–145, 1982.
373. Meyer DJ, Strombeck DR, Stone EA, Zenoble RD, Buss DD: Ammonia tolerance test in clinically normal dogs and in dogs with portosystemic shunts. *J Am Vet Med Assoc* 173:377–379, 1978.
374. Center SA, Baldwin BH, de Lahunta A, Dietze AE, Tennant BC: Evaluation of serum bile acid concentrations for the diagnosis of portosystemic venous anomalies in the dog and cat. *J Am Vet Med Assoc* 186:1090–1094, 1985.
375. Bjorck G, Dyrendahl S, Olsson SE: Hereditary ataxia in smooth-haired fox terriers. *Vet Rec* 69:87–92, 1957.

376. Bjorck G, Mair W, Olsson SE, Sourander P: Hereditary ataxia in fox terriers. *Acta Neuropathol (Berl) 1* (Suppl):45–48, 1962.
377. Hartley WJ, Palmer AC: Ataxia in Jack Russell terriers. *Acta Neuropathol (Berl)* 26:71–74, 1973.
378. Cockrell BY, Herigstad RR, Flo GJ, Legendre AB: Myelomalacia in Afghan hounds. *J Am Vet Med Assoc* 162:362–365, 1973.
379. Averill DR, Bronson RT: Inherited necrotizing myelopathy of Afghan hounds. *J Neuropathol Exp Neurol* 36:734–747, 1977.
380. Cummings JF, de Lahunta A: Hereditary myelopathy of Afghan hounds, a myelinolytic disease. *Acta Neuropathol (Berl)* 42:173–181, 1978.
381. Kramer JW, Hegreberg GA, Bryan GM, Meyers K, Ott RL: A muscle disorder of Labrador retrievers characterized by deficiency of type II muscle fibers. *J Am Vet Med Assoc* 169:817–820, 1976.
382. Kramer JW, Hegreberg GA, Hamilton MJ: Inheritance of a neuromuscular disorder of Labrador retriever dogs. *J Am Vet Med Assoc* 179:380–381, 1981.
383. Braund KG: Hereditory myopathy in Labrador retrievers. *Calif Vet* 39:18–21, 1985.
384. McKerrell RE, Braund KG: An examination of the range of morphological and morphometric abnormalities of muscle seen in Labrador retriever myopathy. In *Proceedings of the 3rd Medical Forum, American College of Veterinary Internal Medicine*, June 1, 1985, p 136.
385. McKerrell RE, Anderson JR, Herrtage ME, Littlewood JD, Palmer AC: Generalized muscle weakness in the Labrador retriever. *Vet Rec* 115:276, 1984.
386. Simpson ST, Braund KG, Sorjonen DC: Muscular dystrophy of Labrador retrievers. In *Scientific Proceedings, American College of Veterinary Internal Medicine*, July 19, 1982, p 78.
387. Palmer AC, Payne JE, Wallace ME: Hereditary quadriplegia and amblyopia in the Irish setter. *J Small Anim Pract* 14:343–352, 1973.
388. Carmichael LE, Squire RA, Krook L: Clinical and pathological features of a fatal virus disease of new-born pups. *Am J Vet Res* 26:803–814, 1965.
389. Percy DH, Munnell JF, Olander HJ, Carmichael LE: Pathogenesis of canine herpesvirus encephalitis. *Am J Vet Res* 31:145–156, 1970.
390. Carmichael LE, Barnes FD, Percy DH: Temperature as a factor in resistance of young puppies to canine herpesvirus. *J Infect Dis* 120:669–678, 1970.
391. Wright NG, Cornwell HJC: Experimental herpes virus infection in young puppies. *Res Vet Sci* 9:295–299, 1968.
392. Percy DH, Olander HJ, Carmichael LE; Encephalitis in the newborn pup due to a canine herpesvirus. *Pathol Vet* 5:135–145, 1968.
393. Ward BC, Jones BD, Rubin GJ: Hexachlorophene toxicity in dogs. *J Am Anim Hosp Assoc* 9:167–169, 1973.
394. Edds GT, Simpson CF: Hexachlorophene-pHisohex toxicity in pups. *Am J Vet Res* 35:1005–1007, 1974.
395. Bath ML; Hexachlorophene toxicity in dogs. *J Small Anim Pract* 19:241–244, 1978.
396. Kimbrough RD: Review of the toxicity of hexachlorophene including its toxicity. *J Clin Pharmacol* 13:439–444, 1973.
397. Hanig JP, Krop S, Morrison JM, Colson SH: Observations on hexachlorophene-induced paralysis in the cat and its antagonism by hypertonic urea (39352). *Proc Soc Exp Biol Med* 152:165–169, 1976.
398. Palmer AC, Medd RK: Hound ataxia. *Vet Rec* 109:43, 1981.
399. Icenogle DA, Kaplan AM: A review of congenital neurologic malformations. *Clin Pediatr* 20:565–576, 1981.
400. MacLachlan NJ, Osburn BI: Bluetongue virus-induced hydranencephaly in cattle. *Vet Pathol* 20:563–573, 1983.
401. Osburn BI, Silverstein AM, Prendergast RA, Johnson RJ, Parshall CJ: Experimental viral-induced congenital encephalopathies. I. Pathology of hydranencephaly and porencephaly caused by bluetongue vaccine virus. *Lab Invest* 25:197–205, 1971.
402. Greene CE, Gorgacz EJ, Martin CL; Hydranencephaly associated with feline panleukopenia. *J Am Vet Med Assoc* 180:767–768, 1982.
403. Selby LA, Hayes HM, Becker SV: Epizootiologic features of canine hydrocephalus. *Am J Vet Res* 40:411–413, 1979.
404. Fankhauser R: Hydrocephalus studien. *Schweiz Arch Tierheilkd* 101:407–416, 1959.
405. Sahar A, Hochwald GM, Kay WJ, Ransohoff J: Spontaneous canine hydrocephalus:

cerebrospinal fluid dynamics. *J Neurol Neurosurg Psychiatry* 34:308–315, 1971.

406. Higgins RJ, Vandevelde M, Braund KG: Internal hydrocephalus and associated periventricular encephalitis in young dogs. *Vet Pathol* 14:236–246, 1977.

407. James AV, Burns B, Flor WF, Strecker E-P, Merz T, Bush M, Price DL: Pathophysiology of chronic communicating hydrocephalus in dogs (canis familiaris). *J Neurol Sci* 24:151–178, 1975.

408. Strecker E-P, Bush M, James AV: Cerebrospinal fluid imaging as a method to evaluate communicating hydrocephalus in dogs. *Am J Vet Res* 34:101–104, 1973.

409. Silson M, Robinson R: Hereditary hydrocephalus in the cat. *Vet Rec* 84:477, 1969.

410. de Lahunta A, Cummings JF: The clinical and electroencephalographic features of hydrocephalus in three dogs. *J Am Vet Med Assoc* 146:954–964, 1965.

411. Prynn RB, Redding RW: Electroencephalogram in occult canine hydrocephalus. *J Am Vet Med Assoc* 152:1651–1657, 1968.

412. Few AB: The diagnosis and surgical treatment of canine hydrocephalus. *J Am Vet Med Assoc* 149:286–293, 1966.

413. Gage ED, Hoerlein BF: Surgical treatment of canine hydrocephalus by ventriculoatrial shunting. *J Am Vet Med Assoc* 153:1418–1431, 1968.

414. Johnson I, Gilday DL, Hendrick EB: Experimental effects of steroids and steroid withdrawal on cerebrospinal fluid absorption. *J Neurosurg* 42:690–695, 1975.

415. Braund KG, Dillon AR, Mikeal RL, August JR: Subclinical myopathy associated with hyperadrenocorticism in the dog. *Vet Pathol* 17:134–148, 1980.

416. Hoskins JD, Nafe LA, Cho DY: Myopathy associated with hyperadrenocorticism in a dog: a case report. *Vet Med Small Anim Clin* 77:760–764, 1982.

417. Greene CE, Lorenz MD, Munnell JF, Prasse KW, White NA, Bowen JM: Myopathy associated with hyperadrenocorticism in the dog. *J Am Vet Med Assoc* 174:1310–1315, 1979.

418. Braund KG, Dillon AR, Mikeal RL; Experimental investigation of glucocorticoid-induced myopathy in the dog. *Exp Neurol* 68:50–71, 1980.

419. Jezyk PF: Hyperkalemic periodic paralysis in a dog. *J Am Anim Hosp Assoc* 18:977–980, 1982.

420. Cummings JF, Cooper BJ, de Lahunta A, van Winkle TJ: Canine inherited hypertrophic neuropathy. *Acta Neuropathol (Berl)* 53:137–143, 1981.

421. English PB, Seawright AA: Deforming cervical spondylosis of the cat. *Aust Vet J* 40:376–381, 1964.

422. Baker JR, Hughes IB: A case of deforming cervical spondylosis in a cat associated with a diet rich in liver. *Vet Rec* 83:44–45, 1968.

423. Lucke VM, Baskerville A, Bardgett PL, Mann PGH, Thompson SY: Deforming cervical spondylosis in the cat associated with hypervitaminosis A. *Vet Rec* 82:141–142, 1968.

424. Fry PD: Cervical spondylosis in the cat. *J Small Anim Pract* 9:59–61, 1968.

425. Clark L, Seawright AA, Gartner RJW: Longbone abnormalities in kittens following vitamin A administration. *J Comp Pathol* 80:113–121, 1970.

426. Caywood DD, Wilson JW, Hardy RM, Shull RM: Pancreatic islet cell adenocarcinoma: clinical and diagnostic features of six cases. *J Am Vet Med Assoc* 174:714–717, 1979.

427. Turnwald GH, Troy GC: Hypoglycemia. Part I. Carbohydrate metabolism and laboratory evaluation. *Comp Cont Educ* 5:932–937, 1983.

428. Turnwald GH, Troy GC: Hypoglycemia. Part II. Clinical aspects. *Comp Cont Educ* 6:115–125, 1984.

429. Prescott CW, Thompson HL: Insulinoma in the dog. *Aust Vet J* 56:502–505, 1980.

430. Steinberg HS: Insulin secreting pancreatic tumors in the dog. *J Am Anim Hosp Assoc* 16:695–698, 1980.

431. Kruth SA, Feldman EC, Kennedy PC: Insulin-secreting islet cell tumors: establishing a diagnosis and the clinical course for 25 dogs. *J Am Vet Med Assoc* 181:54–58, 1982.

432. Shahar R, Rousseaux C, Steiss J: Peripheral polyneuropathy in a dog with functional islet B-cell tumor and widespread metastasis. *J Am Vet Med Assoc* 187:175–177, 1985.

433. Chrisman CL: Postoperative results and complications of insulinomas in dogs. *J Am Anim Hosp Assoc* 16:677–684, 1980.

434. Parker AJ, O'Brien D, Musselman EE: Diazoxide treatment of metastatic insulinoma

in a dog. *J Am Anim Hosp Assoc* 18:315–318, 1982.

435. Leifer CE, Peterson ME, Matus RE, Patnaik AK: Hypoglycemia associated with nonislet cell tumor in 13 dogs. *J Am Vet Med Assoc* 186:53–55, 1985.

436. Done JT: Developmental disorders of the nervous system in animals. *Adv Vet Sci Comp Med* 21:69–114, 1977.

437. Foulkes JA: Myelin and dysmyelination in domestic animals. *Vet Bull* 8:441–450, 1974.

438. Harding JDJ, Done JT, Harbourne JF, Gilbert FR: Congenital tremor type A III in pigs: an hereditary sex-linked cerebrospinal hypomyelinogenesis. *Vet Rec* 92:527–529, 1973.

439. Vandevelde M, Braund KG, Walker TL, Kornegay JN: Dysmyelination of the central nervous system in the chow-chow dog. *Acta Neuropathol (Berl)* 42:211–215, 1978.

440. Vandevelde M, Braund KG, Luttgen PJ, Higgins RJ: Dysmyelination in chow chow dog: further studies in older dogs. *Acta Neuropathol (Berl)* 55:81–87, 1981.

441. Mayhew IG, Blakemore WF, Palmer AC, Clarke CJ: Tremor syndrome and hypomyelination in lurcher pups. *J Small Anim Pract* 25:551–559, 1984.

442. Griffiths IR, Duncan ID, McCulloch M, Harvey MJA: Shaking pups: a disorder of central myelination in the spaniel dog. Part 1. Clinical genetic and light microscopical observations. *J Neurol Sci* 50:423–433, 1981.

443. Greene CE, Vandevelde M, Hoff EJ: Congenital cerebrospinal hypomyelinogenesis in a pup. *J Am Vet Med Assoc* 171:534–536, 1977.

444. Braund KG, Dillon AR, August JR, Ganjam VK: Hypothyroid myopathy in two dogs. *Vet Pathol* 18:589–598, 1981.

445. Cardinet GH: Nemaline rods in neuromuscular disorders of the dog. *Zentralbl Veterinarmed* C13:87, 1984.

446. Braund KG, Dillon AR, Pidgeon GL, August JR: Neuromuscular changes in dogs with spontaneous diabetes mellitus. In *American College of Veterinary Internal Medicine, Scientific Proceedings*, July 20, 1981, p 53.

447. Cardinet GH, Wallace LJ, Fedde MR, Guffy MM, Bardens JW: Developmental myopathy in the canine. *Arch Neurol* 21:620–631, 1969.

448. Cardinet GH, Fedde MR, Tunell GL: Correlates of histochemical and physiologic properties in normal and hypertrophic pectineus muscles of the dog. *Lab Invest* 27:32–38, 1972.

449. Lust G, Craig DH, Ross GE, Geary JC: Studies on pectineus muscles in canine hip dysplasia. *Cornell Vet* 62:628–645, 1972.

450. Braund KG, Luttgen PJ, Sorjonen DC, Redding RW: Idiopathic facial paralysis in the dog. *Vet Rec* 105:297–299, 1979.

451. Renegar WR: Auriculopalpebral nerve paralysis following prolonged anesthesia in a dog. *J Am Vet Med Assoc* 174:1007–1009, 1979.

452. Vandevelde M, Braund KG: Polioencephalomyelitis in cats. *Vet Pathol* 16:420–427, 1979.

453. Schunk KL: Feline polymyopathy. In *Proceedings of the Second Annual Forum, American College of Veterinary Internal Medicine*, Washington, May 17, 1984, pp 197–200.

454. Lane JR, de Lahunta A: Polyneuritis in a cat. *J Am Anim Hosp Assoc* 20:1006–1008, 1984.

455. Bedford PDC: Congenital vestibular disease in the English cocker spaniel. *Vet Rec* 105:530–531, 1979.

456. Chrisman CL: Vestibular diseases. *Vet Clin North Am* 10:103–129, 1980.

457. Lee M: Congenital vestibular disease in a German shepherd dog. *Vet Rec* 113:571, 1983.

458. Braund KG, Shires PK, Mikeal RL: Type 1 fiber atrophy in the vastus lateralis muscle in dogs with femoral fractures treated by hyperextension. *Vet Pathol* 17:164–176, 1980.

459. Shires PK, Braund KG, Milton JL, Liu W: Effect of localized trauma and temporary splinting on immature skeletal muscle and mobility of the femorotibial joint in the dog. *Am J Vet Res* 43:454–460, 1982.

460. Detweiler DK, Ratcliffe ML, Luginbuhl H: The significance of naturally occurring coronary and cerebral arterial disease in animals. *Ann NY Acad Sci* 149:868–881, 1968.

461. Patterson JS, Rusely MS, Zachary JF: Neurologic manifestations of cerebrovascular atherosclerosis associated with primary hypothyroidism in a dog. *J Am Vet Med Assoc* 186:499–503, 1985.

462. Greene CE, Higgins RJ: Fibrocartilaginous emboli as the cause of ischemic myelopathy in a dog. *Cornell Vet* 66:131–142, 1976.

463. Griffiths IR: Spinal cord infarction due to emboli arising from the intervertebral discs in the dog. *J Comp Pathol* 83:225–232, 1973.

464. Hayes MA, Creighton SR, Boysen BG, Holfeld N: Acute necrotizing myelopathy from nucleus pulposus embolism in dogs with intervertebral disk degeneration. *J Am Vet Med Assoc* 169:289–295, 1978.

465. Zaki FA, Prata RG, Kay WJ: Necrotizing myelopathy in five Great Danes. *J Am Vet Med Assoc* 165:1080–1084, 1974.

466. Zaki FA, Prata RG: Necrotizing myelopathy secondary to embolization of herniated intervertebral disk material in the dog. *J Am Vet Med Assoc* 169:222–228, 1976.

467. Zaki FA, Prata RG, Werner LL: Necrotizing myelopathy in a cat. *J Am Vet Med Assoc* 169:228–229, 1976.

468. de Lahunta A: Feline neurology. *Vet Clin North Am* 6:433–452, 1976.

469. Zaki FA, Nafe LA: Ischemic encephalopathy and focal granulomatous meningoencephalitis in the cat. *J Small Anim Pract* 21:429–438, 1980.

470. Appel MJG, Bistner SI, Menegus M, Albert D, Carmichael LE: Pathogenicity of low virulence strains of two canine adenovirus types. *Am J Vet Res* 34:543–550, 1973.

471. Wright NG: Recent advances in canine virus research. *J Small Anim Pract* 14:241–250, 1973.

472. Liu S-K: Acquired cardiac lesions leading to congestive heart failure in the cat. *Am J Vet Res* 31:2071–2088, 1970.

473. Tilley LP, Lord PF, Wood A: Acquired heart disease and aortic thromboembolism in the cat In Kirk RW (ed): *Current Veterinary Therapy V*. Philadelphia, WB Saunders, 1974, p 305.

474. Butler HC: An investigation into the relationship of an aortic embolus to posterior paralysis in the cat. *J Small Anim Pract* 12:141–158, 1971.

475. Olmstead ML, Butler HC: Five-hydroxytryptamine antagonists and feline aortic embolism. *J Small Anim Pract* 18:247–259, 1977.

476. Tilley LP, Liu S-K: Cardiomyopathy and thromboembolism in the cat. *Feline Pract* 5:32–41, 1975.

477. Griffiths IR, Duncan ID: Ischaemic neuromyopathy in cats. *Vet Rec* 104:518–522, 1979.

478. Schunk KL, Averill DR: Peripheral vestibular syndrome in the dog: a review of 83 cases. *J Am Vet Med Assoc* 182:1354–1357, 1983.

479. Roberts SR, Vainisi SJ: Hemifacial spasm in dogs. *J Am Vet Med Assoc* 150:381–385, 1967.

480. Parker AJ, Cusick PK, Park RD, Small E: Hemifacial spasms in a dog. *Vet Rec* 93:514–516, 1973.

481. Oliver JE, Lorenz MD: *Handbook of Veterinary Neurologic Diagnosis*. Philadelphia, WB Saunders, 1983.

482. Reinke JD, Suter PF: Laryngeal paralysis in a dog. *J Am Vet Med Assoc* 172:714–716, 1978.

483. Venker-van Haagen AJ, Hartman W, Goedogebuure SA: Spontaneous laryngeal paralysis in young Bouviers. *J Am Anim Hosp Assoc* 14:714–720, 1978.

484. Venker-van Haagen AJ, Bouw J, Hartman W: Hereditary transmission of laryngeal paralysis in Bouviers. *J Am Anim Hosp Assoc* 17:75–76, 1981.

485. O'Brien JA, Harvey CE, Kelly AA, Tucker JA: Neurogenic atrophy of the laryngeal muscles of the dog. *J Small Anim Pract* 14:521–532, 1973.

486. Gaber CE, Amis TC, LeCouteur RA: Laryngeal paralysis in dogs: a review of 23 cases. *J Am Vet Med Assoc* 186:377–380, 1985.

487. Schaer M, Zaki FA, Harvey HJ, O'Reilly WH: Laryngeal hemiplegia due to neoplasia of the vagus nerve in a cat. *J Am Vet Med Assoc* 174:513–515, 1979.

488. Hardie EM, Kolata RJ, Stone EA, Steiss JE: Laryngeal paralysis in three cats. *J Am Vet Med Assoc* 179:879–882, 1981.

489. Harvey CE, O'Brien JA: Management of respiratory emergencies in small animals. *Vet Clin North Am* 2:243–258, 1972.

490. Harvey CE, Venker-van Haagen AJ: Surgical management of pharyngeal and laryn-

geal airway obstruction in the dog. *Vet Clin North Am* 5:515–535, 1975.
491. Hendricks JC, O'Brien JA: Inherited laryngeal paralysis in Siberian husky crosses. In *Proceedings of the Third Annual Medical Forum, American College of Veterinary Internal Medicine*, San Diego, June 1, 1985, p 143.
492. Zook BC, Carpenter JL, Roberts RM: Lead poisoning in dogs: occurrence, source, clinical pathology, and electroencephalography. *Am J Vet Res* 33:891–902, 1972.
493. Zook BC, Kopito MS, Carpenter JL, Cramer DV, Shwachman H: Lead poisoning in dogs: analysis of blood, urine, hair, and liver for lead. *Am J Vet Res* 33:903–909, 1972.
494. Clarke EGC: Lead poisoning in small animals. *J Small Anim Pract* 14:183–193, 1973.
495. Kowalczyk DF: Lead poisoning in dogs at the University of Pennsylvania Veterinary Hospital. *J Am Vet Med Assoc* 168:428–432, 1976.
496. Kowalczyk DF: Lead poisoning. In Kirk RW (ed): *Current Veterinary Therapy VIII*. Philadelphia, WB Saunders, 1983, p 107.
497. O'Brien DP: Lead toxicity in a dog. *J Am Anim Hosp Assoc* 17:845–850, 1981.
498. Zook BC: The pathologic anatomy of lead poisoning in dogs. *Vet Pathol* 9:310–327, 1972.
499. Gamble DA, Chrisman CL: A leukoencephalomyelopathy of rottweiler dogs. *Vet Pathol* 21:174–180, 1984.
500. Greene CE, Vandevelde M, Braund K: Lissencephaly in two Lhasa apso dogs. *J Am Vet Med Assoc* 169:405–410, 1976.
501. Zaki FA: Lissencephaly in Lhasa apso dogs. *J Am Vet Med Assoc* 169:1165–1168, 1976.
502. Oliver JE, Selcer RR, Simpson S: Cauda equina compression from lumbosacral malarticulation and malformation in the dog. *J Am Vet Med Assoc* 173:207–214, 1978.
503. Tarvin G, Prata RG: Lumbosacral stenosis in dogs. *J Am Vet Med Assoc* 177:154–159, 1980.
504. Denny HR, Gibbs C, Holt PE: The diagnosis and treatment of cauda equina lesions in the dog. *J Small Anim Pract* 23:425–443, 1982.
504a. Hurov L: Laminectomy for treatment of cauda equina syndrome in a cat. *J Am Vet Med Assoc* 186:504–505, 1985.
505. Berzon JL, Dueland R: Cauda equina syndrome: pathophysiology and report of seven cases. *J Am Anim Hosp Assoc* 15:635–643, 1979.
506. Slocum B, Rudy RL; Fractures of the seventh lumbar vertebra in the dog. *J Am Anim Hosp Assoc* 11:167–174, 1975.
507. Lenehan TM: Canine cauda equina syndrome. *Comp Cont Educ* 5:941–951, 1983.
508. Bagshaw RJ, Cox RH, Knight DH, Detweiler DK: Malignant hyperthermia in a greyhound. *J Am Vet Med Assoc* 172:61–62, 1978.
509. Cohen CA: Malignant hyperthermia in a greyhound. *J Am Vet Med Assoc* 172:1254–1255, 1978.
510. Sawyer DC: Malignant hyperthermia. *J Am Vet Med Assoc* 179:341–344, 1981.
511. McGrath CJ, Crimi AJ, Ruff J: Malignant hyperthermia in dogs. *Vet Med Small Anim Clin* 77:218–220, 1982.
512. Short CE: Malignant hyperthermia in the dog. *Anesthesiology* 39:462–463, 1973.
513. De Jong RH, Heavner JE, Amory DW: Malignant hyperpyrexia in the cat. *Anesthesiology* 41:608–609, 1974.
514. O'Brien PJ, Cribb PH, White RJ, Olfert ED, Steiss JE: Canine malignant hyperthermia: diagnosis of susceptibility in a breeding colony. *Can Vet J* 24:172–177, 1983.
515. O'Brien PJ, Rand JS: Canine stress syndrome. *J Am Vet Med Assoc* 186:432–433, 1985.
516. Kirmayer AH, Klide AM, Purvance JE: Malignant hyperthermia in a dog: case report and review of the syndrome. *J Am Vet Med Assoc* 185:978–982, 1984.
517. Bagshaw RJ, Cox RH, Rosenberg H: Dantrolene treatment of malignant hyperthermia. *J Am Vet Med Assoc* 178:1029, 1981.
518. O'Brien PJ, Forsyth GW: Preparation of injectible dantrolene for emergency treatment of malignant hyperthermia-like syndromes. *Can Vet J* 24:200, 1983.
519. O'Brien PJ, Forsyth GW, Olexsen DW, Thatte HS, Addis PB: Canine malignant hyperthermia susceptibility: erythrocyte defects—osmotic fragility, glucose-6-phosphate dehydrogenase deficiency and abnormal Ca^{2+} homeostasis. *Can J Comp Med* 48:381–389, 1984.
520. Burditt LJ, Chotai K, Hirani S, Nugent PG, Winchester BG, Blakemore WF:

Biochemical studies on a case of feline mannosidosis. *Biochem J* 189:467–473, 1980.

521. Walkley SU, Blakemore WF, Purpura DP: Alterations in neuron morphology in feline mannosidosis. *Acta Neuropathol (Berl)* 53:75–79, 1981.

522. Vandevelde M, Fankhauser R, Bischel P, Wiesmann U, Herschkowitz N: Hereditary neurovisceral mannosidosis associated with α-mannosidase deficiency in a family of Persian cats. *Acta Neuropathol (Berl)* 58:64–68, 1982.

523. Whitney JC: Eosinophilic myositis in dogs. *Vet Rec* 67:1140–1143, 1955.

523a. Scott DW, de Lahunta A: Eosinophilic polymyositis in a dog. *Cornell Vet* 64:47–56, 1974.

524. Bullmore CC, Sevedge JP: Canine meningoencephalitis. *J Am Anim Hosp Assoc* 14:387–394, 1978.

525. Hudson MD: Bacterial meningitis. *J Am Anim Hosp Assoc* 12:88–91, 1976.

526. Kornegay JN, Lorenz MD, Zenoble RD: Bacterial meningoencephalitis in two dogs. *J Am Vet Med Assoc* 173:1334–1336, 1978.

527. Chew M: Canine meningo-encephalitis due to *Trypanosoma evansi* infection. A report of two cases. *Vet Rec* 83:663–665, 1968.

528. Brewer NS: Antimicrobial agents. Part II. The aminoglycosides. *Mayo Clin Proc* 52:675–679, 1977.

529. Meric S, Perman V, Hardy R: Corticosteroid responsive meningitis in ten dogs. In *Proceedings of the 3rd Annual Medical Forum, American College of Veterinary Internal Medicine*, June 1, 1985, p 148.

530. Harcourt RA: Polyarteritis in a colony of beagles. *Vet Rec* 102:519–522, 1978.

531. Kelly DF, Grunsell CSG, Kenyon CJ: Polyarteritis in a dog: a case report. *Vet Rec* 92:363, 1973.

532. Hoff EJ, Vandevelde M: Case report: necrotizing vasculitis in the central nervous system of two dogs. *Vet Pathol* 18:219–223, 1981.

533. Haskins ME, Jezyk PF, Desnick RJ, McDonough SK, Patterson DF: Mucopolysaccharidosis in a domestic short-haired cat—a disease distinct from that seen in the Siamese cat. *J Am Vet Med Assoc* 175:384–387, 1979.

534. Cowell KR, Jezyk PF, Haskins ME, Patterson DF: Mucopolysaccharidosis in a cat. *J Am Vet Med Assoc* 169:334–339, 1976.

535. Langweiler M, Haskins ME, Jezyk PF: Mucopolysaccharidosis in a litter of cats. *J Am Anim Hosp Assoc* 14:748–751, 1978.

536. Haskins ME, Bingel SA, Northington JW, Newton GD, Sande RD, Jezyk PF, Patterson DF: Spinal cord compression and hindlimb paresis in cats with mucopolysaccharidosis VI. *J Am Vet Med Assoc* 182:983–985, 1983.

537. Breton L, Guerin P, Morin M: A case of mucopolysaccharidosis VI in a cat. *J Am Anim Hosp Assoc* 19:891–896, 1983.

538. Gambardella PC, Osborne CA, Stevens JB: Multiple cartilaginous exostoses in the dog. *J Am Vet Med Assoc* 166:761–768, 1975.

539. Prata RG, Stoll SG, Zaki FA: Spinal cord compression caused by osteocartilaginous exostoses of the spine in two dogs. *J Am Vet Med Assoc* 166:371–375, 1975.

540. Cummings JF, de Lahunta A, Winn SS: Acral multilation and nociceptive loss in English pointer dogs. A canine sensory neuropathy. *Acta Neuropathol (Berl)* 53:119–127, 1981.

541. Cummings JF, de Lahunta A, Braund KG, Mitchell WJ: Animal model of human disease: hereditary sensory neuropathy: nociceptive loss and acral mutilation in pointer dogs: canine hereditary sensory neuropathy. *Am J Pathol* 112:136–138, 1983.

542. Cummings JF, de Lahunta A, Simpson ST, McDonald JM: Reduced substance P-like immunoreactivity in hereditary sensory neuropathy of pointer dogs. *Acta Neuropathol (Berl)* 63:33–40, 1984.

543. Sanda A, Pivnik L: Die Zehennekrose bei kurzhaarigen Vorstehhunden. *Kleintierpraxis* 9:76–83, 1964.

544. Pivnik L: Zur vergleichenden Problematic einiger akrodystrophischer Neuropathien bei Menschen und Hund. *Schweiz Arch Neurol Neurochir Psychiatr* 112:365–371, 1973.

545. Sova Z: Die Pfotennekrose (neurotrophische erblich bedingte Osteopathie) Eine neue Erkrankung bei Welpen von Vorstehhunden. *Tierarztl Prax* 2:225–230, 1974.

546. Palmer AC, Barker J: Myasthenia in the dog. *Vet Rec* 95:452–454, 1974.

547. Schutt I, Kersten U: Myasthenia gravis pseudoparalytica bei drei Deutschen Schaferhundinnen. *Kleintierpraxis* 22:45–50, 1977.

548. Dawson JR: Myasthenia gravis in a cat. *Vet Rec* 86:562–563, 1970.
549. Mason KV: A case of myasthenia gravis in a cat. *J Small Anim Pract* 17:467–472, 1976.
550. Lennon VA, Palmer AC, Pflugfelder C, Indrieri RJ: Myasthenia gravis in dogs: acetylcholine receptor deficiency with and without anti-receptor antibodies. In Rose NR, Bigazzi PE, Warner NL (eds): *Genetic Control of Autoimmune Diseases.* New York, Elsevier-North Holland, 1978, p 295.
550a. Palmer AC, Lennon VA, Beadle C, Goodyear JV: Autoimmune form of myasthenia gravis in a juvenile Yorkshire terrier × Jack Russell terrier hybrid contrasted with congenital (non-autoimmune) myasthenia gravis of the Jack Russell. *J Small Anim Pract* 21:359–364, 1980.
551. Pflugfelder CM, Cardinet GH, Lutz H, Holliday TA, Hansen RJ: Acquired canine myasthenia gravis: immunocytochemical localization of immune complexes at neuromuscular junctions. *Muscle Nerve* 4:289–295, 1981.
552. Poffenbarger E, Klausner JS, Caywood DD: Acquired myasthenia gravis in a dog with thymoma: a case report. *J Am Anim Hosp Assoc* 21:119–124, 1985.
553. Breton L, Gosselin Y, Couture L: Myasthenie grave chez un jeune chien. *Can Vet J* 22:305–308, 1981.
554. Van Heerden J, Van Schouwenburg SJ: The use of corticosteroids in a dog with myasthenia gravis. *J S Afr Vet Assoc* 54:135–137, 1983.
555. Palmer AC, Goodyear JV: Congenital myasthenia in the Jack Russell terrier. *Vet Rec* 103:433–434, 1978.
556. Johnson RP, Watson ADJ, Smith J, Cooper BJ: Myasthenia in springer spaniel littermates. *J Small Anim Pract* 16:641–647, 1975.
557. Jenkins WL, Van Dyk E, McDonald CB: Myasthenia gravis in a fox terrier litter. *J S Afr Vet Assoc* 47:59–62, 1976.
558. Miller LM, Lennon VA, Lambert EH, Reed SM, Hegreberg GA, Miller JB, Ott RL: Congenital myasthenia gravis in 13 smooth fox terriers. *J Am Vet Med Assoc* 182:694–697, 1983.
559. Cordes DO, Royal WA: Cryptococcosis in a cat. *NZ Vet J* 15:117–121, 1967.
560. Jasmin AM, Carroll JM, Baucom JN, Beusse DO: Systemic blastomycosis in Siamese cats. *Vet Med Small Anim Clin* 64:33–37, 1969.
561. Kurtz HJ, Sharpnack S: *Blastomyces dermatitidis* meningoencephalitis in a dog. *Pathol Vet* 6:375–377, 1969.
562. Palmer AC, Herrtage ME, Kaplan W: Cryptococcal infection of the central nervous system of a dog in the United Kingdom. *J Small Anim Pract* 22:579–586, 1981.
563. Pryor WH, Huizenga CG, Splitter GA, Harwell JF: *Coccidioides immitis* encephalitis in two dogs. *J Am Vet Med Assoc* 161:1108–1112, 1972.
564. Sutton RH: Cryptococcosis in dogs: a report on 6 cases. *Aust Vet J* 57:558–564, 1981.
565. Wagner JL, Pick JR, Krigman MR: *Cryptococcus neoformans* infection in a dog. *J Am Vet Med Assoc* 153:945–949, 1968.
566. Nafe LA, Turk JR, Carter JD: Central nervous system involvement of blastomycosis in the dog. *J Am Anim Hosp Assoc* 19:933–936, 1983.
567. Schaer M, Johnson KE, Nicholson AC: Central nervous system disease due to histoplasmosis in a dog: a case report. *J Am Anim Hosp Assoc* 19:311–315, 1983.
568. Gwin RM, Makley TA, Wyman M, Werling K: Multifocal ocular histoplasmosis in a dog and cat. *J Am Vet Med Assoc* 176:638–642, 1980.
569. Scott DW: Feline dermatology. *J Am Anim Hosp Assoc* 16:349–365, 1980.
570. Wilkinson GT: Feline cryptococcosis: a review and seven case reports. *J Small Anim Pract* 20:749–768, 1979.
571. Prevost E, McKee JM, Crawford P: Successful medical management of severe feline cryptococcosis. *J Am Anim Hosp Assoc* 18:111–114, 1982.
572. Jang SS, Biberstein EL, Rinaldi MG, Henness AM, Boorman GA, Taylor RF: Feline brain abscesses due to *Cladosporium trichoides. Sabouraudia* 15:115–123, 1977.
573. Newsholme SJ, Tyrer MJ: Cerebral mycosis in a dog caused by *Cladosporium trichoides* Emmons 1952. *Onderstepoort J Vet Res* 47:47–49, 1980.
574. Ribas JL, Newton J, Braund KG, Dillehay D, Kwapien RP: Cerebral phaeohyphomycosis: an unusual mycosis of dogs and cats. In *Proceedings of the 3rd Medical Forum, American College of Veterinary Internal Medicine,* June 1, 1985, p 151.
575. Patnaik AK, Liu S-K, Wilkins RJ, Johnson GF, Seitz PE: Paecilomycosis in a dog. *J Am Vet Med Assoc* 161:806–813, 1972.

576. van den Hoven E, McKenzie RA: Suspected paecilomycosis in a dog. *Aust Vet J* 50:368–369, 1974.

577. Patterson JM, Rosendal S, Humphrey J, Teeter WG: A case of dissemiated paecilomycosis in the dog. *J Am Anim Hosp Assoc* 19:569–574, 1983.

578. Sims MA: *Flavobacterium meningosepticum*: a probable cause of meningitis in a cat. *Vet Rec* 95:567–569, 1974.

579. Lincoln SD, Adcock JL: Disseminated geotrichosis in a dog. *Pathol Vet* 5:282–289, 1968.

580. Mullaney TP, Levin S, Indrieri RJ: Disseminated aspergillosis in a dog. *J Am Vet Med Assoc* 182:516–518, 1983.

581. Wentink GH, van der Linde-Sipman JS, Meijer AEF, Kamphuisen HAC, van Vorstenbosch CJ, Hartman W, Hendriks HJ: Myopathy with a possible recessive X-linked inheritance in a litter of Irish terriers. *Vet Pathol* 9:328–349, 1972.

582. Wentink GH, Hartman W, Koeman JP: Three cases of myotonia in a family of chows. *Tijdschr Diergeneeskd* 14:729–731, 1974.

583. Shires PK, Nafe LA, Hulse DA: Myotonia in a Staffordshire terrier. *J Am Vet Med Assoc* 183:229–232, 1983.

584. Duncan ID, Griffiths IR, McQueen A: A myopathy associated with myotonia in the dog. *Acta Neuropathol (Berl)* 31:297–303, 1975.

585. Jones BR, Anderson LJ, Barnes GRG, Johnstone AC, Juby WD: Myotonia in related chow chow dogs. *NZ Vet J* 25:217–220, 1977.

586. Jones BR: Hereditary myotonia in the chow chow. *Vet Annu* 24:286–291, 1984.

587. Farrow BRH, Malik R: Hereditary myotonia in the chow chow. *J Small Anim Pract* 22:451–465, 1981.

588. Simpson ST, Braund KG: Myotonic dystrophy-like disease in a dog. *J Am Vet Med Assoc* 186:495–498, 1985.

589. Mitler MM, Boysen BG, Campbell L, Dement W: Narcolepsy-cataplexy in a female dog. *Exp Neurol* 45:332–340, 1974.

590. Mitler MM, Soave O, Dement WC: Narcolepsy in seven dogs. *J Am Vet Med Assoc* 168:1036–1038, 1976.

591. Knecht CD, Oliver JE, Redding R, Selcer R, Johnson G: Narcolepsy in a dog and a cat. *J Am Vet Med Assoc* 162:1052–1053, 1973.

592. Delashaw JB, Foutz AS, Guilleminault C, Dement WC: Cholinergic mechanisms and cataplexy in dogs. *Exp Neurol* 66:745–757, 1979.

593. Foutz AS, Mitler MM, Dement WC: Narcolepsy. *Vet Clin North Am* 10:65–80, 1980.

594. Boehme RE, Baker TL, Mefford IN, Barchas JD, Dement WC, Ciaranello RD: Narcolepsy: cholinergic receptor changes in an animal model. *Life Sci* 34:1825–1828, 1984.

595. Luginbuhl H: A comparative study of neoplasms of the central nervous system in animals. *Acta Neurochirurg* 10 (Suppl):30–42, 1964.

596. Luginbuhl H: Oligodendrogliomas in animals. *Acta Neurochirurg* 10 (Suppl):173–184, 1964.

597. Braund KG: Neoplasia of the nervous system. *Comp Cont Educ* 6:717–722, 1984.

598. Gieb LW: Ossifying meningioma with extracranial metastasis in a dog. *Pathol Vet* 3:247–254, 1966.

599. Luginbuhl H, Fankhauser R, McGrath JT: Spontaneous neoplasms of the nervous system in animals. *Prog Neurol Surg* 2:85–164, 1968.

600. Cordy DR: Tumors of the nervous system and eye. In Moulton JM (ed): *Tumors in Domestic Animals*, ed 2. Los Angeles, University of California Press, 1961, p 430.

601. Fankhauser R: Tumoren des Zentralnervensystems beim Tier. *Bull Schweiz Akad Med Wiss* 24:168–184, 1968.

602. Fankhauser R, Luginbuhl H, McGrath JT: Tumors of the nervous system. *Bull WHO* 50:53–69, 1974.

603. Hayes KC, Schiefer B: Primary tumors in the CNS of carnivores. *Pathol Vet* 6:94–116, 1969.

604. Palmer AC: Tumours of the central nervous system. *Proc R Coll Med* 69:49–51, 1976.

605. Kornegay JN, Oliver JE, Gorgacz EJ: Clinicopathologic features of brain herniation in animals. *J Am Vet Med Assoc* 182:1111–1116, 1983.

606. Palmer AC: Clinical and pathological features of some tumours of the central nervous system in dogs. *Res Vet Sci* 1:36–46, 1960.

607. Palmer AC: Clinical signs associated with intracranial tumours in dogs. *Res Vet Sci* 2:326–339, 1961.
608. Braund KG, Everett RM, Albert RA: Neurological manifestations of monoclonal IgM gammopathy associated with lymphocytic leukemia in a dog. *J Am Vet Med Assoc* 172:1407–1410, 1978.
609. Luttgen PJ, Braund KG, Brawner WR, Vandevelde M: A retrospective study of twenty-nine spinal tumours in the dog and cat. *J Small Anim Pract* 21:213–226, 1980.
610. Prata RG: Diagnosis of spinal cord tumors in the dog. *Vet Clin North Am* 7:165–185, 1977.
611. Hayes HM, Priester WA, Pendergrass TW: Occurrence of nervous-tissue tumors in cattle, horses, cats and dogs. *Int J Cancer* 15:39–47, 1975.
612. McGrath JT: Intracranial pathology of the dog. *Acta Neuropathol (Berl)* 1 (Suppl) 3–4, 1962.
613. Zaki FA: Spontaneous central nervous system tumors in the dog. *Vet Clin North Am* 7:153–163, 1977.
614. McGrath JT: Morphology and classification of brain tumors in domestic animals. In *Proceedings, Brain Tumors in Man and Animals*, National Institute of Environmental Health Sciences, Research Triangle Park, NC, September 4, 1984.
615. Fankhauser R, Vandevelde M: Zur klinik der tumoren des Nervensystems bei Hund und Katze. *Schweiz Arch Tierheilkd* 123:553–571, 1981.
616. Zaki FA, Nafe LA: Choroid plexus tumors in the dog. *J Am Vet Med Assoc* 176:328–330, 1980.
617. Braund KG, Ribas JL: Brain ventricular tumors. In *Proceedings of the 3rd Annual Medical Forum, American College of Veterinary Internal Medicine*, San Diego, June 1, 1985, p 157.
618. Andrews EJ: Clinicopathologic characteristics of meningiomas in dogs. *J Am Vet Med Assoc* 163:151–157, 1973.
619. Nafe LA: Meningiomas in cats: a retrospective clinical study of 36 cases. *J Am Vet Med Assoc* 174:1224–1227, 1979.
620. Luginbuhl H: Studies on meningiomas in cats. *Am J Vet Res* 22:1030–1040, 1961.
621. Zaki FA, Hurvitz AI: Spontaneous neoplasms of the central nervous system of the cat. *J Small Anim Pract* 17:773–782, 1976.
622. Braund KG, Everett RM, Bartels JE, DeBuysscher E: Neurologic complications of IgA multiple myelomas associated with cryoglobinulinemia in a dog. *J Am Vet Med Assoc* 174:1321–1325, 1979.
623. Wright JA, Bell DA, Clayton-Jones DG: The clinical and radiological features associated with spinal tumours in thirty dogs. *J Small Anim Pract* 20:461–472, 1979.
624. Morgan JP, Ackerman N, Bailey CS, Pool RR: Vertebral tumors in the dog: a clinical, radiologic, and pathologic study of 61 primary and secondary lesions. *Vet Radiol* 21:197–212, 1980.
625. Dorn CR: Epidemiology of canine and feline tumors. *J Am Anim Hosp Assoc* 12:307–312, 1976.
626. Engle GC, Bradey RS: A retrospective study of 395 feline neoplasms. *J Am Anim Hosp Assoc* 5:21–31, 1969.
627. O'Brien D, Parker AJ, Tarvin G: Osteosarcoma of the vertebra causing compression of the thoracic spinal cord in a cat. *J Am Anim Hosp Assoc* 16:497–499, 1980.
628. Northington JW, Juliana MM: Extradural lymphosarcoma in six cats. *J Small Anim Pract* 19:409–416, 1978.
629. Sorjonen DC, Braund KG, Hoff EJ: Paraplegia and subclinical neuromyopathy associated with a primary lung tumor in a dog. *J Am Vet Med Assoc* 180:1209–1211, 1982.
630. Bradley RL, Withrow SJ, Snyder SP: Nerve sheath tumors in the dog. *J Am Anim Hosp Assoc* 18:915–921, 1982.
631. Vandevelde M, Braund KG, Hoff EJ: Central neurofibromas in two dogs. *Vet Pathol* 14:470–478, 1977.
632. Allen JG, Amis T: Lymphosarcoma involving cranial nerves in a cat. *Aust Vet J* 51:155–158, 1975.
633. Rendano VT, de Lahunta A, King JM: Extracranial neoplasia with facial nerve paralysis in two cats. *J Am Anim Hosp Assoc* 16:921–925, 1980.
634. Kay WJ: Diagnosis of intracranial neoplasm. *Vet Clin North Am* 7:145–152, 1977.

635. Palmer AC, Malinowski W, Barnett KC: Clinical signs including papilloedema associated with brain tumors in twenty-one dogs. *J Small Anim Pract* 15:359–386, 1974.

636. Kallfelz FA, de Lahunta A, Allhands RV: Scintigraphic diagnosis of brain lesions in the dog and cat. *J Am Vet Med Assoc* 172:589–597, 1978.

637. Fike JR, Le Couteur RA, Cann CE, Pflugfelder CM: computerized tomography of brain tumors of the rostral and middle fossas in the dog. *Am J Vet Res* 42:275–281, 1981.

638. Fike JR, LeCouteur RA, Cann CE: Anatomy of the canine brain using high resolution computed tomography. *Vet Radiol* 22:236–243, 1981.

639. Le Couteur RA, Fike JR, Cann CE, Pedroia VG: Computed tomography of brain tumors in the caudal fossa of the dog. *Vet Radiol* 22:244–251, 1981.

640. Le Couteur RA, Fike JR, Cann CE, Turrell JM, Thompson JM, Biggart JF: X-ray computed tomography of brain tumors in cats. *J Am Vet Med Assoc* 183:301–305, 1983.

641. Schunk KL: Computed tomography of brain tumors in small animals. In *Proceedings of the 3rd Annual Medical Forum, American College of Veterinary Internal Medicine*, San Diego, June 1, 1985, p 159.

642. Roszel JF, Steinberg SA, McGrath JT: Periodic acid-Schiff-positive cells in cerebrospinal fluid of dogs with globoid cell leukodystrophy. *Neurology* 22:738–741, 1972.

643. Vandevelde M, Spano JS: Cerebrospinal fluid cytology in canine neurologic disease. *Am J Vet Res* 38:1827–1832, 1977.

644. Shell L, Colter SB, Blass CE, Ingram JT: Surgical removal of a meningioma in a cat after detection by computerized axial tomography. *J Am Anim Hosp Assoc* 21:439–442, 1985.

645. Troy GC, Hurov LI, King GK: Successful surgical removal of a cervical subdural neurofibrosarcoma. *J Am Anim Hosp Assoc* 15:477–481, 1979.

646. Turrel JM, Fike JR, LeCouteur RA, Pflugfelder CM, Borchich JK: Radiotherapy of brain tumors in dogs. *J Am Vet Med Assoc* 184:82–86, 1984.

647. Woodard JC, Collins GH, Hessler JR: Feline hereditary neuroaxonal dystrophy. *Am J Pathol* 74:551–560, 1974.

648. Cork LC, Troncoso JC, Price DL, Stanley EF, Griffin JW: Canine neuroaxonal dystrophy. *J Neuropathol Exp Neurol* 42:286–296, 1983.

649. Chrisman CL, Cork LC, Gamble DA: Neuroaxonal dystrophy of rottweiler dogs. *J Am Vet Med Assoc* 184:464–467, 1984.

650. Clark RG, Hartley WJ, Burgess GS, Cameron JS, Mitchell G: Suspected neuroaxonal dystrophy in collie sheep dogs. *NZ Vet J* 30:102–103, 1982.

651. Bardens JW: Congenital malformations of the foramen magnum in dogs. *Southwest Vet* 18:295–298, 1965.

652. Hoerlein BF: *Canine Neurology—Diagnosis and Treatment*, ed 2. Philadelphia, WB Saunders, 1971, p 217.

653. Parker AJ, Park RD: Occipital dysplasia in the dog. *J Am Anim Hosp Assoc* 10:520–525, 1974.

654. Kelly JH: Occipital dysplasia and hydrocephalus. *Vet Med Small Anim Clin* 70:940–941, 1975.

655. Wright JA: A study of the radiographic anatomy of the foramen magnum in dogs. *J Small Anim Pract* 20:501–508, 1979.

656. Ernest JT: Bilateral optic nerve hypoplasia in a pup. *J Am Vet Med Assoc* 168:125–128, 1976.

657. Gelatt KN, Leipold HW: Bilateral optic nerve hypoplasia in two dogs. *Can Vet J* 12:91–96, 1971.

658. Kern TJ, Riis RC: Optic nerve hypoplasia in three miniature poodles. *J Am Vet Med Assoc* 178:49–54, 1981.

659. Barnett KC, Grimes TD: Bilateral aplasia of the optic nerve in a cat. *Br J Ophthamol* 58:663–667, 1974.

660. Saunders LZ: Congenital optic nerve hypoplasia in collie dogs. *Cornell Vet* 42:67–80, 1952.

661. Yakely WL, Wyman M, Donovan EF, Fechheimer NS: Genetic transmission of an ocular fundus anomaly in collies. *J Am Vet Med Assoc* 152:457–461, 1968.

662. Carson TL: Organophosphate and carbamate insecticide poisoning. In Kirk RW (ed): *Current Veterinary Therapy VIII*. Philadelphia, WB Saunders, 1983, p 116.

663. Hatch RC: Organophosphate pesticides. In Booth NH, McDonald LE (eds): *Veteri-*

nary Pharmacology and Therapeutics. ed 5. Ames, Iowa State University Press, 1982, p 984.

664. Liu S-K, Dorfman HD: A condition resembling human localized myositis ossificans in two dogs. *J Small Anim Pract* 17:371–377, 1976.

665. Norris AM, Pallett L, Wilcock B: Generalized myositis ossificans in a cat. *J Am Anim Hosp Assoc* 16:659–663, 1980.

666. Waldron D, Pettigrew V, Turk M, Turk J, Gibson R: Progressive ossifying myositis in a cat. *J Am Vet Med Assoc* 187:64–65, 1985.

667. Warren HB, Carpenter JL: Fibrodysplasia ossificans in three cats. *Vet Pathol* 21:495–499, 1984.

667a. Bone DL, McGavin MD: Myositis ossificans in the dog: a case report and review. *J Am Anim Hosp Assoc* 21:135–138, 1985.

668. Cardinet GH, Holliday TA: Neuromuscular diseases of domestic animals: a summary of muscle biopsies from 159 cases. *Ann NY Acad Sci* 317:290–313, 1979.

669. Griffiths IR, Duncan ID, Swallow JS: Peripheral neuropathies in dogs: a study of five cases. *J Small Anim Pract* 18:101–116, 1977.

670. Tyler HR: Paraneoplastic syndromes of nerve muscle and neuromuscular junction. *Ann NY Acad Sci* 230:348–357, 1974.

671. Kula RW: Neuromuscular disorders associated with systemic neoplastic diseases In Vinken PJ, Bruyn GW (eds): *Handbook of Clinical Neurology* Amsterdam, North-Holland Publishing Co, 1979, vol 41, pp 317–403.

672. Scelsi R, Pinelli P: Subclinical myopathic findings in patients affected by malignant tumors. *Acta Neuropathol (Berl)* 38:103–108, 1977.

673. Luttgen PJ, Crawley RR: Posterior paralysis caused by epidural dirofilariasis in a dog. *J Am Anim Hosp Assoc* 17:57–59, 1981.

674. Mandelker L, Brutus RL: Feline and canine *Dirofilaria* encephalitis. *J Am Vet Med Assoc* 159:776, 1971.

675. Kotani T, Tomimura T, Ogura M, Yoshida H, Mochizuki H, Koreeda T: Cerebral infarction caused by *Dirofilaria immitis* in three dogs. *Nippon Juigaku Zasshi* 37:379–390, 1975.

676. Patton CS, Garner FM: Cerebral infarction caused by heartworms (*Dirofilaria immitis*) in a dog. *J Am Vet Med Assoc* 156:600–605, 1970.

677. Donahoe JMR, Holzinger EA: *Dirofilaria immitis* in the brains of a dog and a cat. *J Am Vet Med Assoc* 164:518–519, 1974.

678. Segedy AK, Hayden DW: Cerebral vascular accident caused by *Dirofilaria immitis* in a dog. *J Am Anim Hosp Assoc* 14:752–756, 1978.

679. Richards MA, Sloper JC: Hypothalamic involvement by "visceral" larva migrans in a dog suffering from diabetes insipidus. *Vet Rec* 76:449–451, 1964.

680. Barron CN, Saunders LZ: Visceral larva migrans in the dog. *Pathol Vet* 3:315–330, 1966.

681. Mason KV, Prescott CW, Kelly WR, Waddell AH: Granulomatous encephalomyelitis of puppies due to *Angiostrongylus cantonensis*. *Aust Vet J* 52:295, 1976.

682. Buick TD, Campbell RSF, Hutchinson GW: Spinal nematodiasis of the dog associated with *Ancylostoma caninum*. *Aust Vet J* 53:602–603, 1977.

683. MacDonald JM, de Lahunta A, Georgi J: *Cuterebra encephalitis in a dog*. *Cornell Vet* 66:372–380, 1976.

684. McKenzie BE, Lyles DI, Clinkscales JA: Intracerebral migration of *Cuterebra* larva in a kitten. *J Am Vet Med Assoc* 172:173–175, 1978.

685. Hatziolos BC: *Cuterebra* larva in the brain of a cat. *J Am Vet Med Assoc* 148:787–793, 1966.

686. Cook JR, Levesque DC, Nuehring LP: Intracranial cuterebral myiasis causing lacteralizing meningoencephalitis in two cats. *J Am Anim Hosp Assoc* 21:279–284, 1985.

687. Georgi JR, de Lahunta A, Percy DH: Cerebral coenurosis in a cat. Report of a case. *Cornell Vet* 59:127–134, 1969.

688. Hayes MA, Creighton SR: A Coenurus in the brain of a cat. *Can Vet J* 19:341–343, 1978.

689. Jauregui PH, Marquez-Monter H: Cysticercosis of the brain in dogs in Mexico City. *Am J Vet Res* 38:1641–1642, 1977.

690. Johnson BJ, Castro AE: Isolation of canine parvovirus from a dog brain with severe necrotizing vasculitis and encephalomalacia. *J Am Vet Med Assoc* 184:1398–1399, 1984.

691. Averill DR: Diseases of the muscle. *Vet Clin North Am* 10:223–234, 1980.

692. Bestetti G, Fatzer R, Fankhauser R: Encephalitis following vaccination against distemper and infectious hepatitis in the dog. An optical and ultrastructual study. *Acta Neuropathol (Berl)* 43:69–75, 1978.

693. Hartley WJ: A post-vaccinal inclusion body encephalitis in dogs. *Vet Pathol* 11:301–312, 1974.

694. Fatzer R, Fankhauser R: Enzephalomyelitis bei jungen Hunden nach Staupe-HCC-Impfung. *Prakt Teirarztl* 57:280–282, 1976.

695. Barnard BJH, Geyer HJ, de Koker WC: Neurologic symptoms in a cat following vaccination with high egg passage Flury rabies vaccine of chicken embryo origin. *Onderstepoort J Vet Res* 44:195–196, 1977.

696. Pedersen NC, Emmons RW, Selcer R, Woodie JD, Holliday TA, Weiss M: Rabies vaccine virus infection in three dogs. *J Am Vet Med Assoc* 172:1092–1096, 1978.

697. Vandevelde M, Fatzer R: Neurologische komplicaties bij drie honden na vaccinatie met een rabiesweefselktuurvaccin. *Vlaams Diergeneeskd Tijdsch* 43:253–259, 1974.

698. Fekadu M, Baer GM: Recovery from clinical rabies of 2 dogs inoculated with a rabies virus strain from Ethiopia. *J Am Vet Med Assoc* 41:1632–1634, 1980.

699. Imes GD, Lloyd JC, Brightman MP: Disseminated protothecosis in a dog. *Onderstepoort J Vet Res* 44:1–6, 1977.

700. Tyler DE, Lorenz MD, Blue JL, Munnell JF, Chandler FW: Disseminated protothecosis with central nervous system involvement in a dog. *J Am Vet Med Assoc* 176:987–993, 1980.

701. Cook JR, Tyler DE, Coulter DB, Chandler FW: Disseminated protothecosis causing acute blindness and deafness in a dog. *J Am Vet Med Assoc* 184:1266–1272, 1984.

702. Hagemoser WA, Kluge JP, Hill HT: Studies on the pathogenesis of pseudorabies in domestic cats following oral inoculation. *Can J Comp Med* 44:192–202, 1980.

703. McCracken RM, McFerran JB, Dow C: The neural spread of pseudorabies virus in calves. *J Gen Virol* 20:10–28, 1973.

704. Gustafson DP: Pseudorabies in dogs and cats. In Kirk RW (ed): *Current Veterinary Therapy VI*. Philadelphia, WB Saunders, 1977.

705. Fankhauser R, Fatzer R, Steck F, Zendali JP: Morbus Aujeszky bei Hund und Katze in der Schweiz. *Schweiz Arch Tierheilkd* 117:623–629, 1975.

706. Knosel H: Zur Histopathologie der Aujeszky' schen Krankheit bei Hund und Katze. *Zentralbl Veterinarmed* B15:592–598, 1968.

707. Hugoson G, Rockborn G: On the occurrence of pseudorabies in Sweden. I. An outbreak in dogs caused by feeding abattoir offal. *Zentralbl Veterinarmed* B19:641–645, 1972.

708. Gore R, Osborne AD, Darke PGG, Todd JN: Aujesky's disease in a pack of hounds. *Vet Rec* 101:93–95, 1977.

709. Whitley RD, Nelson SL: Pseudorabies (Aujeszky's disease) in the canine: two atypical cases. *J Am Anim Hosp Assoc* 16:69–72, 1980.

710. Shell LG, Ely RW, Crandell RA: Pseudorabies in a dog. *J Am Vet Med Assoc* 178:1159–1161, 1981.

711. Taylor D: Epizootic aspects. *Vet Rec* 99:157–160, 1976.

712. Gillespie JH, Timoney JF: Rabies and other rhabdoviruses. In Hagan WA, Bruner DW (eds): *Infectious Diseases of Domestic Animals*, ed 7. Ithaca, NY, Cornell University Press, 1981.

713. Bedford PGC: Diagnosis of rabies in animals. *Vet Rec* 99:160–162, 1976.

714. Fischman HR, Schaeffer M: Pathogenesis of experimental rabies as revealed by immunofluorescence. *Ann NY Acad Sci* 177:78–97, 1971.

715. Schindler R: Studies on the pathogenesis of rabies. *Bull WHO* 25:119–126, 1961.

716. Murphy FA, Bauer SP, Harrison AK, Winn WC: Comparative pathogenesis of rabies and rabies-like viruses. Viral infection and transit from inoculation site to the central nervous system. *Lab Invest* 28:361–376, 1973.

717. Murphy FA: Rabies pathogenesis: brief review. *Arch Virol* 54:279–297, 1977.

718. Tsiang H, Koulakoff A, Bizzini B, Berwald-Netter Y: Neurotropism of rabies virus. An in vitro study. *J Neuropathol Exp Neurol* 42:439–452, 1983.

719. Fekadu M, Shaddock JM, Baer GM: Excretion of rabies virus in the saliva of dogs. *J Infect Dis* 145:715–719, 1982.

720. Minor R: Rabies in the dog. *Vet Rec* 101:516–520, 1977.

721. Troy GC, Vulgamott JC, Turnwald GH: Canine ehrlichiosis: a retrospective study of 30 naturally occurring cases. *J Am Anim Hosp Assoc* 16:181–187, 1980.

722. Green CE, Burgdorfer W, Cavagnolo R, Philip RN, Peacock MG: Rocky Mountain

spotted fever in dogs and its differentiation from canine ehrlichiosis. *J Am Vet Med Assoc* 186:465–472, 1985.

723. Leipold HW, Huston K, Blauch B, Guffy MM: Congenital defects of the caudal vertebral column and spinal cord in Manx cats. *J Am Vet Med Assoc* 164:520–523, 1974.

724. Long SE, Berepubo NA: A 37XO chromosome complement in a kitten. *J Small Anim Pract* 21:627–631, 1980.

725. Todd NB: The inheritance of taillessness in Manx cats. *J Hered* 52:228–232, 1961.

726. Deforest ME, Basrur PK: Malformations and the Manx syndrome in cats. *Can Vet J* 20:304–314, 1979.

727. James CC, Lassman LP, Tomlinson BE: Congenital anomalies of the lower spine and spinal cord in Manx cats. *J Pathol* 97:269–276, 1968.

728. Kitchen H, Murray RE, Cockrell BY: Spina bifida sacral dysgenesis and myelocele. *Am J Pathol* 66:203–206, 1972.

729. Martin AH: A congenital defect in the spinal cord of the Manx cat. *Vet Pathol* 8:232–238, 1971.

730. Frye FL: Spina biffida occulta with sacro-coccygeal agenesis in a cat. *Anim Hosp* 3:238–242, 1967.

731. Meyers KM, Lund JE, Padgett G, Dickson WM: Hyperkinetic episodes in Scottish terrier dogs. *J Am Vet Med Assoc* 155:129–133, 1969.

732. Meyers KM, Dickson WM, Lund JE, Padgett GA: Muscular hypertonicity. *Arch Neurol* 25:61–67, 1971.

733. Meyers KM, Schaub RG: The relationship of serotonin to a motor disorder of Scottish terrier dogs. *Life Sci* 14:1895–1906, 1974.

734. Woods CB: Hyperkinetic episodes in two dalmations. *J Am Anim Hosp Assoc* 13:255–257, 1977.

735. Furber RM: Cramp in Norwich terriers. *Vet Rec* 115:46, 1984.

736. Russo ME: The pathophysiology of epilepsy. *Cornell Vet* 71:221–247, 1981.

737. Oliver JE: Protocol for diagnosis of seizure disorders in companion animals. *J Am Vet Med Assoc* 172:822–824, 1978.

738. Holliday TA: Seizure disorders. *Vet Clin North Am* 10:3–29, 1980.

739. Farnbach GC: Serum concentrations and efficacy of phenytoin, phenobarbital, and primidone in canine epilepsy. *J Am Vet Med Assoc* 184:1117–1120, 1984.

740. Yeary RA: Serum concentrations of primidone and its metabolites phenylethylmalonamide and phenobarbital in the dog. *Am J Vet Res* 41:1643–1645, 1980.

741. Cunningham JG, Haidukewych D, Jensen HA: Therapeutic serum concentrations of primidone and its metabolites phenobarbital and phenylethylmalonamide in epileptic dogs. *J Am Vet Med Assoc* 182:1091–1094, 1983.

742. Bunch SE, Baldwin BH, Hornbuckle WE, Tennant BC: Compromised hepatic function in dogs treated with anticonvulsant drugs. *J Am Vet Med Assoc* 184:444–448, 1984.

743. Bunch SE, Castleman WL, Baldwin BH, Hornbuckle WE: Effects of long-term primidone and phenytoin administration on canine hepatic function and morphology. *Am J Vet Res* 46:105–115, 1985.

744. Schwartz-Porsche D, Loscher W, Frey HH: Therapeutic efficacy of phenobarbital and primidone in canine epilepsy: a comparison. *J Vet Pharmacol Ther* 8:113–119, 1985.

745. Poffenbarger EM, Hardy RM: Hepatic cirrhosis associated with long-term primidone therapy in a dog. *J Am Vet Med Assoc* 186:978–980, 1985.

746. Farnbach GC: Efficacy of primidone in dogs with seizures unresponsive to phenobarbital. *J Am Vet Med Assoc* 185:867–868, 1984.

747. Sanders JE, Yeary RA, Powers JD, de Wet P: Relationship between serum and brain concentrations of phenytoin in the dog. *Am J Vet Res* 40:473–476, 1979.

748. Sanders JE, Yeary RA, Fenner WR, Powers JD: Interaction of phenytoin with chloramphenicol or pentobarbital in the dog. *J Am Vet Assoc* 175:177–180, 1979.

749. Nash AS, Thompson H, Bogan JA: Phenytoin toxicity: a fatal case in a dog with hepatitis and jaundice. *Vet Rec* 100:280–281, 1977.

750. Wouda W, Vandevelde M, Oettle P, van Nes JJ, Hoerlein BF: Sensory neuropathy in dogs: a study of four cases. *J Comp Pathol* 93:437–450, 1983.

751. Carmichael S, Griffiths IR: Case of isolated sensory trigeminal neuropathy in a dog. *Vet Rec* 109:280–282, 1981.

752. Bundza A, Lowden JA, Charlton KM: Niemann-Pick disease in a poodle dog. *Vet*

      Pathol 16:530–538, 1979.

753. Crisp CE, Ringler DH, Abrams GD, Radin NS, Brenkert A: Lipid storage disease in a Siamese cat. *J Am Vet Med Assoc* 156:616–622, 1970.

754. Snyder SP, Kingston RS, Wenger DA: Animal model of human disease: Niemann-Pick disease. Sphingomyelinosis of Siamese cats. *Am J Pathol* 108:252–254, 1982.

755. Wenger DA, Sattler M, Kudoh T, Snyder SP, Kingston RS: Niemann-Pick disease: a genetic model in Siamese cats. *Science* 208:1472–1473, 1980.

756. Wilson JW, Kurtz HJ, Leipold HW, Lees GE: Spina bifida in the dog. *Vet Pathol* 16:165–179, 1979.

757. Pattern B: Overgrowth of the neural tube in young human embryos. *Anat Rec* 113:381–393, 1952.

758. Padget D: Neuroschisis and human embryonic development. *J Neuropathol Exp Neurol* 29:192–216, 1970.

759. Chesney CJ: A case of spina bifida in a Chihuahua. *Vet Rec* 93:120–121, 1973.

760. Clarke L, Carlisle CH: Spina bifida with syringomyelia and meningocoele in a short-tailed cat. *Aust Vet J* 51:392–394, 1975.

761. Frye FL, McFarland LZ: Spina bifida with rachischisis in a kitten. *J Am Vet Med Assoc* 146:481–482, 1965.

762. Furneaux RW, Doige CE, Kaye MM: Syringomyelia and spina bifida occulta in a Samoyed dog. *Can Vet J* 14:317–321, 1973.

763. Jubb KVF, Kennedy PC: *Pathology of Domestic Animals*, ed 2. New York, Adademic Press, 1970, p 344.

764. Parker AJ, Byerly CS: Meningomyelocoele in a dog. *Vet Pathol* 10:266–273, 1973.

765. Shelton MC: A possible mode of inheritance for spinal dysraphism in the dog with a more complete description of the clinical syndrome. MS Thesis, Iowa State University, Ames, 1977.

766. Gieb LW, Bistner SI: Spinal cord dysraphism in a dog. *J Am Vet Med Assoc* 150:618–620, 1967.

767. McGrath JT: Spinal dysraphism in the dog *Pathol Vet* 2 (Suppl):1–36, 1965.

768. Neufeld JL, Little PB: Spinal dysraphism in a dalmation dog. *Can Vet J* 15:335–336, 1974.

769. Engel HN, Draper DD: Comparative prenatal development of the spinal cord in normal and dysraphic dogs: embryonic stage. *Am J Vet Res* 43:1729–1734, 1982.

770. Engel HN, Draper DD: Comparative prenatal development of the spinal cord in normal and dysraphic dogs: fetal stage. *Am J Vet Res* 43:1735–1743, 1982.

771. Confer AW, Ward BC: Spinal dysraphism: a congenital myelodysplasia in the weimaraner. *J Am Vet Med Assoc* 160:1423–1426, 1972.

772. Draper DD, Kluge JP, Miller WJ: Neurologic, pathologic, and genetic aspects of spinal dysraphism in dogs (abstr). *Anat Histol Embryol* 4:369, 1975.

773. Sandefeldt E, Cummings JF, de Lahunta A, Bjorck G, Krook L: Hereditary neuronal abiotrophy in the Swedish Lapland dog. *Cornell Vet* 63 (Suppl 3):1–71, 1973.

774. Sandefeldt E, Cummings JF, de Lahunta A, Bjorck G, Krook LP: Hereditary neuronal abiotrophy in Swedish Lapland dogs. *Am J Pathol* 82:649–652, 1976.

775. Cork LC, Griffin JW, Munnell JF, Lorenz MD, Adams RJ, Price DL: Hereditary canine spinal muscular atrophy. *J Neuropathol Exp Neurol* 38:209–221, 1979.

776. Cork LC, Griffin JW, Adams RJ, Price DL: Hereditary canine spinal muscular atrophy. *Am J Pathol* 100:599–602, 1980.

777. Cork LC, Griffin JW, Choy C, Padula CA, Price DL: Pathology of motor neurons in accelerated hereditary canine spinal muscular atrophy. *Lab Invest* 46:89–99, 1982.

778. Lorenz MD, Cork LC, Griffin JW, Adams RJ, Price DL: Hereditary muscular atrophy in Birttany spaniels: clinical manifestations. *J Am Vet Med Assoc* 175:833–839, 1979.

779. Inada S, Sakomoto H, Haruta K, Miyazono Y, Sasaki M, Yamauchi C, Igata A, Osame M, Fukunaga H: A clinical study on hereditary progressive neurogenic muscular atrophy in pointer dogs. *Jpn J Vet Sci* 40:539–547, 1978.

780. Izumo S, Ikuta F, Igata A, Osame M, Yamauchi C, Inada S: Morphological study on the hereditary neurogenic amyotrophic dogs: accumulation of lipid compound-like structures in the lower motor neurons. *Acta Neuropathol (Berl)* 61:270–276, 1983.

781. Stockard CR: An hereditary lethal factor for localized motor and preganglionic neurons. *Am J Anat* 59:1–53, 1936.

782. Hartley WJ: Lower motor neurone disease in dogs. *Acta Neuropathol (Berl)* 2:334–342, 1963.

783. Vandevelde M, Greene CE, Hoff EJ: Lower motor neuron disease with accumulation

of neurofilaments in a cat. *Vet Pathol* 13:428–435, 1976.

784. de Lahunta A, Shively GN: Neurofibrillary accumulation in a puppy. *Cornell Vet* 65:240–247, 1975.

785. Swaim SF: Biomechanics of cranial fractures, spinal fractures, and luxations. In *Pathophysiology in Small Animal Surgery*. Philadelphia, Lea & Febiger, 1981, pp 774–781.

786. Basinger RR, Bjorling DE, Chambers JN: Cervical spinal luxation in 2 dogs with entrapment of the cranial articular process of C6 over the caudal articular process of C5. *J Am Vet Med Assoc*, in press.

787. Griffiths IR: Trauma of the spinal cord. *Vet Clin North Am* 10:131–146, 1980.

788. Matthiesen DT: Thoracolumbar spinal fractures/luxations: surgical management. *Comp Cont Educ* 5:867–878, 1983.

789. Morgan JP: Spondylosis deformans in the dogs. A morphologic study with some clinical and experimental observations. *Acta Orthop Scand* (Suppl 96), 1967.

790. Morgan JP: Spondylosis deformans in the dog. its radiographic appearance. *J Am Vet Radiol Soc* 8:17–22, 1967.

791. Wright JA: Spondylosis deformans of the lumbosacral joint in dogs. *J Small Anim Pract* 21:45–58, 1980.

792. Larsen JS, Selby LA: Spondylosis deformans in large dogs—relative risk by breed, age and sex. *J Am Anim Hosp Assoc* 17:623–625, 1981.

793. Braund KG, Taylor TKF, Ghosh P, Sherwood AA: Spinal mobility in the dog. A study in chondrodystrophoid and non-chondrodystrophoid animals. *Res Vet Sci* 22:78–82, 1977.

794. Kelly DF, Gaskell CJ: Spongy degeneration of the central nervous system in kittens. *Acta Neuropathol (Berl)* 35:151–158, 1976.

795. Mason RW, Hartley WJ, Randall M: Spongiform degeneration of the white matter in a Samoyed pup. *Aust Vet Pract* 9:11–13, 1979.

796. Richards RB, Kakulas BA: Spongiform leukoencephalopathy associated with congenital myoclonia syndrome in the dog. *J Comp Pathol* 88:317–320, 1978.

797. O'Brien DP, Zachary JF: Clinical features of spongy degeneration of the central nervous system in two Labrador retriever littermates. *J Am Vet Med Assoc* 186:1207–1210, 1985.

798. Osweiler GD: Strychnine poisoning. In Kirk RW (ed): *Current Veterinary Therapy VIII*. Philadelphia, WB Saunders, 1983, p 98.

799. Hatch RC: Poisons causing nervous stimulation or depression. In Booth NH, McDonald LE (eds): *Veterinary Pharmacology and Therapeutics*, ed 5. Ames, Iowa State University Press, 1982, p 994.

800. Bailey EM, Szabuniewicz M: Strychnine poisoning in the dog. *Vet Med Small Anim Clin* 70:170–174, 1975.

801. Beckett SD, Branch CE, Robertson BT: Syncopal attacks and sudden death in dogs: mechanisms and etiologies. *J Am Anim Hosp Assoc* 14:378–386, 1978.

802. Fisher EW: Fainting in boxers—the possibility of vaso-vagal syncope (Adams-Stokes attacks). *J Small Anim Pract* 12:347–349, 1971.

803. Price DL, Griffin J, Young A, Peck K, Stocks A: Tetanus toxin: direct evidence for retrograde intraaxonal transport. *Science* 188:945–947, 1975.

804. Schwab ME, Thoenen H: Electron microscopic evidence for a transsynaptic migration of tetanus toxin in spinal cord motoneurons: an autoradiographic and morphometric study. *Brain Res* 105:213–227, 1976.

805. English PB, Carlisle CH: Tetanus in the dog. *Aust Vet J* 37:62–65, 1961.

806. Killingsworth C, Chiapella A, Veralli P, de Lahunta A: Feline tetanus. *J Am Anim Hosp Assoc* 13:209–215, 1977.

807. Zontine WJ, Uno T: Tetanus in a dog. *Vet Med Small Anim Clin* 63:341–344, 1968.

807a. Matthews BR, Forbes DC: Tetanus in a dog. *Can Vet J* 26:159–161, 1985.

808. Greene CE: Tetanus. In Kirk RW (ed): *Current Veterinary Therapy VIII*. Philadelphia, WB Saunders, 1983, p 705.

809. Everett GM: Observations on the behavior and neurophysiology of acute thiamin deficient cats. *Am J Physiol* 141:439–448, 1944.

810. Jubb KV, Saunders LZ, Coates HV: Thiamine deficiency encephalopathy in cats. *J Comp Pathol* 66:217–227, 1956.

811. Read DH, Jolly RD, Alley MR: Polioencephalomalacia of dogs with thiamine deficiency. *Vet Pathol* 14:103–112, 1977.

812. Read DH, Harrington DD: Experimentally induced thiamine deficiency in beagle

dogs: clinical observations. *Am J Vet Res* 42:984–991, 1981.

813. Munday BL, King SJ: A condition resembling Chastek paralysis in cats. *NZ Vet J* 20:80–81, 1972.

814. Ilkiw JE: Tick paralysis in Australia. In Kirk RW (ed): *Current Veterinary Therapy VII.* Philadelphia, WB Saunders, 1980, pp 777–779.

815. Dubey JP: *Toxoplasma, Hammondia, Besnoitia, Sarcocystis,* and other tissue cyst-forming coccidia of man and animals. In Kreier JP (ed): *Parasitic Protozoa.* New York, Academic Press, 1977 vol 3, pp 101–237.

816. Siim JC, Biering-Sorensen U, Moller T: Toxoplasmosis in domestic animals, *Adv Vet Sci* 8:335–429, 1963.

817. Jones SR: Toxoplasmosis: a review. *J Am Vet Med Assoc* 163:1038–1042, 1973.

818. Desmonts G, Couvreur J: A prospective study of 378 pregnancies. *N Engl J Med* 290:1110–1116, 1974.

819. Fankhuaser R: Toxoplasmose-encephalitis beim Hunde. *Schweiz Arch Neurol Psychiatr* 69:391–397, 1952.

820. Hirth RS, Nielsen SW: Pathology of feline toxoplasmosis. *J Small Anim Pract* 10:213–221, 1969.

821. Koestner A, Cole CR: Neuropathology of canine toxoplasmosis. *Am J Vet Res* 21:831–844, 1960.

822. Hartley WJ, Lindsay AB, Mackinnon MM: *Toxoplasma* meningo-encephalomyelitis and myositis in a dog. *NZ Vet J* 6:124–127, 1958.

823. Moller T, Neilsen SW: Toxoplasmosis in distemper-susceptible carnivora. *Pathol Vet* 1:189–203, 1964.

824. Averill DR, de Lahunta A: Toxoplasmosis of the canine nervous system: clinicopathological findings in four cases. *J Am Vet Med Assoc* 159:1134–1141, 1971.

825. Kyle RJ: *Toxoplasma* encephalitis in a cat. *NZ Vet J* 23:13–14, 1975.

826. Ward JM, Nelson N, Wright JF, Berman E: Chronic nonclinical cerebral toxoplasmosis in cats. *J Am Vet Med Assoc* 159:1012–1014, 1971.

827. Vainisi SJ, Campbell LH: Ocular toxoplasmosis in cats. *J Am Vet Med Assoc* 154:141–152, 1969.

828. Drake JC, Hime JM: Two syndromes in young dogs caused by *Toxoplasma gondii. J Small Anim Pract* 8:621–626, 1967.

829. Holliday TA, Olander HJ, Wind AP: Skeletal muscle atrophy associated with toxoplasmosis: a case report *Cornell Vet* 53:288–300, 1963.

830. Nesbit JW, Lourens DC, Williams MC: Spastic paresis in two littermate pups caused by *Toxoplasma gondii. J S Afr Vet Assoc* 52:243–246, 1981.

831. Suter MM, Hauser B, Palmer DG, Oettli P: Polymyositis-polyradiculitis due to toxoplasmosis in the dog: serology and tissue biopsy as diagnostic aids. *Zentralbl Veterinarmed* A31:792–798, 1984.

832. Walker TL: Ischiadic nerve entrapment. *J Am Vet Med Assoc* 178:1284–1288, 1981.

833. Fanton JW, Blass CE, Withrow SJ: Sciatic nerve injury as a complication of intramedullary pin fixation of femoral fractures. *J Am Anim Hosp Assoc* 19:687–694, 1983.

834. Gilmore DR: Sciatic nerve injury in twenty-nine dogs. *J Am Anim Hosp Assoc* 20:403–407, 1984.

835. Braund KG, Walker TL, Vandevelde M: Fascicular nerve biopsy in the dog. *Am J Vet Res* 40:1025–1030, 1979.

836. Bennett D, Vaughan LC: The use of muscle relocation techniques in the treatment of peripheral nerve injuries in dogs and cats. *J Small Anim Pract* 17:99–108, 1976.

837. Lesser AS: The use of a tendon transfer for the treatment of a traumatic sciatic nerve paralysis in the dog. *Vet Surg* 7:85–89, 1978.

838. Hoelzle RJ: Idiopathic trigeminal neuropathy in a dog. *Vet Med Small Anim Clin* 78:345, 1983.

839. Kaspar LV, Lombard LS: Nutritional myodegeneration in a litter of beagles. *J Am Vet Med Assoc* 143:284–288, 1963.

840. Manktelow BW: Myopathy of dogs resembling white muscle disease of sheep. *NZ Vet J* 11:52–55, 1963.

841. Meier H: Myopathies in the dog. *Cornell Vet* 48:313–330, 1958.

842. Dennis JM, Alexander RW: Nutritional myopathy in a cat. *Vet Rec* 111:195–196, 1982.

4
Diagnostic Techniques

While a tentative diagnosis of a neurological disease can often be made based on history, signalment data, and neurological examination, final confirmation usually requires additional diagnostic testing. This chapter covers the main laboratory diagnostic aids that pertain to neurological diseases; it includes a review of radiographic techniques, electrodiagnostic testing, cerebrospinal fluid analysis, spinal neurosurgical techniques, and surgical procedures for obtaining biopsies of muscle and nerve.

Radiographic Techniques and Interpretation

Radiography is probably the most commonly used ancillary aid in clinical neurological practice. Routine or plain radiographs are used primarily for the detection of bony abnormalities of the vertebral column and skull, such as bone proliferation, bone lysis, abnormalities in the shape of vertebrae or the skull, and vertebral displacement. However, soft tissue structures not normally detected by routine radiography can be visualized and/or outlined through the use of contrast agents and such specialized techniques as computerized axial tomography.

As is the case with other ancillary aids, radiography is used to confirm or rule out a clinical diagnosis. While many vertebral or cranial abnormalities are readily discernible radiographically, subtle lesions can be missed if sufficient attention is not given to good radiographic techniques. Similarly, artifacts arising from poor techniques can create confusion and/or a false diagnosis. Thus, attention must be given to positioning, correct exposure settings, and proper development techniques. In general, animals subjected to spinal or skull radiography should be anesthetized in order to avoid movement artefacts and to facilitate such manipulative procedures as spinal extension or flexion. High-contrast radiographs of skull and spinal column can be attained using high milliamperes and low kilovolt techniques. Radiographic detail is enhanced by use of nonscreen X-ray film or X-ray cassettes with slow intensifying screens. Grids help to reduce scatter radiation reaching the X-ray film.

For spinal radiography, the two basic positions of the animal are the lateral recumbent and ventrodorsal views. These two views together help to establish the spatial relationship and geometry of a given lesion. Attempts should be made to ensure that the spinal column is straight and parallel to the film in order to avoid distortion of the intervertebral spaces. The use of pads or cushions under the neck, head, and nose will facilitate symmetry of the cervical vertebrae and skull structures. Padding under the pelvis will help to straighten out the lumbosacral vertebral column. Only a few vertebrae at a time should be radiographed in order to allow valid comparison of the width of no more than three or four disk spaces on one film, without distortion or superimposition of vertebral bodies. If the suspected lesion can be localized to a specific vertebral region, the three or four vertebrae in this area should be positioned in the center of the X-ray beam. The ventrodorsal view is taken with the animal in a bilaterally symmetrical position. A slight degree of extension and positioning pads will help to avoid curvature and rotation of the spine. A complete spinal series should be performed, consisting of about five lateral and five ventrodorsal views. This will provide information on possible future spinal problems, and also it may demonstrate other lesion(s) not suspected from the clinical examination, e.g., multiple fractured vertebrae, disk extrusions, or diskospondylitic lesions. However, a complete spinal series may not be cost effective. For skull radiography, the two basic positions of the animal are the lateral and ventrodorsal views. In the latter, the mandible should be parallel to the film and the X-ray beam centered just caudal to the eyes. Two other commonly used views are the frontal and open-mouth.

For the frontal view, the animal is positioned in dorsal recumbency with the nose held vertically, and the X-ray beam is centered between the eyes. A frontal view will demonstrate the frontal sinuses and also lateral ventricles in conjunction with a contrast agent. For the open-mouth view, the animal is positioned as for the frontal view and the mouth is held open using gauze strips. The X-ray beam is centered down the throat. This view is used for demonstrating the odontoid process, osseous bullae, and foramen magnum. Occasionally, oblique-lateral views are used to study the osseous bullae and the petrous temporal bone.

Neurological disorders that are readily diagnosed using routine radiography include degenerative (e.g., disk disease, spondylosis deformans), anomalous (e.g., hydrocephalus, occipital dysplasia, atlantoaxial subluxation/odontoid agenesis, cervical malformation-malarticulation, hemivertebra, spina bifida, caudal dysgenesis, congenital stenosis of the lumbosacral canal), infectious (e.g., osteomyelitis, diskospondylitis, otitis media and/or externa), neoplastic (e.g., vertebral neoplasms such as osteosarcoma, multiple myeloma), nutritional (e.g., hypervitaminosis A), and traumatic (e.g., luxations, fractures) disorders.

Sometimes, usually in conjunction with routine radiographic studies, contrast agents are employed. Contrast procedures are used to confirm a suspected lesion(s) that cannot be identified using plain radiographs or to identify the extent or location of a lesion(s) more precisely. The most frequently used contrast procedure is myelography, in which a contrast agent is injected into the spinal subarachnoid space. The contrast agent surrounds the spinal cord, and any focal or multifocal areas of spinal cord compression or expansion will produce a distortion in the contrast column. The type of column distortion may determine if the mass lesion is in an epidural, intradural-extramedullary, or intramedullary location. An extradural mass (e.g., extruded disk material) typically causes as inward thinning (central deviation) of the dye column or complete obstruction to flow. An intradural-extramedullary mass (e.g., meningioma) may appear similar to an extradural mass; however, the cranial and caudal borders of the mass may have a T-shaped outline of contrast material. An intramedullary mass (e.g., astrocytoma) tends to expand the spinal cord, resulting in an outward thinning (peripheral deviation) or obliteration of the dye column. In some instances, contrast material will pool in the subarachnoid space, suggesting focal spinal cord atrophy.

At present, metrizamide is the most commonly used agent for myelography in the dog and cat (1–8). It is a relatively safe agent that can be injected into either the cisterna magna and allowed to flow caudally or into the caudal lumbar ventral subarachnoid space and forced to flow cranially. The procedures used for myelography are identical to those for obtaining CSF for analysis. Metrizamide can be prepared by dissolving 3.5 gm of the analytical grade powder in 8.9 ml of sterile water and filtering it into a sterile, evacuated test tube or vial without preservative or anticoagulant. The solution requires refrigeration and should be discarded if not used within 2 weeks. A suggested dose is 0.26 to 0.35 mg/kg. For very large dogs, a 10- to 12-ml volume is adequate. The contrast obtained with metrizamide usually remains diagnostic for up to 30 minutes.

Myelography is not without risk. Deterioration of clinical neurological signs is not uncommon following myelography, especially in large breed dogs. Approximately 15 to 20% of dogs may have generalized seizures following metrizamide myelography, usually within 1 to 4 hours of injection. The incidence of seizures appears to correlate with the volume of metrizamide injected, body weight, and, to a lesser extent, injection site. Rarely, vomiting, hyperesthesia, pyrexia, and death have been reported as complications of metrizamide myelography in dogs (7). Certain precautions should be taken to reduce the incidence of complications, such as elevating the table at the time of injection or the head of the animal immediately after injection, to prevent flow of contrast agent into the cisterns of the brain. Seizures usually can be controlled with diazepam at a dose of 5 to 10 mg intravenously, to effect. Subclinical arachnoid fibrosis has been reported as a long-term complication of metrizamide myelography (9). More recently, it has been suggested that two other water-soluble contrast agents, iohexol (Omnipaque, Nyegaard) and iopamidol (Niopam, Merck), are superior in radiographic quality to metrizamide and have less undesirable side effects in dogs and cats (9a-11). The recommended intracisternal dosage of iohexol (at 300 mg of iodine/ml) is from 2 to 6.5 ml, according to the breed size.

Spinal neurological disorders that can be diagnosed using myelography include degenerative (e.g., acute disk disease), anomalous (e.g., myelomeningocele), infectious (e.g., extradural abscess), neoplastic (e.g., extradural, intradural-extramedullary, or intramedullary tumors), and traumatic (e.g., spinal cord edema) disorders.

Another contrast procedure that can be readily performed in clinical practice is ventriculography. This procedure delineates the cerebral ventricular system following the injection of air or positive contrast agent such as metrizamide or meglumine iothalamate (Conray). It is one procedure of choice for the diagnosis of hydrocephalus. Following surgical preparation of the scalp, the site of injection into the lateral ventricle is located by finding the halfway point between the external occipital protuberance and lateral canthus of the eye. A line is traced from this point perpendicular to the median plane of the skull. The skull is entered on this perpendicular line 3 to 5 mm from the median plane of the skull (12). A thin (about 20 gauge), sharp intramedullary pin can be used to penetrate the bone through which a 22 gauge, 1.5-inch spinal needle with stilette can be inserted. The needle is slowly forced directly downward for a distance of 1 to 2 cm. The stilette is withdrawn frequently to detect the presence of CSF. The normal lateral ventricle may be difficult to enter; however, a widely dilated ventricle is entered immediately. The intraventricular pressure may be sufficiently low (as a result of brain parenchymal atrophy) to require gentle aspiration to obtain CSF. A small volume of CSF is withdrawn and replaced with air. Frontal and lateral radiographic views will demonstrate the air-filled lateral ventricles. Use of a contrast agent instead of air has the added advantage of determining if a block exists in the ventricular system at the aqueduct or lateral aperture of the fourth ventricle. If the ventricular system is patent, flow of contrast will be seen in the cervical subarachnoid space. Contrast agents are riskier to use than air, and potential complications include seizures and apnea.

A search for less risky and more reliable radiographic tools for the diagnosis and localization of intracranial soft tissue lesions in animals has led to recent clinical trials of radioisotope imaging (synonyms are "scintigraphy," "radionuclide brain scanning") and computerized axial tomography (synonym is "CAT scan"). These techniques are currently available only at some institutions and specialty practices. Radioisotope imaging is a noninvasive radiographic tool that is based upon the uptake of radiopharmaceutical agents, such as technetium-99m, into brain lesions associated with vascular disruption. This technique appears to be most useful in the diagnosis of focal mass lesions (including neoplasms, ischemic degenerative lesions, and focal inflammation) >1 cm in diameter (13, 14); however, images can be difficult to interpret. The technique is ineffective in diagnosing diffuse inflammatory lesions. Imaging involves the use of rectilinear scanners or gamma cameras. After the desired images are obtained, all excreta from animals are saved for 48 to 72 hours before discarding to allow for decay of the radioisotope.

Ventriculography and other intracranial radiographic contrast procedures, such as cerebral angiography and cavernous sinus angiography, have largely been replaced in institutions and specialty practices by the advent of computerized axial tomography (CAT). The procedure is safe, noninvasive, and provides a qualitative and quantitative appraisal of the brain that is unavailable using conventional radiographic techniques, including radionuclide brain scanning (15, 16). It is used to generate cross-sectional images of "slices" of the head and brain. Localization of lesions may be enhanced by intravenous injection of an organic iodide contrast agent, such as meglumine iothalamate or sodium meglumine ioxaglate (17, 18). This procedure has proved to be an excellent tool for the diagnosis of cerebral neoplasia, abscesses, hemorrhage, and hydrocephalus (16, 19–21). Tumors can be characterized on CAT scans by density changes, presence of edema or calcification, and displacement of normal anatomical landmarks, such as the lateral and third ventricles (16, 21, 22). The CAT scan also may provide information pertaining to tumor malignancy.

Electrodiagnostic Techniques and Interpretation

Electrodiagnostic procedures—such as electroencephalography (EEG), nerve conduction velocity studies (NCV), and electromyography (EMG)—can provide useful ancillary support of a tentative clinical diagnosis. It must be emphasized that none of these procedures will provide a definitive diagnosis; rather, they substantiate the presence of an encephalopathy, neuropathy, junctionopathy, or myopathy. The equipment required for electrodiagnostic testing is expensive and usually found only in institutions and some specialty pratices. Correct interpretation of electrodiagnostic data requires training and experience.

The *electroencephalograph* amplifies and graphically records the electrical activity of the brain. While the EEG usually can indicate that cerebral disease is present, its ability to localize a lesion accurately (e.g., hemispheric, superficial, or deep), define a process as being focal or diffuse, acute or chronic, or distinguish between different disease processes appears to be limited. Furthermore, analysis of EEG recordings is subject to many variables, including age of the animal, degree of alertness, stage and type of sedation, and use of local anesthetics to reduce temporalis muscle artifacts during recordings.

The EEG is typically defined in terms of frequency (number of waves per second) or amplitude (vertical height) of wave forms, e.g., the EEG of a normal, alert, mature dog and cat may have a moderate to fast frequency ranging from 15 to 30 Hertz and a low amplitude ranging from 5 to 15 μV. The EEG of dogs and cats under 6 months of age (the age at which EEG maturity is reached) is characterized by slow-wave activity. Changes in frequency or amplitude should always be referenced to the "normal" EEG in any given practice. Reference values should be established for wave frequency and amplitude in dogs and cats at different ages and under standardized conditions, e.g., local anesthesia in temporal muscles, recordings on alert or anesthetized animals, etc. Nearly all sedatives, hypnotics, and anesthetics alter the normal low-amplitude fast activity and produce relatively higher amplitude slow waves, similar to the sleep pattern (23).

Diseases of the brain cause changes in either EEG frequency or amplitude, or both (24). Low-voltage fast activity with spiking has been reported with inflammatory conditions, whereas high-voltage slow activity is suggestive of neuronal death and has been reported in such conditions as hydrocephalus and brain edema (24, 25). Very low-amplitude slow activity has been reported in animals with ischemic encephalopathy. Space-occupying lesions may be characterized by the presence of intermittent high-amplitude slow waves that last from a few to many seconds and/or high-amplitude intermittent spikes. Bursts of high-voltage slow waves may occur with hypocalcemia and hepatic encephalopathy, while very low-voltage moderate frequency can occur in animals with hypothyroidism. A pattern of generalized slow-wave activity with intermittent high-amplitude slow waves reportedly is suggestive of lead poisoning (26, 27). Lack of standardized EEG techniques and too few, detailed EEG-pathological correlative studies continue to hinder the potential progress and interpretation of this ancillary aid. A recent report of EEG abnormalities associated with cervical disk disease in dogs (28) further clouds the reliability and specificity of the EEG to detect intracranial disease.

Electrodiagnostic studies of skeletal muscle and nerve can be used to confirm the presence or absence of a suspected neuromyopathy and may help to differentiate a myopathy from a neuropathy or a junctionopathy. Analyzing *nerve conduction velocity* is the most common test used for determining peripheral nerve change. This simple test is performed by stimulating a nerve at a proximal and a distal site and recording the evoked potential in a muscle innervated by that nerve. The time between nerve stimulation and evoked muscle action potential is called the latency. Dividing the distance between proximal and distal stimulating sites by the difference of the two latency times gives the nerve conduction velocity in meters per second (29, 30). More precisely, this value will represent the motor nerve conduction velocity. Since the majority of peripheral neuropathies in dogs and cats have motor nerve involvement, this test is usually adequate. However, in some instances where sensory pathology is suspected, determination of the sensory nerve conduction velocity can be a useful aid. Sensory nerve conduction studies require different techniques than do measurements of motor nerve conduction velocity, as both stimulation and recording are performed on the nerve. A stimulating electrode is applied to a distal site of a sensory nerve, and the nerve action potential is measured at a more proximal site. To estimate conduction velocity, the distance from stimulating and recording electrodes is divided by the time taken from stimulation to the beginning of the nerve action potential (31). Normal conduction velocities have been determined for many appendicular sensory nerves in dogs and cats (32–34). Motor nerve conduction velocity for most appendicular nerves in adult dogs is usually 50 m/second or greater in dogs, and generally faster in cats (35–37). A value of less than 50 m/second supports a diagnosis of peripheral neuropathy (30, 38); however, the age of the animal needs to be considered. Young animals, less than 6 months of age, have markedly slower conduction velocities than adult animals (39). Motor nerve conduction velocities remain relatively constant in dogs up to 7 years of age. Thereafter, a gradual decline occurs so that by 10 years the velocity is reduced by 10 to 15% (40). Sensory nerve conduction velocities tend to be slightly higher than those for motor nerves.

Nerve conduction velocities are of most diagnostic value in peripheral neuropathies that are characterized by demyelination (29). Apart from slowing of conduction, demyelination can result in a decreased amplitude and an increased duration and/or number of wave forms (temporal dispersion) in the recorded action potential. Velocities may be decreased only slightly in neuropathies characterized by axonal degeneration since nerve conduction velocities actually reflect conduction in the larger diameter myelinated fibers. If the lesion is severe enough to cause the loss of most or all of the myelinated fibers, nerve conduction will not occur. This situation has been reported in various distal symmetrical polyneuropathies (29, 41).

In conjunction with nerve conduction velocity measurements, the electrical activity of muscle (*electromyography*) is usually assessed and performed on the same equipment. As for nerve conduction studies, EMG recordings are usually performed on anesthetized or sedated animals. The electrical activity of a muscle is recorded in an oscilloscope. When a needle is inserted into the belly of a muscle, a large-amplitude discharge will be recorded as a result of excitation of muscle fibers. This so-called **insertional activity** ceases in normal muscle once the motion of the needle has stopped, and there should be no background electrical activity, with the possible exception of end-plate noise which is noted when the needle is in the area of the motor end-plate. It is characterized by many small potentials that have a moderately loud hissing noise. This noise will disappear when the needle is moved to another location within the muscle. In denervated and diseased muscle, however, the electrical activity of the muscle is altered so that spontaneous, abnormal potentials may be recorded. These abnormal potentials are often characterized by distinctive wave forms and sounds. The abnormal waves include fibrillation potentials, positive sharp waves, myotonic potentials, and bizarre high-frequency discharges (37, 42, 43). **Fibrillation potentials** are small (uni-, bi-, or triphasic) waves that have a sound like frying eggs. **Positive sharp waves** are characterized by a large positive deflection and may sound like an idling outboard motor. **Myotonic potentials** are large-amplitude, multiphasic signals that tend to wax and wane. They produce a unique dive bomber sound. **Bizarre high-frequency discharges** can be similar to the myotonic potentials but are of shorter duration and do not wax and wane.

While all of the abnormal potentials, with the exception of myotonic potentials, may be observed in primary muscle diseases as well as in denervated muscle, they are much more obvious in denervation. They occur in muscle approximately 7 days after denervation (44). It should be noted that abnormal potentials are not usually observed in pure demyelinating neuropathies; however, both axonal degeneration and demyelination typically occur together, in varying degrees in most neuropathies. Myotonic potentials tend to occur only in primary myopathies such as myotonic myopathy in chow chows, steroid myopathy, and polymyositis.

Insertional activity can be reduced in duration, amplitude, or both, after long-standing neuropathies and with myopathies (45).

In junctionopathies or disorders of the neuromuscular junction, such as occur with botulism or tick paralysis, an evoked muscle action potential following nerve stimulation may be very depressed or absent, thus making an estimate of conduction velocity difficult (46). In myasthenia gravis, while motor nerve conduction velocities are normal, a decremental response is seen in the amplitude of evoked muscle action potentials after repeated nerve stimulation (47). An intravenous injection of edrophonium chloride (Tensilon) will prevent this response. Spontaneous abnormal potentials are usually not seen in skeletal muscles from dogs with junctionopathies; however, fibrillation potentials and positive sharp waves have been reported in distal limb muscles of dogs with botulism (48).

Cerebrospinal Fluid Collection Techniques and Interpretation

Cerebrospinal fluid (CSF) is largely derived from the choroid plexus of the ventricular system. The formation of CSF by the choroid plexus involves both filtration through the fenestrated capillaries of the choroid plexus into its interstitial spaces and active secretion of this filtrate by the epithelium of the choroid plexus (49). The rate of production (approximately 0.05 ml/minute in dogs and 0.02 ml/minute in cats) appears to be relatively independent of the hydrostatic pressure of the blood but is influenced by the blood osmotic pressure. Hypertonic solutions such as mannitol reduce the rate of formation of CSF, as do corticosteroids.

CSF supports and protects the entire central nervous system. It circulates from the ventricular system to the subarachnoid spaces of the brain and spinal cord via the lateral openings of the fourth ventricle. CSF may enter the central canal of the spinal cord by way of the fourth ventricle or the conus medullaris at the terminal end of the cord. Absorption of CSF occurs mainly through one-way valves in the arachnoid villi within intracranial venous sinuses. Flow is from CSF to blood. These valves are open when CSF pressure exceeds venous pressure, which is normally the case.

Collection of CSF

The best site for CSF collection in dogs and cats is the cisterna magna at the atlanto-occipital junction (12, 50, 50a). With the animal intubated and under general anesthesia, the atlanto-occipital area is surgically prepared. For a right-handed individual, the animal is placed in lateral recumbency with the limbs pointing toward the operator. The head is flexed with the nose perpendicular to the upper cervical vertebrae using an assistant or the operator's left hand. A 20 gauge, 1.5-inch needle is adequate for most cats and dogs. Commercially available spinal needles with stilettes also are available. The needle is inserted in the dorsal midline at a point halfway between the external occipital protuberance and wings of the atlas, and slowly directed at 90° through the dorsal skin and musculature toward the atlanto-occipital membrane. Slight resistance to pressure can be felt as the atlanto-occipital membrane and dura mater are penetrated simultaneously. The needle is now located within the large subarachnoid space that forms the cisterna magna, and flow of CSF will immediately occur. If a spinal needle is used, the stilette must be removed before flow of CSF can occur. The depth of penetration of the needle will vary according to the size of the animal; ranging from ¼ to ½ inch for cats and toy breed dogs, to 1.0 to 1.5 inches for large breed dogs. The CSF can be collected by allowing it to drip into a glass or plastic test tube or vial. Attachment of a syringe to the needle for aspiration should be avoided since excessive suction may damage the cells and can cause hemorrhage. Collection of 1.0 to 2.0 ml of CSF is sufficient for analysis. Flow of CSF can be enhanced by applying digital pressure on the jugular vein.

An alternative but much less satisfactory collection site is at the lumbosacral spinal cord level. Following general anesthesia, the animal is placed in lateral recumbency with the lumbar spine slightly flexed. A 20 gauge, 3.5-inch needle is inserted perpendicularly along the cranial edge of the spinous process of L6 in order to penetrate the interarcuate ligament between L5 and L6. When bone is encountered, the needle can be moved either cranially or caudally until the interarcuate depression is located. The needle is forced through the ligament into the dorsal subarachnoid space or through the middle of the spinal cord or cauda equina so that the needle rests on the floor of the vertebral canal. The needle can be withdrawn slightly to enter the ventral subarachnoid space. In most dogs and cats, the subarachnoid space at the lumbosacral level is too small to allow flow of CSF, and suction using a syringe attached to the hub of the needle is usually necessary. Typically, the volume of CSF collected is small. Alternative penetration sites in the lumbosacral region are L6-L7 or L4-L5 (12, 50). Penetration of the lumbosacral spinal cord is not usually associated with clinical signs.

Complications of CSF Collection

If the needle moves off the midline plane and enters a branch of the vertebral venous plexus which courses close to the atlanto-occipital site, whole blood may appear in the needle. Entering this plexus usually causes no harm to the animal. These vessels are located outside of the spinal cord, and thus CSF in the subarachnoid space will not be contaminated with blood. A fresh needle should be obtained and the procedure repeated.

Sometimes a thin line of blood can appear in the CSF during collection. This is often due to rupture of small blood vessels (e.g., pia-arachnoid vessels) by the procedure. It may clear spontaneously if the CSF is allowed to flow or if the needle is repositioned slightly. Contamination of CSF by small quantities of blood usually does not interfere with CSF analysis or interpretation; however, if the quantity of blood is excessive, the collection should be abandoned and tried again in 24 to 48 hours.

Examination and Interpretation of CSF

Routine CSF examination includes determination of CSF pressure, physical appearance, cellularity, and protein content.

CSF Pressure

Normal CSF pressure in dogs is <180 mm CSF, and in cats is <100 mm CSF (12, 50, 51, 52). Elevated CSF pressure is rather a nonspecific finding, since it has been reported in association with many different conditions, including tumors, brain edema, abscesses, hematomas, hydrocephalus, and meningoencephalitides (12, 53). Elevated CSF pressure is not synonymous with increased intracranial pressure. For example, an expanding intracranial mass will result initially in a reduction in volume of brain tissues and/or CSF volume. This spatial compensation can prevent an increase in intracranial pressure, although CSF pressure will be increased. Once this reserve capacity has been exhausted, intracranial pressure increases rapidly and may reach an end stage in which intrinsic vasomotor tone is lost in arteries and arterioles, capillaries and veins are distended, intracranial pressure becomes equal to systemic arterial pressure, cerebral blood flow ceases, and brain death occurs.

In those instances where CSF pressure measurements are deemed necessary, a manometer with a three-way stopcock can be carefully inserted into the hub of the needle. The opening CSF pressure is recorded when the CSF has reached its maximum height. The stopcock can be redirected for CSF collection. During the maneuver of pressure recording, the needle is easily displaced, which may lead to spinal cord trauma and/or hemorrhage.

The sudden reduction in CSF pressure following CSF collection occasionally may lead to herniation of brain tissue (e.g., herniation of occipital or temporal lobe under the tentorium cerebelli producing acute midbrain compression, or herniation of the cerebellum through the foramen magnum resulting in compression of medullary centers and possible death). The possibility of herniation is very much increased in cases of acute cerebral trauma associated with edema and/or hemorrhage. In such cases, CSF collection is contraindicated. Brain herniation following CSF removal also can occur with space-occupying masses, such as tumors.

Physical Appearance

Normal CSF is a crystal clear, colorless fluid. A red tinge is indicative of recent hemorrhage. The discoloration should clear after centrifugation if the hemorrhage occurred during the tap. If the discoloration persists, there has been recent hemorrhage into the CSF. A yellow tinge in the supernate following centrifugation indicates xanthochromia, which usually is caused by free bilirubin of previous subarachnoid hemorrhage (54). A green coloration suggests a suppurative inflammatory process.

CSF turbidity or cloudiness is caused by increased cellularity (white and/or red blood cells) greater than $500/mm^3$. If turbidity is observed, the sample should be cultured and smears examined using routine stains such as Gram's, Ziehl-Neelsen, or methylene blue. The only organisms that can be identified consistently in CSF are systemic fungi, such as *Cryptococcus neoformans*. India ink staining may enhance their visibility.

Normal CSF does not coagulate. Coagulation occurs if the CSF protein levels, including fibrinogen, are greatly increased, as in acute suppurative meningitis or profuse hemorrhage.

Cellularity

Determinations of total and differential white blood cell (WBC) counts are the most important parts of the CSF examination. Normal cisternal CSF contains fewer than 5 WBCs/mm^3 and no red blood cells (RBCs). Normal lumbar CSF contains less than 1 WBC/mm^3. The normal WBCs present are lymphocytes and mononuclear cells. CSF examination is most valuable in the confirmation of infectious and inflammatory diseases. Bacterial meningoencephalitides typically cause a marked increase in cellularity (pleocytosis), e.g., 500 to 1000 WBCs/mm^3, usually marked by a predominance of neutrophils. Viral and rickettsial (hemobartonellosis, Rocky Mountain spotted fever) disease result in a mild to moderate pleocytosis, e.g., 20 to 60 WBCs/mm^3. Toxoplasmosis and fungal (e.g., cryptococcosis, blastomycosis, and histoplasmosis) encephalomyelitis usually produce a mixed mononculear and polymorphonuclear pleocytosis, ranging from 40 to 100 WBCs/mm^3. Granulomatous meningoencephalomyelitis can be characterized by a mild to pronounced pleocytosis, ranging from 50 to 600 WBCs/mm^3, consisting of cells that are predominately mononuclear (lymphocytes, monocytes, and variable presence of large anaplastic mononuclear cells with abundant lacy cytoplasm).

Neoplastic cells rarely are observed within the CSF; however, immature lymphoid cells can be seen in association with neural lymphosarcoma (55). A moderate, neutrophilic pleocytosis (20 to 40 WBCs/mm^3) may be present in animals with acute vascular infarction. In cases of cerebrospinal vascular diseases or central nervous system trauma, the presence of siderophages or macrophages with engulfed erythrocytes and/or iron pigment within CSF is definitive proof of blood in the CSF at least 1 day before the CSF collection (56). It should be noted that in cases of central nervous system trauma, there is usually no indication for CSF examination, since the cause and degree of damage usually are obvious on neurological examination. CSF cellularity tends to be within normal limits in congenital malformations, metabolic diseases, and nutritional and toxic disorders. With the rare exception of presence of globoid cells within CSF in animals with globoid cell leukodystrophy (57), CSF cellularity also is usually within normal limits in degenerative diseases. Radiographic contrast agents, such as metrizamide and iopamidol, have been reported to produce a transient mild, neutrophilic pleocytosis that returns to normal after about 24 to 48 hours (9a, 58).

Cell counts are readily performed in clinical practice using a hemocytometer. One chamber of the hemocytometer is filled with a few drops of fresh CSF, and cells within all nine squares are counted and multiplied by 1.1, to give a total count per cubic millimeter. With this method, RBCs may also be present, and these cells need to be differentiated from WBCs. The WBCs are larger, more granular, and more refractile than RBCs. If the presence of RBCs poses a problem in the WBC count, RBCs can be lyzed by drawing 1.0 ml of fresh CSF into a pipette with 0.1 ml of crystal violet-acetic acid diluting fluid. This mixture can be added to the other chamber of the hemocytometer and the counting procedure repeated. The number of cells is multiplied by 1.2 to give the total WBC count per cubic millimeter. Various formulae to correct WBC values obtained from CSF contaminated with blood have been shown to be unreliable (59). In fact, blood contamination appears to have little effect on WBC numbers, even though several thousand RBCs may be present. If more than 10,000 RBCs/mm^3 are present, it might be preferable to repeat the tap after 24 hours, at which time the erythrocytes will be removed from the CSF. To determine a differential cell count in clinical practice, approximately 1.0 ml of fresh CSF is centrifuged (1200 rpm for about 10 minutes). The supernate is saved for CSF chemistries, and the sediment is gently smeared onto a glass slide and stained with new methylene blue, Wright's stain, or Giemsa stain. Addition of a drop or two of serum to the sediment following centrifugation can improve the quality of the smear. Alternative but more time-consuming techniques described include sedimentation and Millipore filtration (51, 60, 61).

Protein Content

Normal CSF has a protein content of <30 mg/dl. In a recent study of canine CSF, it was reported that protein levels in lumbar CSF (mean = 28.68 mg/dl) are significantly higher than those in cisternal CSF (mean = 13.97 mg/dl) (62).

Most of this protein is albumin. Levels of IgG in normal CSF are very low. Minimum or negative concentrations of third component of complement, IgM, and IgA are present in normal CSF (63). Globulin levels can be increased from local production within the CNS (64) and, along with albumin, may be elevated following disruption of the blood-brain barrier. Mild contamination of CSF with blood appears to have little effect on CSF protein (59).

As for cellularity, protein levels typically are elevated in inflammatory and infectious diseases. The highest protein levels are usually seen with bacterial meningoencephalomyelitides, and may exceed 1000 mg/dl. Moderate increases in protein levels, e.g., 60 to 100 mg/dl, in conjunction with pleocytosis may occur with viral, protozoal (toxoplasmosis), fungal, and rickettsial CNS diseases. CSF protein may also increase without a concomitant increase in cells, and this situation has been termed "albuminocytologic dissociation." It has been observed in several conditions, including CNS neoplasia, cerebrovascular diseases, spinal cord compression, and sometimes in certain autoimmune conditions, such as coonhound paralysis (polyradiculoneuritis). CSF protein levels are reportedly increased following repeated spinal taps in dogs (58). A similar increase was not observed in cats (65). In clinical practice, accurate quantitative determination of CSF proteins usually requires the services of a reference laboratory, since the procedure necessitates the use of a spectrophotometer and/or other specialized equipment, such as electrophoretograms, electroimmunodiffusion, or rocket immunoelectrophoresis. The cell-free fraction of CSF, derived from the supernate following centrifugation, can be frozen and dispatched to a reference laboratory for analysis. One indication of excessive protein in the CSF is the appearance and persistence of foam on top of the CSF following agitation. In normal CSF, the small amount of foam present will disappear within 5 minutes. Also, the presence of any coagulation in CSF is an indication of excessive protein content. Simple qualitative tests for increased globulin levels are available for use in clinical practice. The simplest available is the Pandy test. A few drops of CSF are added to 1.0 ml of Pandy reagent (10 mg of carbolic acid crystals brought to a volume of 100 ml with distilled water) in a test tube and shaken thoroughly. Normal CSF will be clear or only slightly hazy, whereas pathological CSF will develop a definitive white turbidity which will be proportional to the amount of globulin present. Another qualitative procedure that can be used in practice is the Nonne-Apelt test, in which 1.0 ml of saturated ammonium sulfate is placed in a small test tube, overlaid with 1.0 ml of CSF, and allowed to stand for 3 minutes. No ring forms in normal CSF, while a white to gray ring at the contact zone indicates the presence of globulins in increased amounts.

Other Studies

Concentrations of sodium, chloride, and magnesium are greater in CSF than in plasma, whereas CSF has less glucose, potassium, and calcium. Decreased levels of glucose in CSF (hypoglycorrhachia) can occur in acute pyogenic infections. Several studies of CSF enzyme concentrations, including creatine phosphokinase (CPK), glutamic oxaloacetic transaminase, glutamic pyruvic transaminase, and lactate dehydrogenase, have been reported in an attempt to define possible diagnostic and/or prognostic indexes of CNS disease (66–68). The results suggest that most enzyme assays lack specificity for a particular disease entity. However, high concentrations of CPK in CSF from animals with neurological disease may indicate a guarded to poor prognosis (69). CSF β-glucuronidase activity is reportedly significantly elevated with dogs with distemper encephalitis (70).

Neurosurgical Techniques

Spinal neurosurgical techniques in dogs and cats have been developed for the management of spinal cord attenuation by extruded disk material, spinal tumors, or vertebral instabilities, such as may occur with spinal fractures, luxations, or malformations. Thus, surgical management of spinal neurological disorders is primarily aimed at providing spinal cord decompression with concomitant removal of the disk or tumor mass and/or vertebral reduction and stabilization. Brain surgery generally remains restricted to institutions and specialty practices; however, craniectomies for the relief of compressive fractures can be performed successfully in clinical practice.

There are many spinal surgical techniques than have been described that allow access to the neuraxis in dogs and cats (53). Some of these are modifications of established procedures (71, 72), while others are more radical (73–76). The eight techniques described in this section represent well-established, clinically tested procedures (53, 77–90). These eight different techniques have been matched with eight surgically treatable diseases that are most commonly seen in practice (Table 4.1).

Special instrumentation that will facilitate these procedures includes the following:

Periosteal elevator (×1)
Hand-held retractors (×2)
Self-retaining retractors (Frazier ×1), (Gelpi ×2)
Rongeur forceps (Lampert; Mastoid)
   small (×1)
   medium (×2)
   large (×2)
Bone-cutting forceps (×1)
Power drill and bits
Tartar scrapers (×4)
Hand-held trephine (×1)

Intervertebral Disk Disease

Disk disease primarily occurs in thoracolumbar and cervical spinal regions. Two well-established decompressive techniques are available that utilize different surgical approaches to the disk and spinal cord.

Dorsolateral Thoracolumbar Approach (Dorsolateral Hemilaminectomy)

Following general anesthesia, the animal is positioned and maintained in sternal recumbency using small pads or towels on either side of the chest and abdomen. Two strips of surgical tape placed over the thorax and pelvis and attached to each side of the table will also ensure immobility during surgical procedure. The dorsal thoracolumbar area is surgically prepared with the site of the lesion (albeit disk, tumor, or fracture) in the center of the surgical field. A dorsal midline incision is made through the skin and dorsolumbar fascia of sufficient length to encompass about three vertebrae on either side of the lesion in question. Using a periosteal elevator or scalpel handle, the musculature is retracted from one side of the spinous processes of five or six vertebrae down to

Table 4.1. Spinal Neurosurgical Approaches and Techniques for Specific Neurological Disorders

Disorder	Regional Site	Surgical Approach	Surgical Technique
Disk disease	1. Thoracolumbar	Dorsolateral	Dorsolateral hemi-laminectomy
	2. Cervical	Ventral	Slot decompression
Lumbosacral stenosis	Lumbosacral	Dorsal	Dorsal laminectomy
Cervical malformation-malarticulation	Cervical (C3-C7)	1. Vental	Slot decompression with stabilization
		2. Dorsal	Dorsal laminectomy with stabilization
Atlantoaxial luxation	Cervical (C1-C2)	Dorsal	Dorsal atlantoaxial stabilization
Spinal fractures and luxations	1. Thoracolumbar	Dorsolateral	Dorsolateral hemi-laminectomy with stabilization
	2. Lumbosacral	Dorsal	Dorsal laminectomy with stabilization
Spinal tumors	1. Cervical	Dorsal	Dorsal laminectomy
	2. Thoracolumbar	Dorsolateral	Dorsolateral hemi-laminectomy
	3. Lumbosacral	Dorsal	Dorsal laminectomy

the level of the transverse (lateral) processes of lumbar vertebrae or rib heads of thoracic vertebrae. Muscle is removed from the interspinous ligaments, and muscular attachments to the vertebral articular and accessory processes are carefully cut in order to avoid the ventrally located spinal vessels and nerves emerging from their intervertebral foraminae. In this fashion, all muscle can be retracted away from the lateral aspects of the vertebral bodies using self-retaining retractors (e.g., Frazier laminectomy retractors). The last rib and/or first lateral process (of L1 vertebra) can be used for establishing landmarks for lesions in the area of the thoracolumbar junction. A rongeur or bone-cutting forceps is used to remove the articular process over the proposed site of decompression and those of vertebrae on either side (Fig. 4.1). In small animals, the spinal canal can be entered by nibbling away bone at the level of the accessory process (using sharp, fine-tipped rongeurs) and extending the hemilaminectomy in rostrad and caudad directions to the level of the articular processes of the adjacent vertebrae. The bony lamina should be removed from the floor of the canal to a level just dorsal to the spinal cord. In larger animals, the hemilaminectomy may be facilitated by using a high-speed air drill or laminectomy trephine (Figs. 4.2–4.4). The site where the articular processes are removed provides a flat surface for drilling or trephining. Both of these procedures require experience and careful handling so as to avoid cord trauma. Frequent rocking of the trephine will help to determine the looseness of the plug. Drilling should be done using a feathering, back-and-forth motion. The depth of the defect can be gauged by visualizing three distinct layers during the drilling process. First, the hard, outer cortical layer is penetrated to expose the softer, more hemorrhagic marrow layer. Finally, the inner cortical layer is observed. The depth can also be checked using a thin-blade, claw type tartar scraper. When the periosteal lining of the canal is exposed, it is safer to complete the hemilaminectomy using rongeurs (Fig. 4.5). The spinal cord may

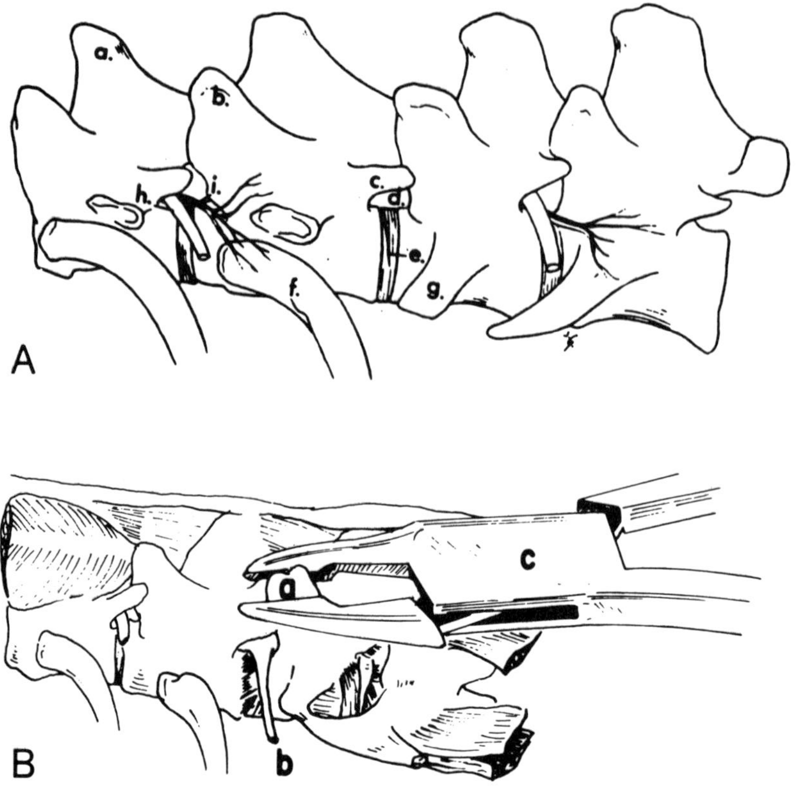

Figure 4.1. (*A*) Anatomical structures encountered during spinal surgery. *a*, Dorsal spine; *b*, articular process; *c*, accessory process; *d*, intervertebral foramen; *e*, intervertebral disk; *f*, rib; *g*, lateral (transverse) process; *h*, spinal nerve; *i*, spinal artery and vein. Notice that the disk is located slightly rostral to the place at which the lateral process or rib joins the body of the vertebra. (*B*) Dorsolateral hemilaminectomy. The articular process (*a*) is being removed to produce a flat surface for trephination or burring; *b*, intervertebral nerves and vessels; *c*, rongeur. (From Hoerlein BF: *Canine Neurology*. Philadelphia, WB Saunders, 1978.)

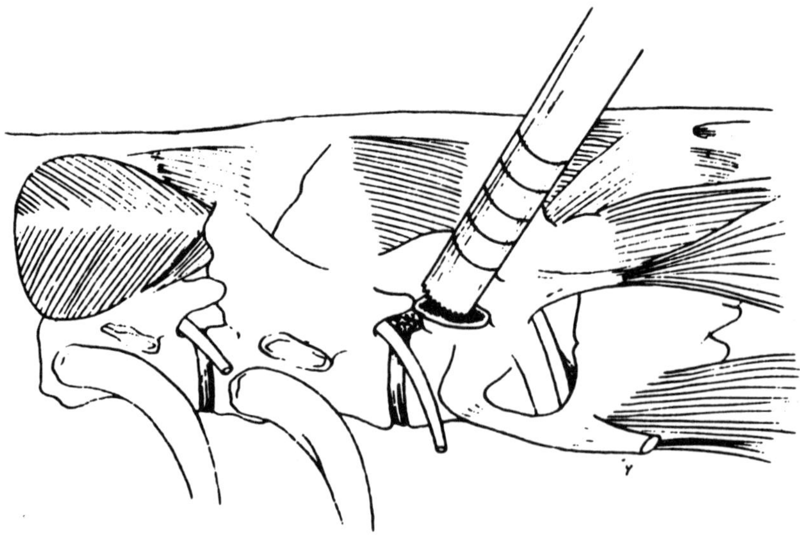

Figure 4.2. (*A*) Michelle laminectomy trephine is used to expose the epidural space and spinal cord. (From Hoerlein BF: *Canine Neurology*. Philadelphia, WB Saunders, 1978.)

be safely exposed over two, and sometimes, three vertebrae. In animals with disk disease, hemilaminectomy extending over two vertebral bodies is usually adequate. If the surgery is performed on the correct side, extruded disk material may be visualized and gently removed (Figs. 4.6 and 4.7). Sometimes, epidural matter can be firmly attached to the dura mater, requiring sharp dissection. A herniated disk can be curetted to remove any remaining degenerated nuclear material. Intervertebral disks are located immediately rostral to the lateral vertebral processes or rib heads. Curettage is accomplished by cutting the outer fibrous layers of the lateral part of the disk with a scalpel blade and inserting a fine hooked tartar scraper or small curette and removing the central parts of the disk by scraping in a downward and outward direction. In animals with disk diseases, two or three disks on either side of the extruded disk can also be fenestrated. Vessels and nerves should be retracted rostrally during disk curettage.

The laminectomy defect can be filled with absorbable gelatin sponge or a full fat graft. The dorsolateral fascia is sutured securely with the material of choice in a simple interrupted pattern. Subcutaneous tissues and skin are routinely closed.

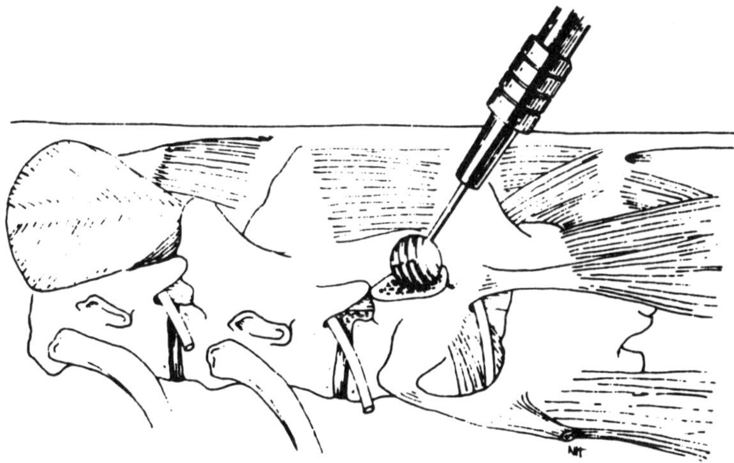

Figure 4.3. An air drill and burr can be used instead of a trephine and rongeurs to create the bone defect. (From Hoerlein BF: *Canine Neurology.* Philadelphia, WB Saunders, 1978.)

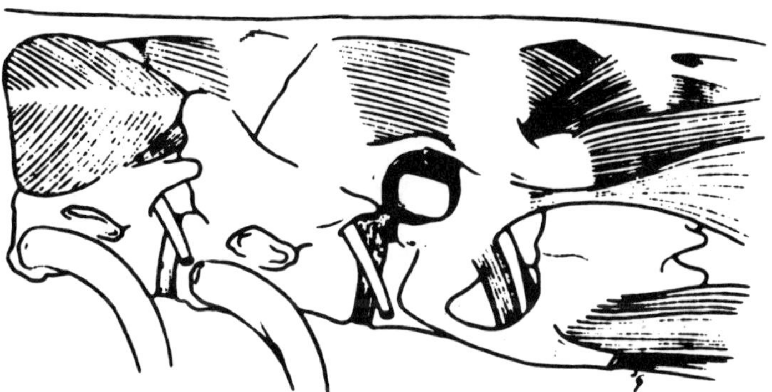

Figure 4.4. Initial exposure of spinal cord following trephination or burring. Protruding or extruded disk material may be observed. (From Hoerlein BF: *Canine Neurology.* Philadelphia, WB Saunders, 1978.)

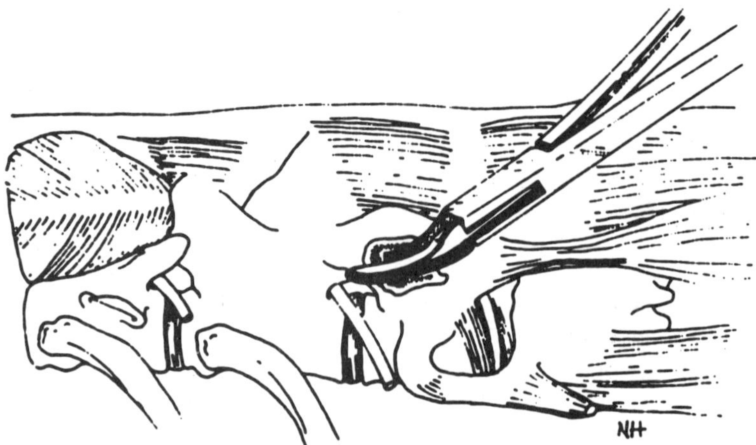

Figure 4.5. Enlargement of the bony defect using rongeurs. (From Hoerlein BF: *Canine Neurology.* Philadelphia, WB Saunders, 1978.)

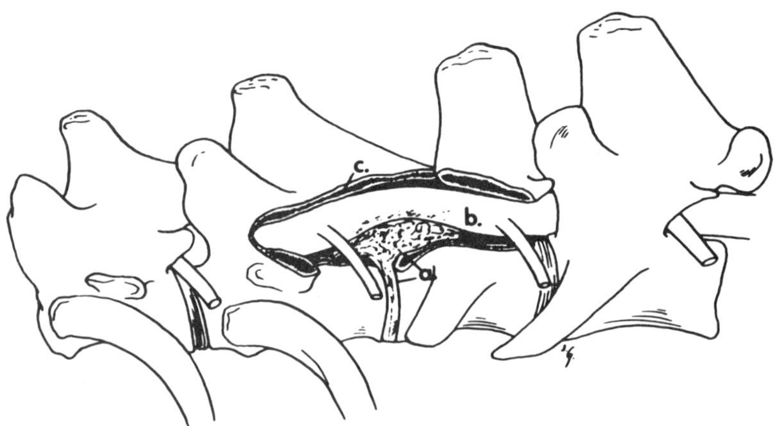

Figure 4.6. Completion of the hemilaminectomy. *a*, Extruded disk material; *b*, spinal cord; *c*, edge of hemilaminectomy. (From Hoerlein BF: *Canine Neurology.* Philadelphia, WB Saunders, 1978.)

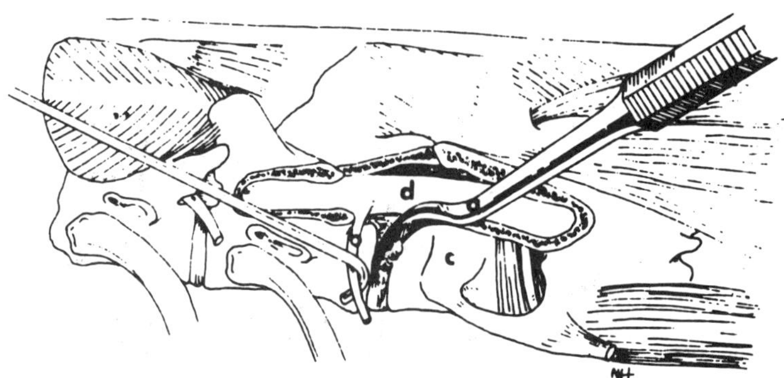

Figure 4.7. The disk material can be removed using a tartar scraper (*a*). *b*, Spinal nerve and vessels; *c*, transverse (lateral) process; *d*, spinal cord. (From Hoerlein BF: *Canine Neurology.* Philadelphia, WB Saunders, 1978.)

Ventral Cervical Approach (Slot Decompression)

The animal is placed in dorsal recumbency with the neck extended over a sandbag and the thoracic limbs pulled back lateral to the chest. A ventral midline incision extends from the level of the atlas to the manubrium sternum. The sternohyoideus muscles are divided along the midline to expose the trachea. The trachea, esophagus, and carotid sheath are carefully retracted laterally to expose the longus colli muscles. The vertebrae or disks required are identified by palpating the markedly pointed prominence located on the midline of the dorsal aspect of the atlas (C1) or by palpating the caudal border of the wing of the atlas into the midline and then the ventral process of each vertebra caudally. The longus colli muscles are separated, their attachments to the ventral processes are cut, and the muscle is retracted laterally from the vertebral bodies on either side of the affected disk (Fig. 4.8).

The lip of the ventral spinous process adjacent to the disk is removed using bone rongeurs (Fig. 4.9), and a high-speed air drill is used to cut a longitudinal slot in two adjacent vertebrae, extending through the disk from the caudal one-third of the cranial vertebra to the cranial one-third of the caudal vertebra. The slot is continued through the bone, disk, and dorsal longitudinal ligament to the floor of the vertebral canal (Fig. 4.10). Disk material may be visualized and removed using the point of a tartar scraper (Fig. 4.11). A potential complication is rupture of the vertebral venous sinus during manipulation of the tartar scraper along the floor of the canal. Bleeding is usually controlled by packing a surgical sponge into the slot and waiting a few minutes.

Adjacent disks can be isolated and fenestrated. The simplest method is to incise the ventral annulus and scoop out as much nucleus pulposus as possible. A claw tartar scraper or a small curette may be used for this purpose.

The longus colli muscles are opposed with simple interrupted sutures of 3-O gut. The trachea, esophagus, and carotid sheath are returned to their normal

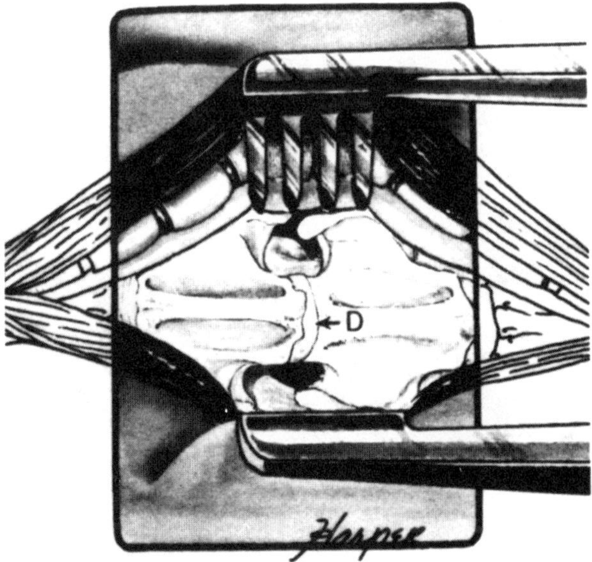

Figure 4.8. The ventral surface of two adjacent cervical vertebrae, with the intervening disk (*D*). (From Swaim SF: Ventral decompression of the cervical spinal cord in the dog. *J Am Vet Med Assoc* 164:491–495, 1974.)

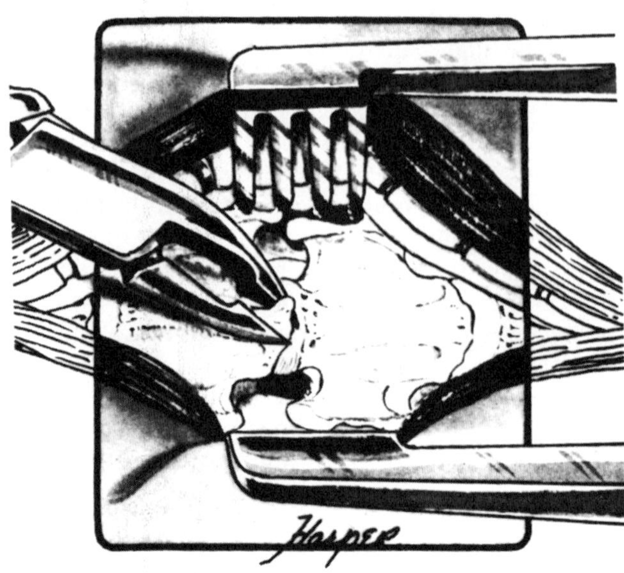

Figure 4.9. The ventral spinous process of the rostral vertebra is removed using rongeurs. (From Swaim SF: Ventral decompression of the cervical spinal cord in the dog. *J Am Vet Med Assoc* 164:491–495, 1974.)

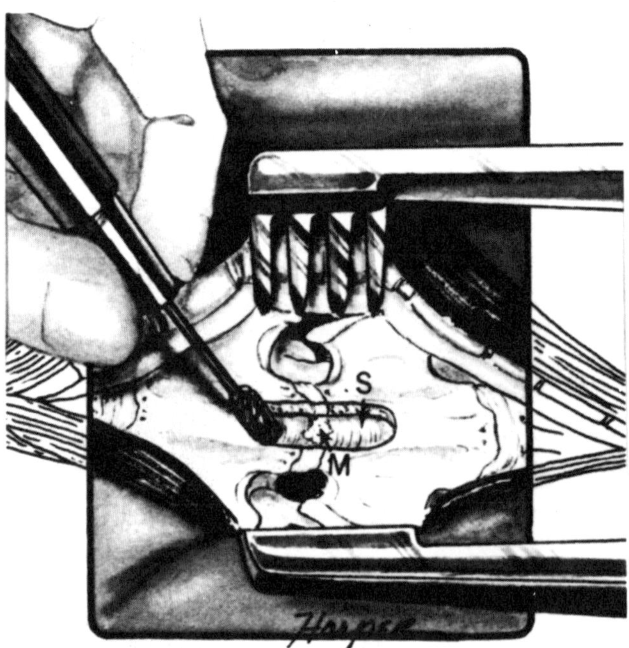

Figure 4.10. A longitudinal slot is made in the two adjacent vertebrae using a high-speed air drill and oblong burr. *S,* Exposed ventral surface of the spinal cord; *M,* extruded disk material within spinal canal. (From Swaim SF: Ventral decompression of the cervical spinal cord in the dog. *J Am Vet Med Assoc* 164:491–495, 1974.)

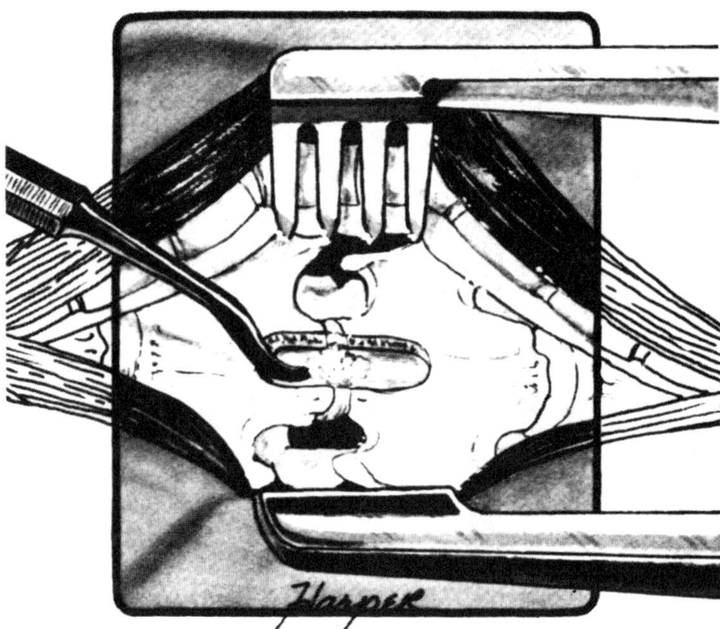

Figure 4.11. A tartar scraper can be used to remove extruded disk material from the spinal canal. (From Swaim SF: Ventral decompression of the cervical spinal cord in the dog. *J Am Vet Med Assoc* 164:491–495, 1974.)

positions. The muscle fascia and skin are closed routinely. Bandaging is not usually required. Animals are encouraged to walk and exercise the day after surgery.

Lumbosacral Stenosis

The lumbosacral canal can be best explored by dorsal laminectomy using a dorsal lumbosacral approach. The animal is placed in sternal recumbency with a sandbag under the pelvic area, and the pelvic limbs are retracted caudally. After surgical preparation, a skin incision is made on the dorsal midline from the dorsal process of the sixth lumbar vertebra to the end of the sacrum (Fig. 4.12). The subcutaneous tissue is incised to the lumbodorsal fascia. An incision is made through the fascia on the midline to reveal the longissimus dorsi and multifidus lumborum muscles which are divided in the midline and retracted laterally, after cutting the fascial attachments to the dorsal spines of the last lumbar vertebra and the sacrum (Fig. 4.13). The dorsal surfaces of these vertebrae are cleared of muscle using a periosteal elevator. The interarcuate ligament (ligamentum flavum) at the lumbosacral joint is identified and carefully removed with a scalpel to reveal the epidural fat covering the cauda equina. The dorsal spines of the last lumbar vertebra and the first sacral segment are removed with bone cutters. Dorsal laminectomy is performed using rongeurs (Fig. 4.14). The length of the laminectomy defect is about half the length of the last lumbar vertebra and the first sacral segment. The width of the laminectomy is usually limited to the level of the dorsal articular processes. This exposure will allow inspection of the lumbosacral disk, allow removal of a mass lesion (tumor or disk material), and permit lumbosacral disk curettage in the event of diskospondylitis (Fig. 4.15). Facetectomy or removal of the articulating processes can be performed if osteophytes developing from these processes result in compression of the cauda equina

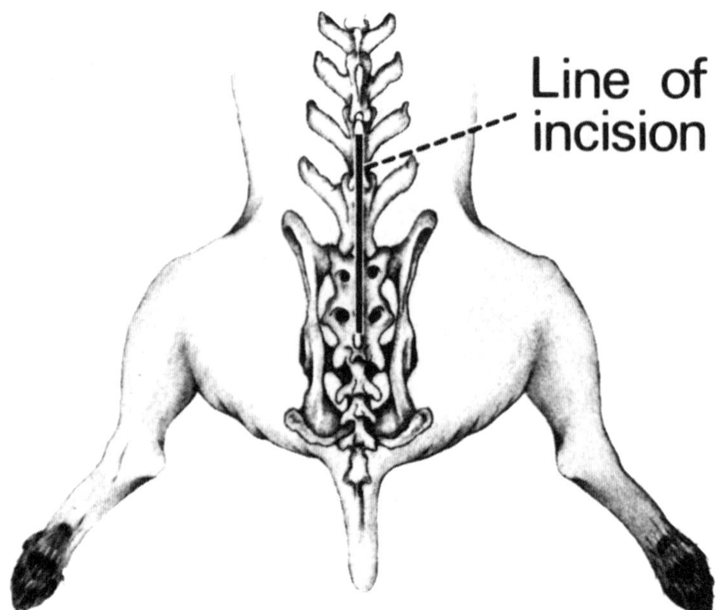

Figure 4.12. A skin incision is made on the midline from L6 to S3. (From Bojrab MJ (ed): *Current Techniques in Small Animal Surgery 1.* Philadelphia, Lea & Febiger, 1975.)

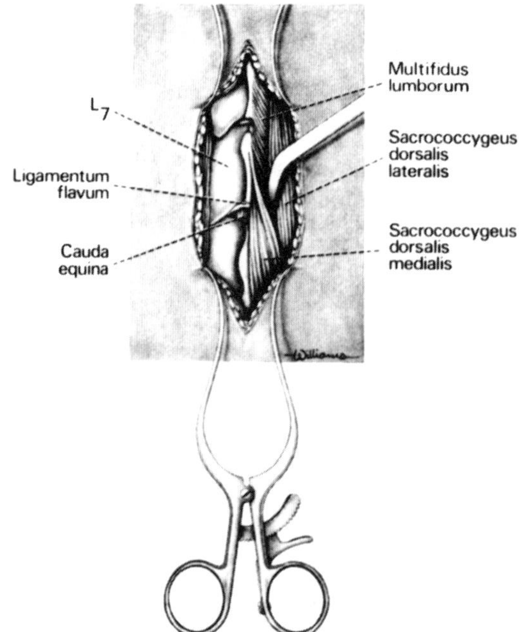

Figure 4.13. The superficial fascia is reflected on the right, exposing the musculature. The epaxial muscles have been reflected from the dorsal spinous processes and laminae to the level of the articular processes on the left. The ligamentum flavum has been partially excised at L7 to S1. (From Bojrab MJ (ed): *Current Techniques in Small Animal Surgery 1.* Philadelphia, Lea & Febiger, 1975.)

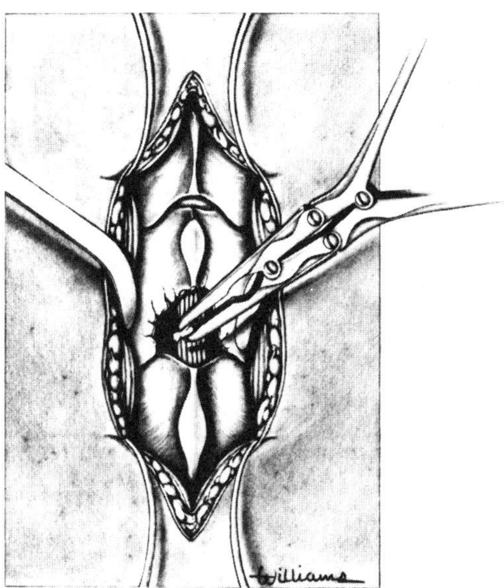

Figure 4.14. The dorsal lamina is carefully removed with a rongeur or air drill. Epidural fat normally fills the spinal canal but is not illustrated. (From Bojrab MJ (ed): *Current Techniques in Small Animal Surgery 1*. Philadelphia, Lea & Febiger, 1975.)

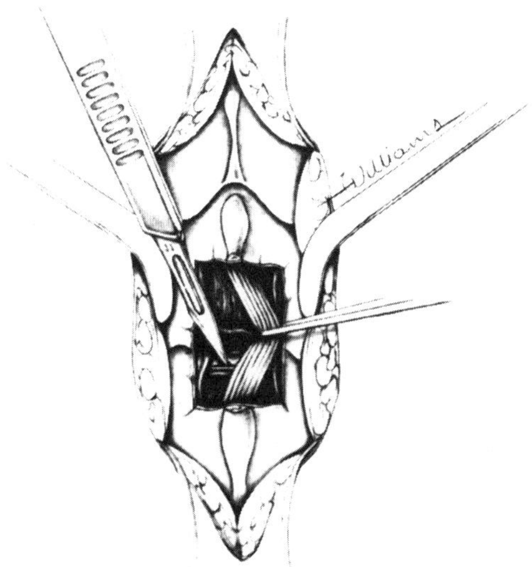

Figure 4.15. Retraction of the cauda equina to allow inspection of the lumbosacral canal. The tip of the scalpel blade is inserted into the dorsal annulus of the lumbosacral disk. The prominent venous sinuses should be avoided. (From Bojrab MJ (ed): *Current Techniques in Small Animal Surgery 1*. Philadelphia, Lea & Febiger, 1975.)

or seventh lumbar nerve root. The laminectomy defect can be filled with a full fat graft. Muscle, lumbodorsal fascia, subcutaneous tissue, and skin layers are routinely closed.

Cervical Malformation-Malarticulation

This disorder can be surgically managed using a ventral cervical approach or a dorsal laminectomy. Each approach lends itself to vertebral stabilizing techniques.

Ventral Cervical Approach (Ventral Slot Decompression/Stabilization)

A surgical approach used for affected dogs is a ventral slot, a corticocancellous bone graft, and ventral plating of the involved interspace (89). The ventral neck, sternum, and both proximal humeri are surgically prepared. The animal is placed and secured in dorsal recumbency, and a standard ventral approach to the affected interspace is made. A ventral slot is performed across the affected interspace extending about 75% through the vertebrae (traction obviates the need to enter the spinal canal and remove the dorsal longitudinal ligament and/or redundant dorsal annulus fibrosus) (Fig. 4.16). The slot is approximately 1 cm^2 for large breed dogs such as Doberman pinschers. The exact length of the bone graft is determined by measuring the length of the slot following rigid longitudinal traction of the cervical spine. This is accomplished using two assistants, one pulling gently on the head (at the base of the skull) and the other pulling on the thoracic limbs. With traction, the slot should approximately double in length. Rigid bone grafts that have been used include pelvic autografts, tibial allografts from a frozen bone bank, and bovine heterografts. Hollow tibial grafts can be packed tightly with fresh, autogenous cancellous bone (e.g., from the proximal humerus) to ensure rigidity. After the graft has been measured and cut to size, it is tapped into place while longitudinal traction is applied to the neck (Fig. 4.17). A medium-sized plastic Lubra plate is placed across the interspace and secured by two cortical, 3.5-mm screws in each vertebral body (Fig. 4.18). The screw holes are drilled at angles away from the vertebral canal. The depth of the holes and length of the screws can be determined from a lateral radiograph.

Closure of soft tissues is routine. A neck brace that attempts to immobilize the

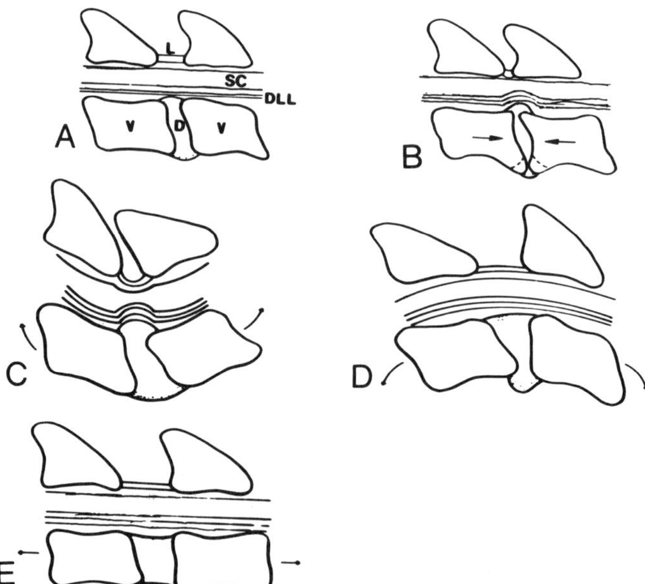

Figure 4.16. (*A*) Normal anatomy of related cervical structures. *L*, ligamentum flavum; *SC*, spinal cord; *DLL*, dorsal longitudinal ligament; *V*, vertebrae; *D*, intervertebral disk. (*B*) A collapsed interspace and spondylitic changes on the ventral ends of the vertebrae are considered to occur in fewer than half the cases seen. (*C*) Hyperextension of the neck accentuates the compression both dorsally and ventrally and must be done with caution. (*D*) Ventral flexion of the neck usually alleviates the compression. (*E*) Linear traction also alleviates compression and is considered the key to therapy. (From Bojrab MJ (ed): *Current Techniques in Small Animal Surgery 2.* Philadelphia, Lea & Febiger, 1983.)

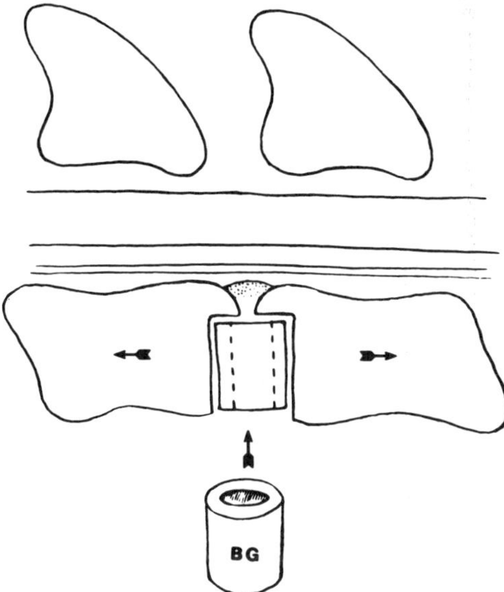

Figure 4.17. Schematic drawing showing how a bone graft (*BG*) is fitted into a ventral cervical slot with the interspace distracted. (From Bojrab MJ (ed): *Current Techniques in Small Animal Surgery 2.* Philadelphia, Lea & Febiger, 1983.)

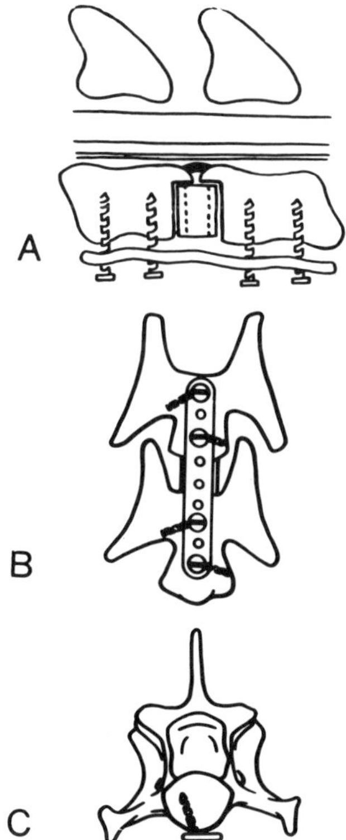

Figure 4.18. (*A*) Postoperative view with plastic plate, screws, and bone graft in place. (*B*) Plate and screws as seen from ventral aspect. (*C*) Cross-sectional view showing appropriate angulation of screws to avoid injury to the spinal cord. (From Bojrab MJ (ed): *Current Techniques in Small Animal Surgery 2.* Philadelphia, Lea & Febiger, 1983.)

neck and thoracic cage as a unit is advocated (Fig. 4.19). If tolerated, the brace should be maintained until there is radiographic evidence of interbody fusion (i.e., from 2 to 3 months).

Currently, results are pending on an alternative surgical technique using Steinmann pins and methyl methacrylate in lieu of the Lubra plates (HB Seim, unpublished information).

Patients with dorsal compression are treated ventrally if traction relieves the compressive forces ("dynamic" lesion), or dorsally via dorsal decompressive laminectomy if the lesion is static. The static or dynamic nature of a lesion is determined using myelography in conjunction with strong linear traction.

Dorsal Cranial Approach (Dorsal Laminectomy with Stabilization)

The dog is positioned in sternal recumbency with a sandbag under the neck, and the dorsal aspect of the neck from the dorsal spine of the axis to the second thoracic dorsal spine is surgically prepared. A 12- to 16-cm skin incision is made along the dorsal midline, with the site of the vertebral lesion approximately in the center of the surgical field. The subcutaneous tissue is incised, exposing the platysma muscle and a median raphe. The incision is continued on the midline through the dorsal cervical muscles until the yellowish nuchal ligament is exposed. The dorsal spinous processes of the cervical vertebrae can be palpated under the nuchal ligament. The nuchal ligament and dorsal muscles are retracted laterally using Frazier laminectomy retractors, and muscle is removed from the dorsal arches of the vertebrae using a periosteal elevator or scalpel handle. A

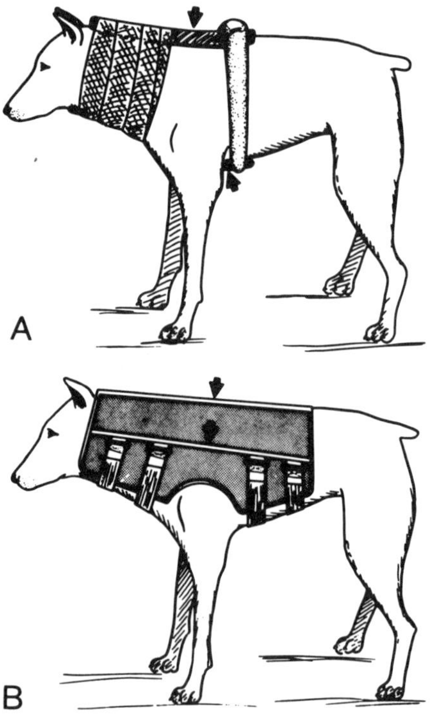

Figure 4.19. Various types of neck braces have been used. (*A*) Plaster splints (*arrows*) supplemented with bandage material may be used. (*B*) A human orthopaedic knee brace with steel rods (*arrows*) may also be adapted for use. (From Bojrab MJ (ed): *Current Techniques in Small Animal Surgery 2*. Philadelphia, Lea & Febiger, 1983.)

dorsal laminectomy is begun by removing the dorsal spinous processes over the decompression area with rongeurs. The dorsal lamina are removed with rongeurs or a drill to allow complete removal of the ligamentum flavum (interarcuate ligament) and effect spinal cord decompression. The length of the defect is about three-quarters the length of each vertebra but can extend the whole length if needed. The width of the laminectomy is limited by the medial aspect of the dorsal articular processes. If it is required, vertebral immobilization can be obtained by bilateral placement of a lag screw (e.g., Bechtol radial-fluted point buttress-threaded bone screws) in the heaviest portion of the overlapping articular processes of the involved vertebrae (53) (Fig. 4.20). The laminectomy defect can be filled with a free fat graft and the incision closed routinely.

Atlantoaxial Luxation

Surgical stabilization of the spinal cord is usually necessary for permanent correction of atlantoaxial luxation (Figs. 4.21–4.23).

The animal is placed in sternal recumbency with a sandbag under the head. A dorsal midline skin incision is made from the occipital protuberance to the third or fourth cervical vertebra. The muscles are incised through the median raphe and carefully elevated from the dorsal arch of the atlas and dorsal spine of the axis. Dissection of the cranial and caudal margins of the arch of the atlas exposes the spinal cord. The dura may be adhered to the cranial margin of the arch of the atlas and should be gently teased free. Reduction of the luxation with immobilization provides adequate decompression. Hemilaminectomy can reduce the stability of the fixation, especially in small animals, and is considered unnecessary (90).

The atlantoaxial luxation can be reduced by depressing the axis ventrally. The

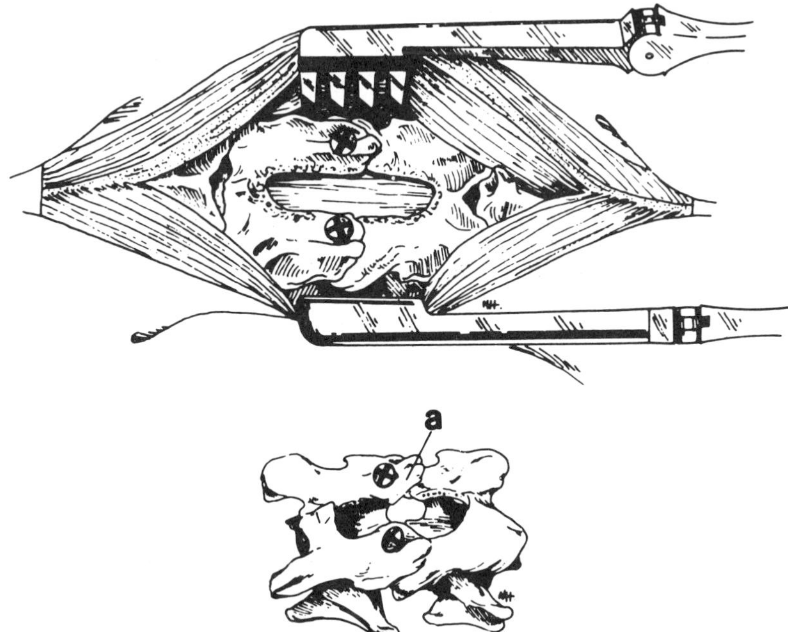

Figure 4.20. Following dorsal laminectomy, immobilization can be achieved by bilateral placement of Bechtol radial-fluted point buttress threaded screws in the heaviest portion of the overlapping articular processes (*a*) of the involved vertebrae. Note the angulation of the screws in the inset drawing. (Courtesy of Dr. SF Swaim.)

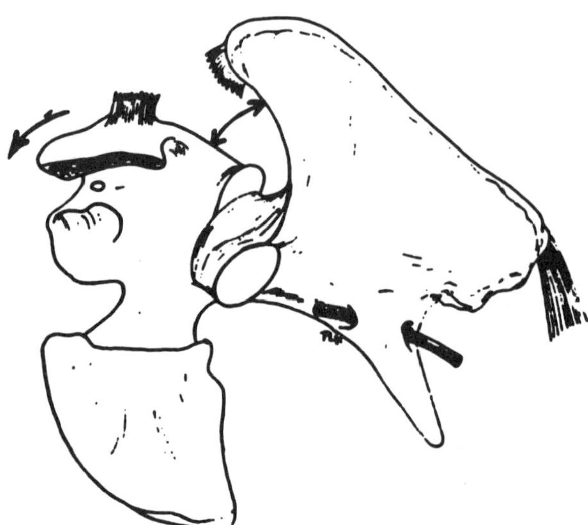

Figure 4.21. Congenital absence of the odontoid process (dens) with lack of joint support and luxation. (From Bojrab MJ (ed): *Current Techniques in Small Animal Surgery 1.* Philadelphia, Lea & Febiger, 1975.)

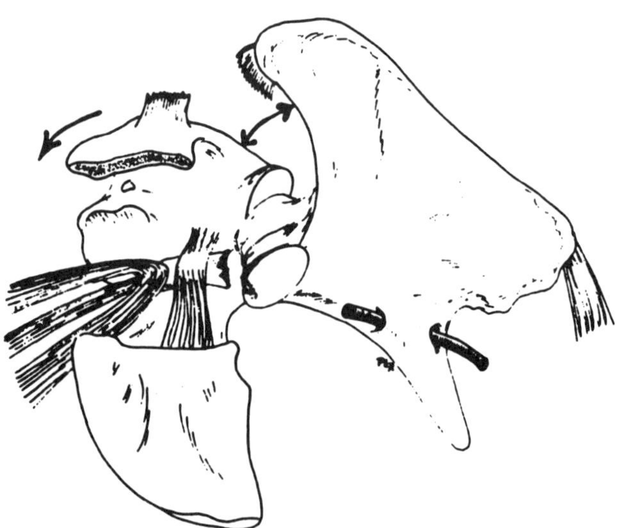

Figure 4.22. Fractured odontoid process (dens) with subsequent luxation of the joint. (From Bojrab MJ (ed): *Current Techniques in Small Animal Surgery 1.* Philadelphia, Lea & Febiger, 1975.)

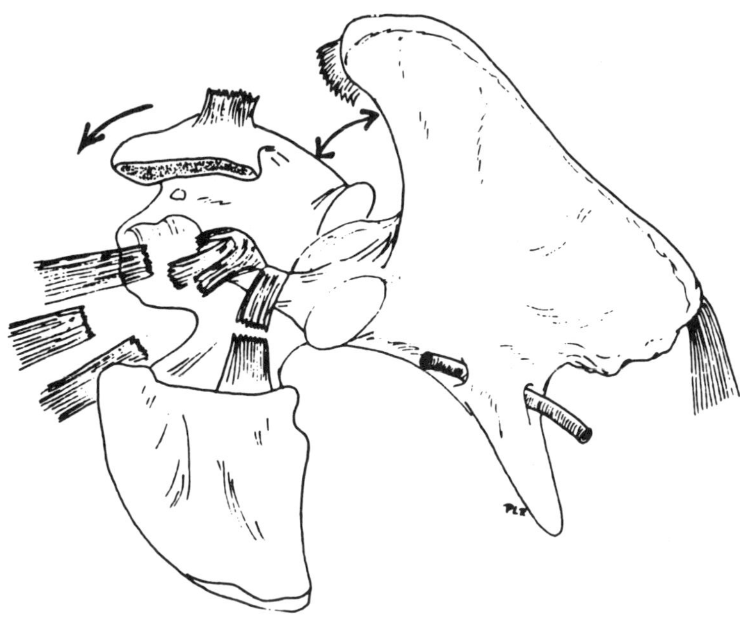

Figure 4.23. Rupture of the joint ligaments with luxation of the atlantoaxial joint. (From Bojrab MJ (ed): *Current Techniques in Small Animal Surgery 1*. Philadelphia, Lea & Febiger, 1975.)

reduction must be maintained throughout the procedure. Two holes are drilled in the dorsal spine of the axis. A loop of orthopaedic wire (20 to 24 gauge) is passed ventral to the dorsal arch of the atlas (Figs. 4.24 and 4.25). Flexion of the head and removal of the caudal aspect of the occipital bone or cranial arch of the atlas with rongeurs may facilitate passage of the wire. The wire loop is retrieved from the atlanto-occipital space, folded back to the axis, and cut in the center. The strands of wire from the atlantoaxial space are tightened through the cranial hole. The tissues are approximated in individual layers for closure. Postoperative radiographs should be taken to evaluate the reduction. A head and neck bandage can be used for 2 to 3 days to provide additional support, and exercise should be restricted for at least 1 month following surgery.

Spinal Fractures/Luxations

The most common sites of spinal fractures are at the thoracolumbar and lumbosacral junctions. Animals with spinal fractures and/or luxations often require spinal cord decompression and internal spinal stabilization.

Dorsolateral Thoracolumbar Approach (Dorsolateral Hemilaminectomy with Stabilization)

Decompression in the thoracolumbar region can be obtained using a dorsolateral hemilaminectomy approach as described for thoracolumbar disk disease. The hemilaminectomy will allow removal of traumatically extruded disk material or depressed bone fragments and of epidural hemorrhage, and will provide prognostic exploration of a swollen cord.

An excellent method of obtaining vertebral stabilization is through the use of vertebral body plates. Unlike the spinous processes, vertebral bodies appear to be more mechanically and physiologically suited for spinal immobilization. Exposure and vertebral size limit the technique to the caudal thoracic area and the midlumbar region (T12 to L4).

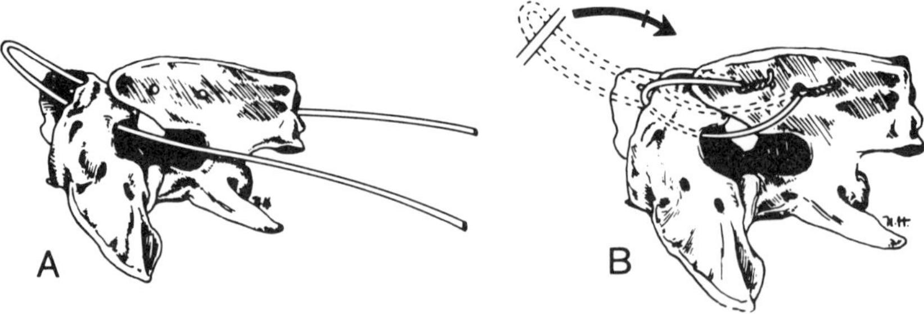

Figure 4.24. (*A*) A double strand of wire is passed under the arch of the atlas. (*B*) After cutting the loop, both of these strands are threaded through the drilled holes and tied as illustrated. (From Swaim SF: Surgical approaches to spinal cord disease of small animals. *Proc Am Anim Hosp Assoc* 1:317, 1975.)

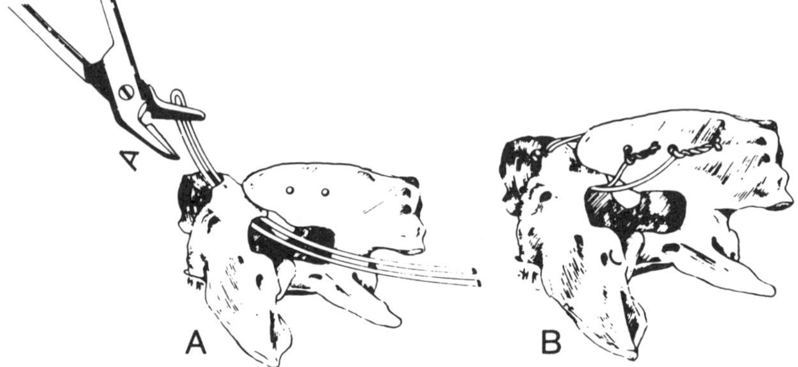

Figure 4.25. This figure illustrates an alternative method of atlantoaxial fixation. (*A*) A double strand of wire is passed under the arch of the atlas. (*B*) After cutting the loop, the cranial and caudal pairs are tied together in their respective drill holes. This forms a bilaterally symmetrical sling. (From Swaim SF: Surgical approaches to spinal cord disease of small animals. *Proc Am Anim Hosp Assoc* 1:317, 1975.)

Following hemilaminectomy, the plate is positioned so that it rests at the junction of the transverse process and vertebral body, just below the hemilaminectomy defect. The spinal nerve and vessels leaving the involved interspace are severed near the intervertebral foramen to prevent entrapment by the plate. A plate size is selected that allows two holes cranial and two holes caudal to the fracture or luxation. Using a drill with a 2-mm bit, holes are drilled through the plate holes in a ventrolateral direction (Fig. 4.26). A depth gauge is used to measure the depth of the hole and the appropriate self-tapping screws are inserted (Fig. 4.27).

In the caudal thoracic area, rib heads are separated with bone cutters and retracted ventrally to allow plate application. When decompression and plating are complete, the rib heads can be elevated back to their original levels by passing a length of orthopaedic wire through predrilled holes in the ribs and through a hole drilled in the corresponding spinous process (81) (Figs. 4.28 and 4.29).

Dorsal Lumbosacral Approach (Dorsal Laminectomy with Stabilization)

Luxation of the lumbosacral joint usually results in a cranioventral displacement of the sacrum (85) with variable compromise of the S1 to S3 nerve roots. When these roots are severed, normal urinary and fecal control are irreversibly

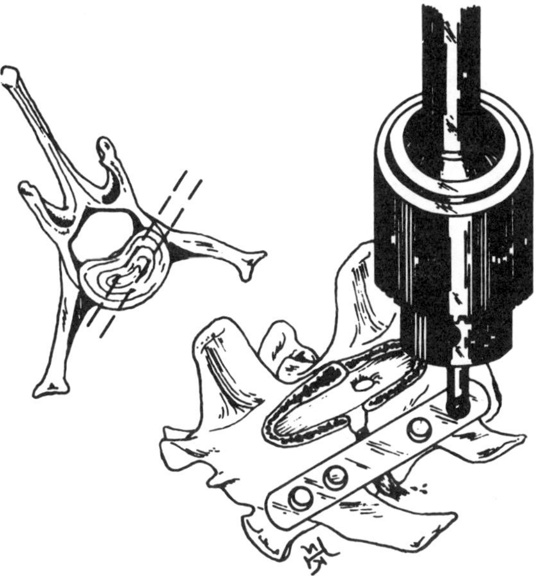

Figure 4.26. After spinal cord decompression by hemilaminectomy, two holes are drilled in each vertebra with the plate in place. The path of the drill holes is depicted. (From Bojrab MJ (ed): *Current Techniques in Small Animal Surgery 1.* Philadelphia, Lea & Febiger, 1975.)

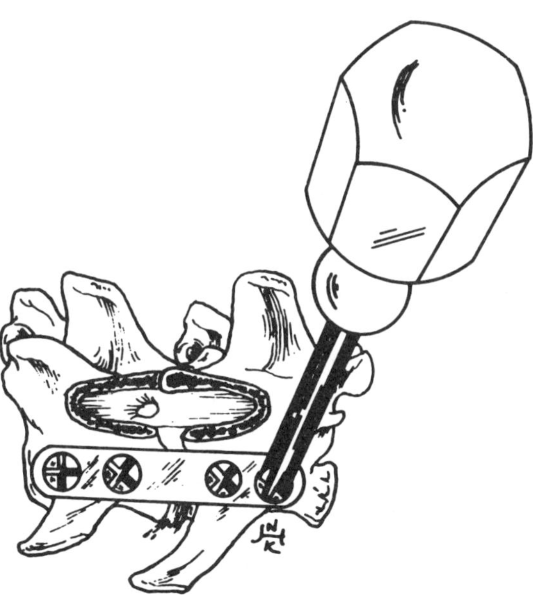

Figure 4.27. Bechtol radial-fluted screws are inserted firmly so that there will be no movement of the plate. A depth gauge is used to select the correct length for the screw. (From Bojrab MJ (ed): *Current Techniques in Small Animal Surgery 1.* Philadelphia, Lea & Febiger, 1975.)

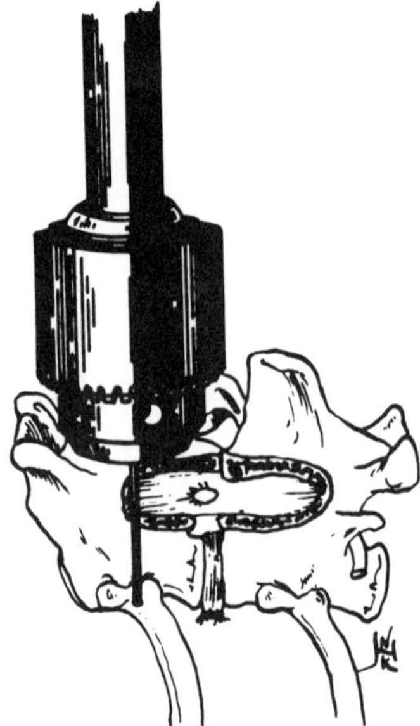

Figure 4.28. In the thoracic area, the ribs must be removed to place the plates. A dorsoventral hole is drilled in the ribs prior to disarticulation of the ribs from the vertebrae. (From Bojrab MJ (ed): *Current Techniques in Small Animal Surgery 1.* Philadelphia, Lea & Febiger, 1975.)

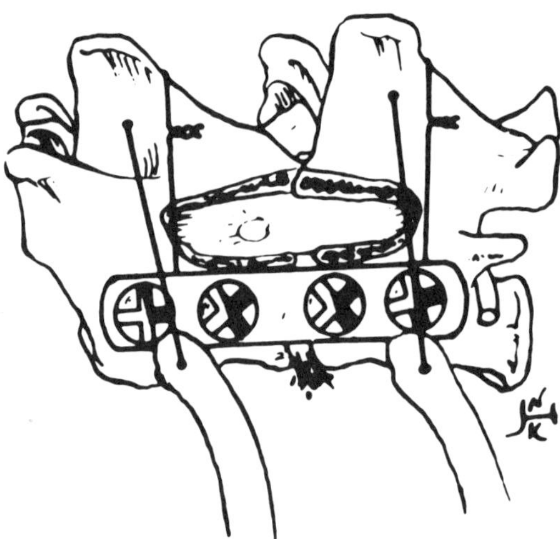

Figure 4.29. Following application of the body plate, the ribs are elevated and wired in place as shown to hold them in their original position. (From Bojrab MJ (ed): *Current Techniques in Small Animal Surgery 1.* Philadelphia, Lea & Febiger, 1975.)

lost. Less severe damage, as indicated by a partial anal reflex or pain perception in the anal or tail area, is an indication for luxation repair.

Exposure of the lumbosacral region is via a dorsal approach, identical to that described for lumbosacral stenosis. The luxation can be reduced by caudal and dorsal distraction of the sacrum and pelvis. Reduction is maintained by a transilial Steinmann pin which is placed between the wings of the ilia and contacts the dorsal surface of L7. The transilial pin can be secured by bending its ends flush with the ilia or by using a threaded pin and nut at each end. Once reduction has been completed, the nerves of the cauda equina can be explored by removing the interarcuate ligament covering the dorsal lumbosacral space. Layers of muscle, fascia, subcutaneous tissue, and skin are routinely closed.

Spinal Tumors

Exploration of the spinal cord for presence and removal of tumors can be accomplished using one of the following regional techniques:

1. Thoracolumbar region: dorsolateral hemilaminectomy (as described for disk disease).

2. Lumbosacral region: dorsal laminectomy (as described for lumbosacral stenosis).

3. Cervical: dorsal laminectomy (as described for cervical malformation-malarticulation).

Muscle and Nerve Biopsy Techniques

Sample biopsies of muscle and nerve are useful ancillary procedures for the diagnosis of neuromyopathies and can be performed easily in clinical practice. The biopsy samples can be mailed to a reference laboratory or institution for processing and examination.

Skeletal Muscle Biopsy

Most muscles of the limbs and head are readily accessible to sample biopsy. In the author's laboratory, biopsy samples usually are obtained from selected pelvic and/or thoracic limb muscles for which baseline qualitative and quantitative data have been established (91–93). These muscles and their usual sampling sites include the following:

Pelvic limb muscles: Biceps femoris (distal one-third); vastus lateralis (distal one-third); lateral head of gastrocnemius (proximal one-third); cranial tibial (proximal one-third).

Thoracic limb muscles: Long head of triceps brachii (distal one-third); medial head of triceps brachii (distal one-third); superficial digital flexor (proximal one-third).

The surgical site for biopsy of the common peroneal and ulnar nerves (see "Nerve Biopsy" below) will permit sampling of the biceps femoris and gastrocnemius muscles in the pelvic limb, and of the medial head of the triceps brachii and superficial digital flexor muscles in the thoracic limb, respectively.

In most instances, muscle biopsies are performed immediately after electrodiagnostic procedures (electromyography, nerve conduction velocity determinations, etc), during which time the animal is under general anesthesia. In older or high-risk animals, Numorphan (oxymorphone hydrochloride) and acepromazine (acetyl promazine) are used for sedation, followed by local infiltration of the skin at the biopsy site with 2% lidocaine (Xylocaine). The biopsy site is surgically prepared and an incision (approximately 5 cm in length) is made through the skin and fascia to expose the muscle. A segment of muscle is grasped with tooth forceps, and a sample is removed by cutting a cylinder (approximately 1.5 cm long, 1 cm wide, and 0.5 cm thick) with a pair of sharp scissors. Multiple samples may be taken from the same area (to reduce the chances of missing a focal pathological change). After the biopsy, the fascia and subcutaneous tissues are sutured with absorbable material, and the skin is then closed.

No attempt is made to maintain the muscle under stretch for routine histology and histochemistry. However, maintaining the muscle at a slightly stretched length is very important for electron microscopy. For this purpose, special biopsy clamps are used.

In contrast with percutaneous needle biopsy, the biopsy procedure described above permits adequate tissue sampling and facilitates orientation for freezing and sectioning.

The muscle sample is rinsed for a few seconds in saline and placed in a tightly closed vial moistened with saline (10 to 20 drops). The vial can be put into a styrofoam container filled with *normal* ice. The container should arrive at the laboratory within 24 hours of mailing (94).

Nerve Biopsy

In conjunction with clinical and electrophysiological evaluation, nerve biopsies are being used increasingly for the investigation of neuromuscular disorders.

The complete examination of a nerve biopsy specimen is a complex and time-consuming procedure that is best performed at centers where there is an interest in peripheral nerve disorders.

Fascicular nerve biopsies are used whenever possible, thereby leaving the majority of the nerve trunk intact (95). This technique preserves the neurological and electrophysiological integrity of the parent nerve and permits data to be compiled on histological, ultrastructural, biochemical, and teased-fiber studies.

Nerves that are routinely examined by biopsy in the author's laboratory include the common peroneal nerve, the ulnar nerve, and the tibial nerve together with its plantar branches.

Common Peroneal Nerve

This is a mixed nerve with motor fibers innervating muscles that flex the hock and extend the digits. It is sensory to the skin of the craniodorsal surface of the paw, hock, and stifle.

When combined nerve and muscle biopsy is desired, biopsy of the nerve at the stifle level will provide exposure for biopsy of the underlying gastrocnemius muscle (lateral head) and distal biceps femoris muscle.

The common peroneal nerve is the nerve favored for biopsy. It is a flat nerve in which individual fascicles are easily identified. Its long subcutaneous course over the stifle, without branching, allows removal of ample lengths (2 to 5 cm), if needed. In addition, well-established, normal electrophysiological data (35, 40, 43, 95) and normal age-related, statistically evaluated morphometric data (96, 97) are available. However, the superficial location of the nerve as it crosses the lateral aspect of the stifle joint renders the nerve vulnerable to trauma.

Biopsy Technique. Following general anesthesia, the animal is positioned in lateral recumbency, and the stifle area is surgically prepared (shaved, scrubbed, disinfected, and draped). A 6- to 8-cm skin incision is made in oblique fashion over the lateral femoral condyle. The nerve is located as it crosses the lateral head of the gastrocnemius muscle and is carefully isolated from surrounding areolar tissue. A 5-O silk suture with a swaged-on noncutting needle is placed in the nerve at its caudal border to include approximately one-third of its width (Fig. 4.30). With gentle retraction of the suture, a pair of fine, sharp scissors is used to divide longitudinally 30% of the nerve fascicles from the parent trunk approximately 3 to 5 cm distally. The nerve fascicles are removed from the parent trunk by a transverse incision, stretched on a tongue depressor, maintained in place using pins, and immersed in 10% buffered neutral formalin solution. The fascial and subcutaneous tissues are closed with absorbable suture, and skin

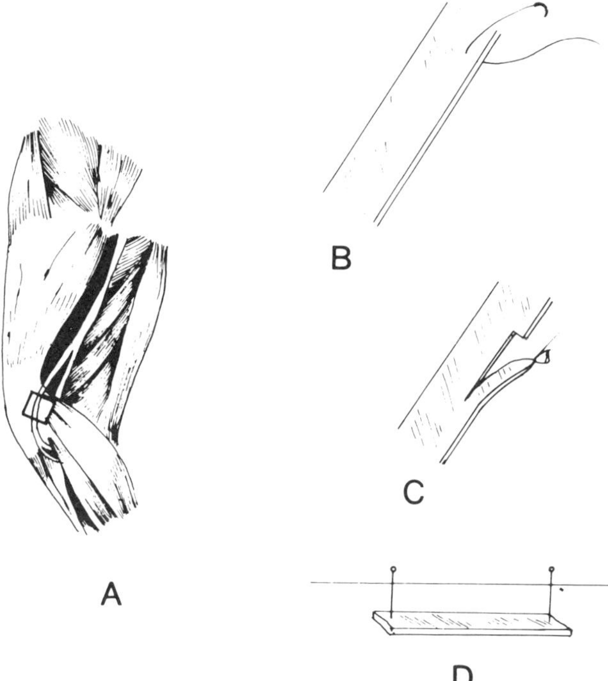

Figure 4.30. Fascicular nerve biopsy technique of the common peroneal nerve. The nerve is isolated as it crosses the lateral head of the gastrocnemius muscle (*inset*) (*A*). A suture is placed in the proximal portion of the nerve to be excised (*B*). With gentle traction the nerve is divided longitudinally and cut approximately 3 to 5 cm distally (*C*), stretched on a tongue depressor (*D*), and placed in fixative.

closure is completed. A dry dressing is applied and held in place with a 10-cm elastic bandage. Activity of the animal should be limited during the immediate postoperative period. The nerve samples are transferred to fluid-tight containers and mailed to the reference laboratory.

Ulnar Nerve

This a mixed nerve with motor branches to the flexors of the carpus and digits. Sensory branches supply the caudal surface of the antebrachium. When combined nerve and muscle biopsy is desired, a combination biopsy of ulnar nerve at the level of the elbow with biopsy of the medial head of the triceps brachii and superficial digital flexor muscles has proven satisfactory. There are no muscular branches that leave the ulnar nerve as it traverses the brachium. Quantitative, electrophysiological, and morphometric data are also available for the ulnar nerve. There are a few disadvantages to use of the ulnar nerve for biopsy: (*a*) it is closely associated with the collateral ulnar vessels; (*b*) individual fascicles cannot be identified; and (*c*) fascicles are difficult to separate in this cylindrical nerve.

Biopsy Technique. Following general anesthesia and positioning, the medial surface of the thoracic limb is surgically prepared extending from the axilla to the metacarpal region. A 6- to 8-cm long skin incision centered midway between the point of the olecranon and the medial condyle of the humerus is made in a slightly oblique fashion. The incision is continued by blunt dissection so as to expose the ulnar nerve as it crosses parallel to the medial head of the triceps brachii muscle. The nerve is isolated from adipose tissue, fascia, and accompanying collateral ulnar artery and vein. A fascicular biopsy may then be obtained by using the technique described for the common peroneal nerve. The wound is closed with close attention to hemostasis and accurate approximation of the fascia, subcutaneous tissue, and skin.

Tibial Nerve and Plantar Branches

In some instances, sampling of more distal nerves may be indicated (e.g., with distal axonopathies). In this situation, biopsy of the distal tibial nerve and its branches (medial and lateral plantar nerves) enables comparison of distal and proximal changes. All three nerves may be sampled from a single incision.

The mixed tibial nerve supplies motor branches to muscles that extend the hock and flex the digits. It is sensory to the skin and footpads of the plantar surface of the paw and metatarsus. At about the middle of the crus near the medial surface, the tibial nerve comes into relationship with the plantar branch of the saphenous artery and vein. Approximately 1 cm proximal to the tibiotarsal joint, the tibial nerve bifurcates into medial and lateral plantar nerves. The medial plantar nerve is smaller, more medial, and more superficial than the lateral plantar nerve.

There are several disadvantages to use of these nerves for biopsy: (*a*) potential bleeding from the branches of the saphenous vessels; (*b*) insufficient morphometric data (98) and no electrophysiological data available for the plantar nerves; (*c*) plantar nerves are not readily accessible to conduction velocity determinations; (*d*) fascicles of tibial nerve are difficult to separate; and (*e*) the lateral plantar nerve is more deeply situated than the more cutaneous medial plantar nerve, and it is difficult to obtain adequate lengths of nerve if needed for special study.

Biopsy Technique. The caudomedial surface of the metatarsus is surgically prepared extending from the stifle to the digits. A 4- to 6-cm long skin incision centered midway between the tuber calcanei and the medial malleolus of the tibia is made. The incision is continued by blunt dissection so as to expose the distal tibial nerve and its bifurcation into medial and lateral plantar nerves. The tibial nerve is isolated from dense fascia and closely associated plantar branches of the saphenous artery and vein. A fascicular biopsy is performed as described for the common peroneal nerve. The plantar branches are isolated from their respective plantar vessels and, at a level approximately 2 to 3 cm distal to the bifurcation of the tibial nerve, whole-nerve biopsies of each nerve are performed. This procedure does not result in clinical sensory or motor deficits. The entire nerve is removed as described for the fascicular biopsy.

References

1. Lord PF, Olsson S-E: Myelography with metrizamide in the dog: A clinical study on its use for the demonstration of spinal cord lesions other than those caused by intervertebral disk protrusions. *J Am Vet Radiol Assoc* 18:42–50, 1976.
2. Funkquist B: Myelographic localization of spinal cord compression in dogs. *Acta Vet Scand* 16:269–287, 1975.
3. Bartels JE, Braund KG, Redding RW: An experimental evaluation of a non-ionic agent "Amipaque" (metrizamide) as a neuroradiologic medium in the dog. *J Am Vet Radiol Soc* 18:117–123, 1977.
4. Wright JA, Bell DA, Clayton-Jones DG: The clinical and radiological features associated with spinal tumours in thirty dogs. *J Small Anim Pract* 20:461–472, 1979.
5. Wright JA, Clayton-Jones DG: Metrizamide myelography in sixty-eight dogs. *J Small Anim Pract* 22:415–435, 1981.

6. Stowater JL, Kneller SK: Clinical evaluation of metrizamide as a myelographic agent in the dog. *J Am Vet Med Assoc* 175:191–195, 1979.

7. Adams WM, Stowater JL: Complications of metrizamide myelography in the dog: summary of 107 clinical case histories. *Vet Radiol* 22:27–34, 1981.

8. Northington JW: Metrizamide myelography in five dogs and two cats with suspected spinal cord neoplasms. *Vet Radiol* 21:149–155, 1980.

9. Bartels JE, Braund KG: Experimental arachnoid fibrosis produced by metrizamide in the dog. *Vet Radiol* 21:78–81, 1980.

9a. Spencer CP, Chrisman CL, Mayhew IG, Kaude JV: Neurotoxicologic effects of the nonionic contrast agent iopamidol on the leptomeninges of the dog. *Am J Vet Res* 43:1958–1962, 1982.

10. Wheeler SJ, Davies JV: Iohexol myelography in the dog and cat: a series of one hundred cases and a comparison with metrizamide and iopamidol. *J Small Anim Pract* 26:247–256, 1985.

11. Wheeler SJ, Clayton-Jones DG, Wright JA: Myelography in the cat. *J Small Anim Pract* 26:143–152, 1985.

12. de Lahunta A: *Veterinary Neuroanatomy and Clinical Neurology*, ed 2. Philadelphia, WB Saunders, 1983.

13. Kallfelz FA, de Lahunta A, Allhands RV: Scintigraphic diagnosis of brain lesions in the dog and cat. *J Am Vet Med Assoc* 172:589–597, 1978.

14. Parker AJ, Devous MD, Twardock AR, O'Brien DP: Scintigraphic imaging of acute unilateral lesions in the brain parenchyma of three dogs. *J Am Anim Hosp Assoc* 18:926–932, 1982.

15. Fike JR, LeCouteur RA, Cann CE: Anatomy of the canine brain using high resolution computed tomography. *Vet Radiol* 22:236–243, 1981.

16. Fike JR, LeCouteur RA, Cann CE, Pflugfelder CM: Computerized tomography of brain tumors of the rostral and middle fossas in the dog. *Am J Vet Res* 42:275–281, 1981.

17. Fike JR, Cann CE: Contrast medium accumulation and washout in canine brain tumors and irradiated normal brain: a CT study of kinetics. *Radiology* 151:115–120, 1984.

18. Fike JR, Cann CE, Norman D, Turrel JM, LeCouteur RA, Pflugfelder CM, Borchich JK: Relative uptake of low- and high-osmolality contrast media in CT of brain tumors. *Am J Neuroradiol* 5:413–417, 1984.

19. LeCouteur RA, Fike JR, Cann CE, Turrel JM, Thompson JM, Biggart JF: X-ray computed tomography of brain tumors in cats. *J Am Vet Med Assoc* 183:301–305, 1983.

20. Shell L, Coulter SB, Blass CE, Ingram JT: Surgical removal of a meningioma in a cat after detection by computerized tomography. *J Am Anim Hosp Assoc* 21:439–442, 1985.

21. Loden D, Norton F, Wolfla LH, Ford RB: Diagnosis of intracranial lesions by computerized tomography in three dogs. *J Am Anim Hosp Assoc* 19:303–308, 1983.

22. Schunk KL: Computerized tomography of brain tumors in small animals. In *Proceedings of the American College of Veterinary Internal Medicine, 3rd Annual Medical Forum*, June 1, 1985, p 159.

23. Redding RW, Knecht CE: *Atlas of Electroencephalography in the Dog and Cat.* New York, Praeger, 1984.

24. Klemm WR, Hall CL: Current status and trends in veterinary encephalography. *J Am Vet Med Assoc* 164:529–532, 1974.

25. Klemm WR, Hall CL: Electroencephalograms of anesthetized dogs with hydrocephalus. *Am J Vet Res* 32:1859–1864, 1971.

26. Zook BC, Carpenter JL, Roberts RM: Lead poisoning in dogs: occurrence, source, clinical pathology and electroencephalography. *Am J Vet Res* 33:891–902, 1972.

27. Knecht CD, Crabtree J, Katherman A: Clinical clinicopathologic and electroencephalographic features of lead poisoning in dogs. *J Am Vet Med Assoc* 175:196–201, 1979.

28. Sorjonen DC, Knecht CD: Electroencephalographic abnormalities associated with cervical intervertebral disk extrusion in four dogs. *J Am Anim Hosp Assoc* 21:275–278, 1985.

29. Duncan ID: Peripheral nerve disease in the dog and cat. *Vet Clin North Am* 10:177–211, 1980.

30. Chrisman CL: *Problems in Small Animal Neurology.* Philadelphia, Lea & Febiger, 1982.

31. Farnbach GC: Clinical electrophysiology in veterinary neurology. Part II. Peripheral nerve testing. *Comp Cont Educ* 2:843–849, 1980.

32. Holliday TA, Ealand BG, Weldon NE: Sensory nerve conduction velocity: technical requirements and normal values for branches of the radial and ulnar nerves of the dog. *Am J Vet Res* 38:1543–1551, 1977.

33. Redding RW, Ingram JT, Colter SB: Sensory nerve conduction velocity of cutaneous afferents of the radial, ulnar, peroneal, and tibial nerves of the dog: reference values. *Am J Vet Res* 43:517–521, 1982.

34. Redding RW, Ingram JT, Colter SB: Sensory nerve conduction velocity of cutaneous afferents of the radial, ulnar, peroneal, and tibial nerves of the cat: reference values. *Am J Vet Res* 45:1042–1045, 1984.

35. Walker TL, Redding RW, Braund KG: Motor nerve conduction velocity and latency in the dog. *Am J Vet Res* 40:1433–1439, 1979.

36. Lee AF, Bowen JM: Evaluation of motor nerve conduction velocity in the dog. *Am J Vet Res* 31:1361–1366, 1970.

37. Chrisman CL: Electromyography in animals. In Bojrab MJ (ed): *Pathophysiology in Small Animal Surgery.* Philadelphia, Lea & Febiger, 1981, p 831.

38. Griffiths IR, Duncan ID, Swallow JS: Peripheral neuropathies in dogs: a study of five cases. *J Small Anim Pract* 18:101–116, 1977.

39. Sims MH, Redding RW: Maturation of nerve conduction velocity and the evoked muscle potential in the dog. *Am J Vet Res* 41:1247–1252, 1980.

40. Swallow JS, Griffiths IR: Age related changes in the motor nerve conduction velocity in dogs. *Res Vet Sci* 23:29–32, 1977.

41. Braund KG, Luttgen PJ, Redding RW, Rumph PF: Distal symmetrical polyneuropathy in a dog. *Vet Pathol* 17:422–435, 1980.

42. Farnbach GC: Clinical electrophysiology in veterinary neurology. Part I. Electromyography. *Comp Cont Educ* 2:791–797, 1980.

43. Bowen JM: Peripheral nerve electrodiagnostics, electromyography, and nerve conduction velocity. In Hoerlein BF (ed): *Canine Neurology—Diagnosis and Treatment,* ed 3. Philadelphia, WB Saunders, 1978, p 254.

44. Griffiths IR, Duncan ID: Some studies of the clinical neurophysiology of denervation in the dog. *Res Vet Sci* 17:377–383, 1974.

45. Steinberg HS: A review of electromyographic and motor nerve conduction velocity techniques. *J Am Anim Hosp Assoc* 15:613–619, 1979.

46. Chrisman CL: Differentiation of tick paralysis and acute idiopathic polyradiculoneuritis in the dog using electromyography. *J Am Anim Hosp Assoc* 11:455–458, 1975.

47. Palmer AC, Barker J: Myasthenia in the dog. *Vet Rec* 95:452–454, 1974.

48. van Nes JJ, van der Most van Spijk D: Electrophysiologic evidence of peripheral nerve dysfunction in six dogs with botulism type C. *Res Vet Sci,* in press.

49. Miller JD, Adams JH: The pathophysiology of raised intracranial pressure. In Adams JH, Corsellis JAN, Duchen LW (eds): *Greenfield's Neuropathology,* ed 4. New York, John Wiley & Sons, 1984, p 53.

50. Kornegay JN: Cerebrospinal fluid collection examination and interpretation in dogs and cats. *Comp Cont Educ* 3:85–94, 1981.

50a. Wright JA: Evaluation of cerebrospinal fluid in the dog. *Vet Rec* 103:48–51, 1978.

51. Mayhew IG, Beal CR: Techniques of analysis of cerebrospinal fluid in the dog. *Vet Clin North Am* 10:155–176, 1980.

52. Oliver JE, Lorenz MD: *Handbook of Veterinary Neurologic Diagnosis.* Philadelphia, WB Saunders, 1983.

53. Hoerlein BF: *Canine Neurology—Diagnosis and Treatment,* ed 3. Philadelphia, WB Saunders, 1978.

54. Roost KT, Pimstone NR, Diamond MD, Schmid R: The formation of cerebrospinal fluid xanthochromia after subarachnoid hemorrhage. *Neurology* 22:973–977, 1972.

55. Vandevelde M, Spano JS: Cerebrospinal fluid cytology in canine neurologic disease. *Am J Vet Res* 38:1827–1832, 1977.

56. Veuger AJLM, Kortbeek LHTS, Booij AC: Siderophages in differentiation of blood in cerebrospinal fluid. *Clin Neurol Neurosurg* 80:46–56, 1977.

57. Roszel JF, Steinberg SA, McGrath JT: Periodic acid-Schiff-positive cells in cerebrospinal fluid of dogs with globoid cell leukodystrophy. *Neurology* 22:738–741, 1972.

58. Carakostas MC, Gossett KA, Watters JW, MacWilliams PS: Effects of metrizamide myelography on cerebrospinal fluid analysis in the dog. *Vet Radiol* 24:267–270, 1983.

59. Wilson JW, Stevens JB: Effects of blood contamination on cerebrospinal fluid analysis. *J Am Vet Med Assoc* 171:256–258, 1977.
60. Roszel JF: Membrane filtration of canine and feline cerebrospinal fluid for cytologic evaluation. *J Am Vet Med Assoc* 160:720–725, 1972.
61. Steinberg SA, Vandevelde M: A comparative study of two methods of cytological evaluation of spinal fluid in domestic animals. *Folia Vet Latina* 4:235–250, 1974.
62. Bailey CS, Higgins RJ: Comparison of total white blood cell count and total protein content of lumbar and cisternal cerebrospinal fluid of healthy dogs. *Am J Vet Res* 46:1162–1165, 1985.
63. Krakowka S, Fenner W, Miele JA: Quantitative determination of serum origin cerebrospinal fluid proteins in the dog. *Am J Vet Res* 42:1975–1977, 1981.
64. Cutler RWP, Averill DR: Cerebrospinal fluid gamma globulins in canine distemper encephalitis. *Neurology* 19:1111–1114, 1969.
65. Yaksh TL, Fedele LA, Yamamura HI: Effects of repeated withdrawal of cerebrospinal fluid by cisternal puncture on cisternal protein levels in the unanesthetized cat. *Physiol Behav* 10:149–151, 1973.
66. Wright JA: Cerebrospinal fluid enzyme estimation in the diagnosis of central nervous system damage in the dog. *Vet Rec* 106:54–57, 1980.
67. Wilson JW, Wiltrout SK: Cerebrospinal fluid phosphokinase in the normal dog. *Am J Vet Res* 37:1099–1100, 1976.
68. Wilson JW: Clinical application of cerebrospinal fluid creatine phosphokinase determination. *J Am Vet Med Assoc* 171:200–202, 1977.
69. Indrieri RJ, Holliday TA, Keen CL: Critical evaluation of creatine phosphokinase in cerebrospinal fluid of dogs with neurologic disease. *Am J Vet Res* 41: 1299–1303, 1980.
70. Long JF, Jacoby RO, Olson M, Koestner A: Beta-glucuronidase activity and levels of protein and protein fractions in serum and cerebrospinal fluid of dogs with distemper associated demyelinating encephalopathy. *Acta Neuropathol (Berl)* 25:179–187, 1973.
71. Trotter EJ: Modified dorsal laminectomy and selective regional spinal cord hypothermia in the treatment of thoracolumbar disk disease. In Bojrab MJ (ed): *Current Techniques in Small Animal Surgery.* Philadelphia, Lea & Febiger, 1975, p 406.
72. Braund KG, Taylor TKF, Ghosh P, Sherwood AA: Lateral spinal decompression in the dog. *J Small Anim Pract* 17:583–592, 1976.
73. Swaim SF, Vandevelde M: Clinical and histologic evaluation of bilateral hemilaminectomy and deep dorsal laminectomy for extensive spinal cord decompression in the dog. *J Am Vet Med Assoc* 170:407–413, 1977.
74. Trotter EJ, Brasmer TH, de Lahunta A: Modified deep dorsal laminectomy in the dog. *Cornell Vet* 65:402–427, 1975.
75. Funquist B: Thoracolumbar disc protrusion with severe cord compression in the dog. III. Treatment by decompressive laminectomy. *Acta Vet Scand* 3:344–366, 1962.
76. Funquist B, Shantz B: Influence of extensive laminectomy on the shape of the spinal canal. *Acta Orthop Scand* 56(Suppl):1–50, 1962.
77. Hoerlein BF: Further evaluation of the treatment of disc protrusion paraplegia in the dog. *J Am Vet Med Assoc* 129:495–502, 1956.
78. Hoerlein BF: *Canine Neurology—Diagnosis and Treatment*, ed 2. Philadelphia, WB Saunders, 1971.
79. Hoerlein BF: The status of various intervertebral disc surgeries for the dog in 1978. *J Am Anim Hosp Assoc* 14:563–570, 1978.
80. Popovic NA, VanderArk G, Kempe L: Ventral approach for surgical treatment of cervical disk disease in the dog. *Am J Vet Res* 32:1155–1161, 1971.
81. Swaim SF: Vertebral body plating for spinal immobilization. *J Am Vet Med Assoc* 158:1683–1695, 1971.
82. Swaim SF: Ventral decompression of the cervical spinal cord in the dog. *J Am Vet Med Assoc* 164:491–495, 1974.
83. Prata RG, Stoll SG: Ventral decompression and fusion for the treatment of cervical disc disease in the dog. *J Am Anim Hosp Assoc* 9:462–472, 1973.
84. Prata RG: Neurosurgical treatment of thoracolumbar disks: the rationale and value of laminectomy with concomitant disk removal. *J Am Anim Hosp Assoc* 17:17–26, 1981.
85. Slocum B, Rudy RL: Fractures of the seventh lumbar vertebra in the dog. *J Am Anim Hosp Assoc* 11:167–174, 1975.
86. Swaim SF, Hyams D: Clinical observations and client evaluation of ventral decompres-

sion for cervical intervertebral disk protrusion. *J Am Vet Med Assoc* 181:259–260, 1982.

87. Denny HR, Gibbs C, Holt PE: The diagnosis and treatment of cauda equina lesions in the dog. *J Small Anim Pract* 23:425–443, 1982.

88. Denny HR, Gibbs C, Gaskell CJ: Cervical spondylopathy in the dog—a review of thirty-five cases. *J Small Anim Pract* 18:117–132, 1977.

89. Withrow SJ, Seim HB: Caudal cervical spondylopathy and myelopathy in large breed dogs. In Bojrab MJ (ed): *Current Techniques in Small Animal Surgery*, ed 2. Philadelphia, Lea & Febiger, 1983, p 541.

90. Cook JR, Oliver JE: Atlantoaxial luxation in the dog. *Comp Cont Educ* 3:242–252, 1981.

91. Braund KG, Hoff EJ, Richardson KEY: Histochemical identification of fiber types in canine skeletal muscle. *Am J Vet Res* 39:561–565, 1978.

92. Braund KG, Lincoln CE: Histochemical differentiation of fiber types in neonatal canine skeletal muscle. *Am J Vet Res* 42:407–415, 1981.

93. Braund KG, McGuire JA, Lincoln CE: Observations on normal skeletal muscle of mature dogs: a cytochemical, histochemical, and morphometric study. *Vet Pathol* 19:577–595, 1982.

94. Heene R, Haar F: Mailing muscle biopsy samples for histochemical processing. Conditions and morphometric approach to the alterations induced by storage. *J Neurol* 231:176–181, 1984.

95. Braund KG, Walker TL, Vandevelde M: Fascicular nerve biopsy in the dog. *Am J Vet Res* 40:1025–1030, 1979.

96. Braund KG, McGuire JA, Lincoln CE: Age-related changes in peripheral nerves of the dog. I. A morphologic and morphometric study of single-teased fibers. *Vet Pathol* 19:365–378, 1982.

97. Braund KG, McGuire JA, Lincoln CE: Age-related changes in peripheral nerves of the dog. II. A morphologic and morphometric study of cross-sectional nerve. *Vet Pathol* 19:379–398, 1982.

98. Braund KG, Steiss JE: Distal neuropathy in spontaneous diabetes mellitus in the dog. *Acta Neuropathol (Berl)* 57:263–269, 1982.

Glossary

abiotrophy. The mechanism of premature degeneration of cells due to an inherent lack of trophic or nutritive factor.

anisocoria. Inequality of the diameters of the pupils.

annulus fibrosus. A fibrocartilaginous structure that forms the major part of the intervertebral disk. It consists of bands of parallel fibers that run obliquely between vertebral bodies.

anosmia. Absence of the sense of smell.

ataxia. Incoordination; irregularity of muscle action.

atrophy. Wasting away or diminution in the size of cell, tissue, organ, or part. Denervation muscle atrophy results from dysfunction of the motor nerve supplying the muscle.

axonotmesis. Damage to peripheral nerve fibers resulting in degeneration; however, the endoneurial and Schwann cell sheaths remain intact and provide a framework for axonal regeneration.

brachycephalic. Having a short, wide head.

cauda equina. Sheath of lumbosacral (and coccygeal) nerve roots that pass in the lumbosacral canal to their site of emergence between the vertebrae.

caudal (caudad). Denoting a position more toward the cauda or tail than some specified point of reference.

chondrodystrophoid. Pertaining to breeds of dogs that are characterized by varying degrees of short-limbed dwarfism and accelerated degeneration of intervertebral disk.

clonus. A spasm in which rigidity and relaxation alternate in rapid succession.

coma. State of unconsciousness from which the patient cannot be aroused, even by powerful stimulation.

consensual. Similar reaction of both pupils to a stimulus applied to only one.

contralateral. Situated on or pertaining to the opposite side.

craniectomy. Excision of a part of the skull.

craniotomy. Any operation on the cranium.

decompression. Removal of pressure.

dermatome. The area of skin supplied with sensory nerve fibers by a single dorsal spinal root.

disk disease. Clinical manifestation of disk protrusion or disk extrusion.

disk extrusion. Rupture of the dorsal layers of the disk with extrusion of disk material into the vertebral canal.

disk protrusion. Dorsal bulging of the outer layers of the disk into the vertebral canal without rupturing.

diskospondylitis. Intervertebral disk infection with concurrent osteomyelitis in contiguous vertebral bodies.

dolicocephalic. Having a long, narrow head.

dying-back disease. A neurological disorder characterized by degeneration of the distal aspects of central and/or peripheral cell processes. Also known as "distal axonal degeneration" and "central-peripheral axonopathy."

dysmetria. Disturbance of the power to control the range of muscular movements.

dysphonia. Impairment of vocalization.

embolus. A clot or other plug brought by the blood from another vessel and forced into a smaller one, thus obstructing the circulation.

fenestration. Disk fenestration is the removal of intervertebral disk material by perforation of the annulus fibrosus and curettage of the intervertebral disk space.

flaccid. Weak or soft.

fontanelle. A soft spot, such as one of the membrane-covered spaces remaining in an incompletely ossified skull.

fucosidosis. Storage disease resulting from a deficiency of the enzyme α-L-fucosidase. Storage substrate is probably α-L-fucose.

gangliosidosis. Storage disease resulting from a deficiency of either β-galactosidase (GM1), hexosaminidase A (GM2 type 1), or hexosaminidase A and B (GM2 type 2). Storage substrates are gangliosides and complex metabolites.

globoid leukodystrophy. Storage disease resulting from a deficiency of the enzyme β-galactosidase. Also known as "Krabbe's disease." Storage substrate is galactocerebroside.

glucocerebrosidosis. Storage disease resulting from a deficiency of the enzyme β-glucosidase. Also known as "canine Gaucher disease." Storage substrate is glucocerebroside.

glycogenosis. Storage disease resulting from a deficiency of either acid α-glucosidase (glycogenosis type 2) or amylo-1,6-glucosidase (glycogenosis type 3). Storage substrate is glycogen.

hemilaminectomy. Removal of the vertebral laminae on one side only.

hemiparesis. Muscular weakness affecting one side of the body.

hemiplegia. Paralysis of one side of the body.

hemivertebra. Developmental anomaly characterized by incomplete development of one side of a vertebra.

hepatic encephalopathy. A complex metabolic disturbance of the central nervous system that results from diminished hepatic function, urea cycle enzyme deficiency, or shunting of portal blood around the liver. Toxic substances that have been incriminated include ammonia, amino acids, short-chain fatty acids, mercaptan, and various biogenic amines, indoles, and skatoles.

hydranencephaly. Complete or almost complete absence of the cerebral hemispheres, the space they normally occupy being filled with cerebrospinal fluid.

hydrocephalus. Abnormal accumulation of fluid within the cranial vault, often accompanied by enlargement of the head, atrophy of the brain, and severe mental impairment.

hypalgesia. Diminished sensitivity to pain.

hyperalgesia.   Excessive sensitivity to pain.

hyperesthesia.   Abnormally increased sensitivity of the skin.

hypermetria.   Form of dysmetria in which voluntary muscular movement (usually of the thoracic limbs) overreaches the intended goal.

hypertonus.   Excessive tone or tension; usually pertaining to skeletal muscle.

hypervitaminosis A.   Crippling degenerative and proliferative bony disorder that primarily affects cervical and thoracic vertebrae and various long bones in cats fed whole liver diets.

hypesthesia.   Abnormally decreased sensitivity of the skin.

hypomyelinogenesis.   Severe myelin deficiency and/or abnormal myelin formation.

hypoplasia.   Defective or incomplete development.

idiopathic.   Of unknown cause.

incontinence.   Inability to control excretory functions such as defecation (fecal incontinence) or urination (urinary incontinence).

incoordination.   Lack of harmonious muscular activity; ataxia.

infarction.   Area of necrosis in a tissue due to local ischemia resulting from obstruction of circulation to the area. Usually caused by a thrombus or an embolus.

intention tremor.   A tremor that arises or is intensified when a voluntary movement is attempted. Usually pertains to the head.

interarcuate ligament (ligamentum flavum; yellow ligament).   Thin, elastic membranous sheets located between arches of adjacent vertebrae.

ipsilateral.   Situated on or pertaining to the same side of the body.

ischemia.   Deficiency of blood in a part due to impaired circulation.

kyphosis.   Abnormally increased dorsal convexity in the curvature of the spine (usually pertaining to the thoracic spine).

labyrinthitis.   Inflammation of the cavities or canals of the inner ear. Also known as otitis interna.

laminectomy.   Excision of the dorsal arch of a vertebra.

leuko-.   Denotes relationship to the white matter of the central nervous system.

leukodystrophy.   Disturbance of the white matter of the central nervous system. Also known as leukoencephalomyelopathy.

lissencephaly.   A malformation in which the brain is characteristically smooth or marked by few convolutions.

lordosis.   Abnormally increased ventral concavity in the curvature of the spine (usually pertaining to the thoracolumbar spine).

lower motor neuron.   Neurons whose cell bodies lie within the brainstem and spinal cord and whose axons form outside the central nervous system to innervate muscular structures (usually skeletal muscles).

luxation.   Dislocation with major displacement.

malacia.   Pathological softening of an area (usually pertaining to the central nervous system).

mannosidosis.   Storage disease resulting from a deficiency of the enzyme acidic α-D-mannosidase. Storage substrate is mannose-rich material.

meningitis.   Inflammation of the meninges.

meningocele.   Hernial protrusion of the meninges through a defect in the skull or vertebral column.

meningomyelocele.   Hernial protrusion of a part of the meninges and substance of the spinal cord through a defect in the vertebral column.

micturition.   Passage of urine; urination.

miosis.   Excessive contraction of the pupil.

mucopolysaccharidosis.   Storage disease resulting from a deficiency of either α-L-iduronidase (mucopolysachharidosis 1) or arylsulfatase B (mucopolysaccharidosis 6). Storage substrates are mucopolysaccharides (glycosaminoglycans).

mydriasis.   Excessive dilation of the pupil.

myelitis.   Inflammation of the spinal cord.

myelocele.   Hernial protrusion of the substance of the spinal cord through a defect in the bony spinal canal.

myelodysplasia.   Defective development of any part of the spinal cord.

myelomalacia.   Pathological softening of the spinal cord.

myoclonus.   Shock-like contractions of a portion of a muscle, an entire muscle, or a group of muscles.

myositis.   Inflammation of a muscle.

myotonia.   Increased muscular irritability and contraction with decreased power of relaxation. Tapping such muscle can produce a dimple contracture.

myringotomy.   Surgical incision of the tympanic membrane.

narcolepsy/cataplexy.   Excessive sleepiness and/or sudden, paroxysmal attacks of flaccid paralysis.

neuroaxonal dystrophy.   Degenerative disease characterized by accumulation of membrane-filled swellings ("spheroids") of distal axons within the central nervous system.

neuroma.   Tumor growing from nerve.

neuron.   Any of the conducting cells of the nervous system.

neuronopathy.   A type of peripheral nerve disease in which the primary changes appear in the nerve cell body.

neuropraxia.   Interruption in the function and conduction of a nerve in the absence of structural changes.

neurotmesis.   Nerve injury in which there is complete severence of all structures of the nerve.

nucleus pulposus.   Gelatinous material that forms the central portion of the intervertebral disk. It contains large amounts of mucopolysaccharides (glycosaminoglycans) and is primarily responsible for dissipation of spinal axial forces.

nystagmus.   Involuntary rapid movement of the eyeball that may be horizontal, vertical, rotatory, or mixed.

opisthotonus.   Form of tetanic spasm in which the head and neck are bent backward, the limbs are extended, and the spine may be held in a position of lordosis.

palmar.   Pertaining to the ventral surface of the front paw.

papilledema.   Edema of the optic disk.

paraneoplasia.   Tumor-induced organ dysfunction not directly attributable to malignant invasion of the organ by the tumor.

paraplegia. Paralysis of the pelvic limbs.

paresis. Slight or incomplete paralysis; weakness.

paresthesia. Abnormal sensation, such as burning or pricking.

paroxysm. Sudden recurrence or intensification of clinical signs.

polio. Denotes relationship of the gray matter of the central nervous system.

polyradiculoneuritis. Inflammation involving multiple nerve roots and possibly multiple peripheral nerves.

porencephaly. Congenital disorder characterized by cysts or cavities in the brain cortex which communicate with the ventricular system.

proprioception. Information concerning position and movements of the body and its parts. Proprioceptive receptors are located primarily in skeletal muscles, joints, and labyrinth of the inner ear.

ptosis. Drooping of the upper eyelid resulting from paralysis of the third cranial nerve (oculomotor) or from disrupted sympathetic innervation.

pyrexia. Abnormal elevation in body temperature.

radiculopathy. Disease of the nerve roots.

risus sardonicus. Grinning expression produced by spasm of the facial muscles.

rostral (rostrad). Denoting a position more toward the nose than some specified point of reference.

sacrococcygeal dysgenesis. Defective development of the sacrococcygeal spinal cord and/or vertebrae.

seizure. Paroxysmal disorder of the nervous system that has a tendency to recur. Also known as "convulsion", "epilepsy", or "fit."

spastic. Denotes increased muscular tension and stiffness; often characterized by hypertonia and exaggerated reflexes.

sphingomyelinosis. Storage disease resulting from a deficiency of the enzyme sphingomyelinase. Storage substrate is sphingomyelin.

spina bifida. Developmental anomaly characterized by defective closure of the bony encasement of the spinal cord, through which the spinal cord and meninges may or may not protrude.

spinal muscular atrophy. Premature degeneration and death (abiotrophy) of various neuronal cell populations in the spinal cord and/or brainstem.

stenosis. Narrowing or stricture of a duct or canal.

storage diseases. Inherited defects of lysosomal hydrolase enzymes that result in accumulation or "storage" of that enzyme's substrate within lysosomes.

strabismus. Deviation of the eyeball.

stupor. State of partial unconsciousness.

subluxation. Dislocation with minor displacement.

syncope. Sudden loss of consciousness usually associated with impaired cerebral circulation and deprivation of oxygen and glucose.

syndrome. A set of clinical signs that occurs together; the sum of signs of any diseased state.

syringomyelia. Fluid-filled cavities in the substance of the spinal cord.

tetraparesis. Muscular weakness in all four limbs.

tetraplegia (quadriplegia). Paralysis of all four limbs.

tone. As it pertains to muscle, the resistance to passive elongation or stretch.

trismus. Difficulty in opening the mouth (lockjaw).

upper motor neuron. Motor neurons whose cell bodies and axons lie totally within the central nervous system, the axons forming the descending tracts or fasciculi.

xanthochromia. Yellowish discoloration.

Index

Page numbers followed by "t" denote tables.